HEALTHCARE TECHNOLOGIES SERIES 24

Mobile Technologies for Delivering Healthcare in Remote, Rural or Developing Regions

IET Book Series on e-Health Technologies – Call for Authors

Book Series Editor: Professor Joel P. C. Rodrigues, the National Institute of Telecommunications (Inatel), Brazil and Instituto de Telecomunicações, Portugal

While the demographic shifts in populations display significant socio-economic challenges, they trigger opportunities for innovations in e-Health, m-Health, precision and personalized medicine, robotics, sensing, the Internet of Things, cloud computing, Big Data, Software Defined Networks, and network function virtualization. Their integration is however associated with many technological, ethical, legal, social and security issues. This new Book Series aims to disseminate recent advances for e-Health Technologies to improve healthcare and people's wellbeing.

Topics considered include Intelligent e-Health systems, electronic health records, ICT-enabled personal health systems, mobile and cloud computing for eHealth, health monitoring, precision and personalized health, robotics for e-Health, security and privacy in e-Health, ambient assisted living, telemedicine, Big Data and IoT for e-Health, and more.

Proposals for coherently integrated International multi-authored edited or co-authored handbooks and research monographs will be considered for this Book Series. Each proposal will be reviewed by the Book Series Editor with additional external reviews from independent reviewers. Please email your book proposal for the IET Book Series on e-Health Technologies to: Professor Joel Rodrigues at joeljr@ieee.org or joeljr@inatel.br

Mobile Technologies for Delivering Healthcare in Remote, Rural or Developing Regions

Edited by
Pradeep Kumar Ray, Naoki Nakashima, Ashir Ahmed, Soong-Chul Ro and Yasuhiro Soshino

The Institution of Engineering and Technology

Published by The Institution of Engineering and Technology, London, United Kingdom

The Institution of Engineering and Technology is registered as a Charity in England & Wales (no. 211014) and Scotland (no. SC038698).

First published 2020

The Institution of Engineering and Technology
Michael Faraday House
Six Hills Way, Stevenage
Herts, SG1 2AY, United Kingdom

www.theiet.org

British Library Cataloguing in Publication Data
A catalogue record for this product is available from the British Library

ISBN 978-1-83953-047-0 (hardback)
ISBN 978-1-83953-048-7 (PDF)

Typeset in India by MPS Ltd

Contents

About the editors

Pradeep Kumar Ray is the Director of the Centre For Entrepreneurship, University of Michigan-Shanghai Jiao Tong University Joint Institute, China, and currently leads the international initiative mHealth for Belt and Road region (mHBR) involving more than ten countries. Pradeep works on a range of innovative projects on eHealth and mHealth (jointly with industry, governments and global bodies like WHO, EU and IEEE) in eHealth and mHealth across the Asia Pacific region. He founded the WHO Collaborating Centre for eHealth in UNSW-Australia. He also co-founded IEEE Healthcom, premier international event held annually since 1999.

Naoki Nakashima is a professor and Director at the Medical Information Center of Kyushu University Hospital, and also a visiting professor of National Institute of Informatics, Japan. He is the leader for mHealth for Parkinsons Disease in mHBR. He is vice-president of the Japan Association for Medical Informatics (JAMI). He is also a founding member (2003) and past-vice director (2012) of the Telemedicine Development Center of Asia (TEMDEC) in Kyushu University.

Ashir Ahmed is an associate professor at the department of advanced information technology in Kyushu University, Japan and director of Global Communication Centre (GCC) projects at Grameen Communications, Bangladesh. Ashir leads the Portable Health Clinic project in mHBR. His research aims to produce and promote ICT-based social services for remote communities in the world.

Soong-Chul Ro is an associate professor and leader of the Bangladesh Challenge Project at the Centre For Entrepreneurship, University of Michigan-Shanghai Jiao Tong University Joint Institute (UM-SJTU JI), People's Republic of China. He also leads the Global Challenge project of mHBR. He has created and overseen several CSR projects, in partnership with NGOs and private companies. He is an honorary member of the Korean Diakonia Welfare Foundation.

Yasuhiro Soshino is the director of the International Medical Relief at Japan Red Cross Kumamoto Hospital, Japan. He also leads the Drones project at mHBR. He works closely with governments and industry in reaching medical relief in disaster affected areas using drones and has extensive experience in leading Red Cross disaster relief missions following natural disasters. He has been working on a range of disaster relief technologies including photovoltaics, IoT and drones.

Acknowledgements

This book is a result of a collaboration among ongoing projects of highly diverse nature, held together by a common interest in mobile health technologies for furthering sustainable development. Other than this common interest, however, the projects contained in this book have different origins, are at different stages of development, often work with multiple partners, sponsors and funding. Editors would like to thank the University of Michigan-Shanghai Jiao Tong University Joint Institute for supporting the idea of *Technology Entrepreneurship for Sustainable Development (TESD)* that has been the main motivation for the launch of the mhealth for Belt and Road Initiative (mHBR) that brought together many researchers and authors from several countries across several continents Asia, Australia and Europe to write this book. It would be quite impossible to name all the individuals and institutions that helped the projects here and the list will be tedious. Authors of each chapter have their acknowledgements incorporated in their chapter. Editors would like to express special gratitude to Mr. Hanrunyu Yan, who provided vital support in carefully collecting manuscripts from the authors, screening and standardizing them in preparation for this book.

Introduction

Healthcare is probably the most important social entrepreneurship sector that can benefit from the innovation and zeal of young entrepreneurs and public–private partnership both of which are being actively promoted in healthcare worldwide. China's Belt and Road Initiative (BRI) can be leveraged in promoting technology entrepreneurship in the social sector in general and in healthcare in particular. The United Nations has recognized the need for a holistic approach of sustainable development where health, environment and social wellbeing are being targeted together through the new global Sustainable Development Goals (SDGs). In the healthcare sector, Universal Health Coverage (UHC) is the platform that seeks to overcome inequality in tackling the gap in the service provision and finance that populations face.

The role of ICT (Information and Communication Technologies) to build the essential building blocks of UHC has been widely accepted. The proliferation of mobile technologies in developing countries has improved access to quality healthcare in a cost-effective manner. Mobile technologies (phones, drones, robots, Apps, wearable monitoring devices, etc.) are instrumental to socio-economic and healthcare development in many disadvantaged sections of the population. Mobile technologies are now being exploited to transform the face of health service delivery across the globe. Widely referred to as 'mHealth', 'mobile communication devices, in conjunction with internet and social media, present opportunities to enhance disease prevention and management by extending health interventions beyond the reach of traditional care' and the World Health Organization (WHO) has announced that m-health has the 'potential to transform the face of health service delivery across the globe' [1]. However, achieving UHC through mHealth presents some challenges, particularly from the perspective of sustainability and management. Entrepreneurship in mHealth services provide some mechanisms to overcome these challenges [2].

On the other hand, China has undertaken a major initiative called Belt and Road Initiative (BRI) for the development of the region from the western and southern regions of China through the adjacent countries towards Europe and Africa. This initiative involves developing regions (e.g., Yunnan and Guanxi provinces) of China and other neighbouring countries (Pakistan, Bangladesh, Myanmar, Kazhakastan, Uzbekistan, etc.) [3]. The BRI scheme mainly funds the infrastructure development of the Belt and Road region and countries through public collaboration; however, once the infrastructure projects are done, it is important to build comprehensive social development utilizing increased connectivity through people-to-people collaboration along the BRI countries and region. For this latter part, entrepreneurship has important roles to play in channelling the benefits of infrastructure and technology to the currently under-developed regions. In view of similarities in the problems for populations in this region, it may be possible to share some cost-effective solutions as well, making such collaboration all the more significant. In addition, although under-represented in the discussions on healthcare so far, entrepreneurship has much potential in increasing its significance in relation to healthcare in general and mHealth in particular.

This book evolved from a new multi-country and multi-disciplinary initiative called mHealth for Belt and Road region (mHBR). The project involves the application of a range of mHealth technologies (e.g., mobile phones, drones, robots, etc.) for healthcare across the BRI region involving China and neighbouring countries. This project was launched at the first Entrepreneurship Week in September 2018 at the University of Michigan-Shanghai Jiao Tong University (UMJI), Shanghai, China [4]. More than 20 investigators from more than 10 countries (including Bangladesh, China, Thailand, Japan, Australia, Nepal, India and Europe) have been working together on this project and this book is the first major outcome of the project that was discussed again in Entrepreneurship Week 2019, hosted by the Asian Institute of Technology, Bangkok.

A systematic survey was carried out by UMJI team on the role of entrepreneurship in mHealth in terms of four emerging major issues: sustainability, evaluation, social media and interoperability. Sustainability in mHealth projects has become an issue because there are many pilot projects in mHealth without leading to any large scale deployment with the exception of some specialized medical devices incorporating mHealth features. There is also an issue of evaluation surrounding the debate on the suitability of expensive, time-consuming randomized controlled trials, a gold standard evaluation methodology for healthcare intervention. Some researchers are questioning this gold standard for mHealth project evaluation given the rapid obsolescence on mHealth technologies. The rapid proliferation of mobile technologies in social media, on the other hand, offers increasing number of options for mHealth solutions but since mHealth represents a class of solutions based on multi-disciplinary knowledge involving many complex technologies, often mHealth solutions do not work together, leading to interoperability problems and hence the lack of effective interventions. This survey is an attempt to link the emerging issues on mHealth with the strong interest amongst entrepreneurs on the development of medical devices based on mobile technology [2].

The project encompasses multiple disciplines including software, healthcare, mobile communications, entrepreneurship, business and social development. Students, faculty and researchers, in these different institutions and disciplines, are cooperatively investigating the technical and entrepreneurship aspects of mobile technologies (such as phones, robots, drones, etc.) for healthcare development in the specified BRI regions and countries. Bangladesh has been selected as a major partner in this project because of its pioneering status in commercializing mHealth (healthcare using mobile phones) through services, such as Health Hotline 789. Guangxi province has been selected as a part of the developing BRI Region in

China. The works in this mHBR project can be an illustrative example of the multi-country, multi-stakeholder collaborative approach to the development of BRI region through entrepreneurship in a popular technology (mobile) application particularly in healthcare sector. Other groups can use this as a model for future development, especially in social entrepreneurship (entrepreneurship to help disadvantaged section of the population, e.g., poor, disabled, elderly, etc.).

The book is organized into five sections as follows:

I. Global Challenge
II. Portable Health Clinic
III. Sustainable and Resilient mHealth Services
IV. mHealth for the Elderly
V. mHealth for Chronic Illnesses

These sections are summarised next.

Section I – Global Challenge

The Global Challenge section examines the perspectives of different stakeholders of the mHealth intervention. Broadly defined, stakeholders are individuals and organizations that influence or are influenced by mHealth systems or intervention. WHO (2016) recognizes the importance of identifying engaging stakeholders early on for the successful scale-up mHealth projects (p.18) [1]. This is especially so, given the innate interdisciplinary nature of mHealth technologies. In addition, any project along the Belt and Road region targets clients and beneficiaries from different cultural backgrounds, necessitating a variety of operational models under diverse social and political contexts. Therefore knowing the stakeholders – who they are, what they can do for mHealth projects, what motivates them to contribute – is at the core properly responding to the global challenge of extending universal healthcare coverage (UHC) and sustainable development through technology.

There are other chapters in this book that contain important narratives relating to stakeholders in relation to a particular technology or health issue. This section, however, focuses on the perspectives of stakeholders and explores how they could be involved in mHealth projects. It is impossible to start this inquiry by drawing up a comprehensive list of stakeholders or even key stakeholders. Instead, the following five chapters examine five stakeholders somewhat neglected in the literature on mHealth.

Chapter 1 opens the discussion by examining the role of the university for sustainable development. It provides an overview of the current debates on this topic and examines the potential for entrepreneurial outreach activities to be used as the main channel through which universities can actively make visible impacts on sustainable development. Chapter 2 extends this agenda by examining the role of entrepreneurship ecosystem that creates connections among various other stakeholders across different regions in response to the fast-developing technological environment. Both of these chapters contain case studies to illustrate the points and draw lessons for broader application.

Following two chapters deal with specific issues relating to particular clients or beneficiaries of the mHealth intervention. Chapter 3 examines the specific needs of the expat community who also face limited access to the healthcare system but often neglected in the literature on UHC. The Bangladeshi community in China and the Chinese community in Bangladesh are examined through a survey to illustrate the expat communities' special needs. This chapter also demonstrates how understanding of the needs of beneficiary could lead to an innovative mHealth application. Chapter 4, on the other hand, studies the perception and behaviour of the one-child-policy generation in China who face having to support a larger number of ageing members of the family than those who have siblings. It demonstrates how particular circumstances of clients affect their perception, and in turn create different pattern of behaviour regarding available healthcare options.

Section II – Portable Health Clinic

The Portable Health Clinic (PHC), developed by Kyushu University-Japan, is a practical example of mHealth for the Primary care in remote developing regions in the world. This involves a divergence from the role of the typical healthcare professional, who operate from hospitals, clinics, laboratories or other institutions, who otherwise lack an incentive to travel to remote regions to provide their services. Doing this is costly, time-consuming and inefficient. Instead, PHC uses local health workers that already reside in these unreached communities to provide preventative primary care, with the option to consult a doctor using video call technology. To improve upon gender equality and female employment in these underdeveloped regions, the job of these local health assistants are designated to women. They own and operate a portable briefcase consisting of medical diagnostic equipment and sensors necessary to carry out health checkups. The medical records are archived in a software system, 'GramHealth', which doctors at a medical call centre can access to provide e-prescriptions and diagnoses following a reviewal of the patient's medical records and a consultation using the video conferencing tool included within the briefcase. In short, as opposed to a traditional model by which patients see doctors, PHC involves a local health worker to function as a liaison between patient and doctor to provide primary healthcare to the poor. This section is devoted to various aspects of PHC and related matter.

The lack of healthcare access the rural regions of SARC and ASEAN countries along the Belt and Road Region therefore serves not only as a major impediment in development, poverty alleviation and the wellbeing of their people, but also a violation of a basic human right. Chapter 6 of this section discusses the general motivation and mHealth services for primary care in remote South Asian communities from the perspective of preventive healthcare services.

Chapter 7 presents the Concept, Design and Implementation of PHC from the standpoint of technical and social challenges.

Portable Health Clinic (PHC) has been designed for providing primary healthcare service to the rural communities by telemedicine with the support of remote doctor. However, when the health workers visit rural areas with PHC for primary care, they face many patients who needs secondary or tertiary level of treatment for various diseases. That leads for the modular expansion with various specialized features of the basic PHC system. Besides, adding new healthcare features for specific diseases, PHC also aims to add new service approaches for better treatment in PHC. Thus, the concept of self-reported health outcomes is to be added in PHC and this chapter gives a light on it. Also, the living environment as well as the working habit highly influences the health status. Thus, the occupational and environmental health becomes so important. Chapter 8 discusses the modular expansion of PHC that has been deployed in Bangladesh by Grameen Communications.

Chapter 9 introduces the case studies of remote healthcare services in India, China, Cambodia and Pakistan. For the purpose of the Non-communicable diseases (NCDs) prevention, India, Cambodia, Pakistan utilize customized or modified PHC to fit into local needs of various targeted populations, while China utilize the government initiated systems. Case studies from each country describe processes in a different stage of designing, planning, implementing, monitoring and evaluating the remote healthcare services as well as challenges and future courses.

Personal Health Record (PHR) is known not only as a self-healthcare/disease management tool by the citizens/patients, but also as a communication tool between patients and the medical staff. Moreover, recently PHR has been considered as an indispensable tool for patient engagement in the area of non-communicable diseases (NCD) and has gained importance. In Chapter 10, we aim to introduce Asian PHR especially focusing on those in Japan, China and Bangladesh, in three different situations.

Telemedicine refers to medicine-related activities performed remotely using communication technology such as the Internet. Demand for telemedicine has been growing in various fields of medicine because it reduces time and cost. In addition, telemedicine is efficient and scalable, as it can be easily repeated and allows participants from multiple locations. Chapter 11 discusses the role of telemedicine for the development medical education in remote rural regions of developing countries.

Section III – Sustainable and Resilient mHealth Services

In the twenty-first century Asia became the most populated region in the world. Whilst the population dramatically increases, challenges remain in coping with natural disasters and better access to health. In reality, Asia is the most disaster-prone region in the world. In the twenty-first century, thousands of people lost their lives in the Gujarat Earthquake (India), Bam Earthquake (Iran), Indonesia Tsunami, Pakistan Earthquake, Cyclone Nargis (Myanmar), the Great East Japan Earthquake/Tsunami, Typhoon Haiyan (Philippines) and Nepal Earthquake.

In these catastrophic disasters, humanitarian services were provided for saving lives and protecting the human dignity of the disaster affected people. Nowadays, the innovative information and communication technologies (ICT) are having a significant impact on humanitarian services in the emergency response. In disaster response, the emergency response teams are required to provide rapid and real-time communication using available tools to collect important information from the disaster affected areas. However, disasters often disrupt the internet connections which results in the delays for vital information to reach the command post in time. Therefore, Chapter 12 proposes the novel and resilient solution to the network problem in disaster environments.

In the rural areas of developing countries, people have difficulties in accessing local health services. Furthermore, in rural areas, proper medical logistics still remain a challenge. Drones are attracting a lot of attention in transporting small amount of medical items such as bloods, samples, serum and medicines. Therefore, Chapter 13 globally reviews the applications of the medical drones in developing countries.

Whilst a lot of studies pointed out the effectiveness of drone operations for humanitarian purposes, there are still challenges in localization of proper technology in developing countries. In fact, the drone uses for humanitarian and developing activities require the global cooperation and collaboration among various stakeholders. In addition, the generation of local drone business plays a vital role in providing the sustainable solutions in developing countries. Therefore, the formulation of the platform/ecosystem for 'the drones for social good' is crucial to share the benefit of humanitarian technologies with the people in the challenging situations. Therefore, Chapter 14 presents the development of the drone ecosystem by the Nepal Flying Labs after the 2015 Nepal Earthquake.

In terms of developed countries in Asia, Japan is facing with two different types of disasters. One of them is what we call 'the silent disaster,' and another is 'the National Catastrophe.' The silent disasters in Japan include the ongoing super aging society, the population decrease, the aging of infrastructure and the increase of the chronic diseases. The symptoms of these silent disasters are particularly seen in the rural and remote areas of Japan. On the other hand, in 30 years, the occurrences of mega-disasters, which can be described as the National Catastrophe and Tokyo Inland Earthquake, are expected in Japan. For example, Nankai Trough Earthquake/Tsunami can cause more than 300,000 fatalities in the western part of Japan. To cope with these silent disasters and the national catastrophes, building the resilient communities is crucial especially in the rural areas. Innovation plays the key role in building the resilient communities. Among innovative technologies, drones are the future main players in the disaster management and the community development.

Therefore, Chapter 15 discusses the sustainable community development by drones in rural town of Minami-Oguni, Kumamoto Japan. The town of Minami-Oguni also faces with both silent disasters and sudden onset disasters. The town has been trying to build up the resilient communities by operating drones both for the community development and for the capacity building against natural disasters.

The past studies pointed out that there is the similarity between the technical needs in rural areas of developed and those in developing countries. By discussing the drone use in rural areas of Japan, this chapter also aims to propose the sustainable drone use model in the rural areas of developing countries.

Section IV – mHealth for the Elderly

Chapter 16 of this section explores how experiences of isolation and loneliness in remote areas can be mitigated through social robots' emotional care. We first discuss the concept of *being social* and how that notion is changing with rapid digitalization. The research for this chapter zooms in the context of remote regions, characterized by vast geographical distances between cities, public services and people's homes, in concrete, in northern and southern European regions. Then, the chapter discusses the Scandinavian term 'welfare technology', and investigate different technological advances aiming towards bridging the gap loneliness poses. We propose the use and development of social robots equipped with emotional care support as a way of mitigating loneliness, given that the users do not experience the implementation of the technology into their daily life as paternalistic. We close the article with reflections on the consequences of such a sensible choice.

As life expectancy of people has increased, it creates a huge demand of care needs for elderly people. By developing elder care robots, researchers and the governments in developed countries want to address this issue, and subsequently want to enhance the quality of life of the elderly people. In Chapter 17, an integrative review study has been conducted to review the scope of the application of robot-assisted services, their use cases and barriers in adopting robot-assisted services or care robots. Based on this study, the authors find that today robots are deemed as social entity, the relationship with humans is entangled with various ethical concerns (e.g. dignity, privacy and consent). Thus, to address this concern, the enhancement of the robots' social skills, adaptability, non-verbal communication and apt behaviour are significant for efficient human-to-robot relationship and coexistence.

Ageing population is a prominent problem worldwide, especially in developing countries, which leads to urgent demand of high quality but low-cost care services for the elderly. Robots are one of the promising solutions which can help with various tasks, including companionship, cognitive and physical assistance, safety protection, and health and activity monitoring. However, building one robot with all functionalities will be costly with respect to both the usage and maintenance. Therefore, in Chapter 18, we propose to transform a robot to a hub which openly hosts multiple wearable devices as plugins for various functionalities. Moreover, wearable devices can be used to enable automatic and remote user authentication, which is vital to implement one-to-many servicing mode between the robot and users. With this design, the average cost per capita can be dramatically reduced because (1) multiple users share the robot to reduce the usage cost, and (2) robots themselves become standard and open units to reduce the design and build cost. Moreover, information-centric services, such as health and activity monitoring, become more customisable, convenient and reliable due to the distributed and wireless deployment of wearables. Finally, a maturity model for robot usage in aged care is proposed to identify potential levels of information utilisation. It demonstrates that the integration of wearable devices helps to promote robot applications into more advanced reactive and proactive categories.

Chapter 19 investigates if smart speakers had utility for seniors and if they would be willing to adopt this new technology. Google Home allows for a hands-free and streamlined approach for tasks such as: answering questions, listening to music and radio, reading from various sources from the internet and other tools commonly found on a mobile device. This technology has been identified as a potential tool that can be readily used and obtained to assist seniors daily, offering an improvement of quality of life and adoption of a new emerging technology. The plan was to give a senior (over 65 years old) a smart speaker for a month and see if they used the speaker throughout the month once the initial novelty wore off. This is a case study of systematic investigation of the adoption and use of ever-increasing mobile technologies by the Elderly.

Section V – mHealth for Chronic Illnesses

As reported recently in Lancet (the top international medical journal), the disease burden has been shifting from infectious diseases (e.g., TB, HIV-AIDS etc.) to Non-Communicable chronic diseases (like diabetes, asthma, cancer and neuro-psychological diseases, such as Parkinsons, dementia, etc.) that require lifestyle changes and management. Hence this section is devoted to a range of techniques that leverage mHealth for the management of chronic illnesses.

The main contribution of Chapter 20 is in analysing mHealth as a *Service*. The explosive growth of mobile wireless communications is offering a compelling healthcare delivery alternative for developing countries. There is a compelling need to understand the comparative nature of healthcare service delivery systems including the emerging mobile health. Service quality is important to meet the patients' expectations and to retain them. However, the antecedents to service quality i.e., service operation and designs are even more important to deliver a quality healthcare service. Healthcare service providers can rely on Information Technology Infrastructure Library to continually deliver optimal services. House of Quality framework with an insight of alternate service delivery systems comparison can help in designing efficient and effective services to meet the patients' expectations and fulfil their care needs and help in raising the bar of healthcare services in developing countries.

The use of online health communities (OHCs) for informational and emotional social support seeking is on the rise. However, still little is known about type of exchanges in these communities. In Chapter 21, authors draw on and contribute to the digital health literature by critically studying online support exchanges in a major Australia online health community for cancer patients. Authors examine about 2,500 messages from 2009 to 2018, and develop a novel annotation scheme of support topics that comprise of five overarching themes: informational support provision, emotional support provision, request for help, self-reflection and disclosures, and conversational cues. Findings revealed that members of OHCs overwhelmingly disclose personal reflections to bond with the community, and many members actively post to the community solely to provide informational and emotional support to others.

Chapter 22 presents the legal and business analysis based on the use cases of the EU 6th Framework project AU2EU involving Australia, Netherlands, Germany, UK, France and Switzerland. A conceptual framework is developed for legal and business analysis that is then applied to all the six use cases. The legal analysis involves two components: the evolving regulatory environment in the countries involved and their implications for the e-Authentication and e-Authorisation related to sensitive information of the AU2EU use cases in general. Sensitive information, also referred to as data in this document, have been classified as regulated data, confidential data and public data. These data may belong to individuals, organisations or government bodies. While the actors and activities relate to the handling of these different types of data, the impact mostly relates to the risk assessment and mitigation in the context of each use case.

The business analysis uses the conceptual framework to analyse in detail the value proposition for introducing an electronic platform with e-Authentication and e-Authorisation to replace the existing process. It compares the current situation (e.g., manual record handling) with the proposed e-Authentication and e-Authorisation strategy. The value proposition has been analysed mainly from the perspectives of cost, productivity and risk.

Chapter 23 is on Promises and Challenges related to the applications of Machine Learning techniques in the diagnosis of Parkinson's Disease. Parkinson's Disease (PD) is the second most common neurodegenerative disorder, after Alzheimer's, affecting between 2% and 3% of the population aged 55 or older. More than 60% of PD prevalence in the world is in developing countries (especially China). Major symptoms of PD include tremor, bradykinesia and freezing of gaits. Despite recent advances in medical diagnostic technology, the precise diagnosis of PD, especially at its early stages, remains a challenge for modern clinicians. This is mainly because there are no objective measurements that can be used in the diagnosis and the physicians have to rely primarily on clinical profiles of the patients. The difficulty to differentiate PD from other neurodegenerative disorders is extremely difficult due to the overlapping manifestations of symptoms with other disorders. Although clinical diagnosis primarily rests on the presence of bradykinesia and other cardinal motor features, PD is associated with a plethora of non-motor symptoms adding to its overall disability. Recent research into diagnosis of PD at its early stages has taken advantage of technological advancements in machine learning. In the stream of applying machine learning for data analysis, several studies have been shown to accurately diagnose PD patients using striatal binding ratio (SBR) values. Furthermore, with deep learning techniques, several neuroimaging modalities, like SPECT and PET, have been shown to aid early and differential diagnosis of PD. In Chapter 23, authors comprehensively review research on relevant machine learning algorithms, provide deep analysis of their limitations and advantages.

People living in the most densely populated countries/regions have been most affected by the destructive impacts of natural hazards. To date, natural disasters have caused enormous damage to property and public infrastructure as well as major loss of human life. Governments must develop and implement an emergency response plan for minimizing the growing impacts of natural disasters. This can be done through vulnerability assessment, which involves three steps: (a) creating vulnerability metrics; (b) evaluating statistical analysis results and (c) interpreting spatial analysis results. In Chapter 24, the authors have present a deeper understanding about the connection between the medical and social vulnerability indices, based on a case study in the state of Victoria, Australia. The deeper understanding enables emergency response plans to be customized to respond to an effected communities' medical needs.

References

[1] WHO Global Observatory for eHealth (2011) New horizons for health through mobile technologies. Geneva: World Health Organization. Available: http://www.who.int/goe/publications/ ehealth_series_vol3/en/. Accessed 15 January 2013.

[2] P. Ray and C. Zhang, Role of Entrepreneurship in Universal Health Coverage (UHC) using mHealth, Proceedings of the IEEE Technology and Engineering Management Society Conference (TEMSCON2017) June 2017, Santa Clara, USA.

[3] T. W. Lim, H. Chan, K. Tseng, China's One Belt One Road Initiative, Imperial College Press, 2016, ISBN: 1783269294.

[4] S. Ro, D. Brian, P. Ray, Entrepreneurship Week2018, IEEE LEADER, November 2018, http://www.ieee-tems.org/2018/11/25/entrepreneurship-week-2018/. Accessed 12 March 2019.

Section I

Global challenge

Chapter 1

Role of the university for sustainable development

Soong-Chul Ro[1], Sohel Ahmed[2], Andy Hsiao[1] and Yulei Fu[3]

1.1 Introduction

UN sustainable development goal (SDG) regards universal health coverage as integral to achieving SDG 3 'good health and well-being' and ending poverty and reducing inequalities. Yet, in responding this global challenge, UN also reports, 'the world is off-track': progress has been uneven between countries; and even within countries that have made gains, there is a significant number of people being left behind [1]. It is in this respect that mobile health (mHealth) intervention is being looked upon as a way of extending health coverage to those left behind. Applied for this purpose, mHealth intervention combines technological innovation with entrepreneurial ventures for sustainable development. As all sustainable development applications, this requires the engagement of multiple stakeholders as partners on a global scale. The world is more interconnected than ever and the mobile technology increases both the width and depth of the interconnection, making it both necessary and possible to create a multi-stakeholder partnership to move the world into the sustainable future. As the Goal 17 of the SDG stipulates, sustainability is only possible when various institutions of the world work together in partnership and the same is true for the successful application of mHealth for low resource countries and regions.

University, of course, has a very important role to play in the application of mHealth for sustainable development. It is as a leading institution of the world deeply involved in technological innovation and in the education of future talents and leaders. These two aspects, research and education, can be said to be the traditional roles of the university. From the 1990s, however, there has been rising discussions regarding an additional role of the university, coinciding with the rising interest in sustainability at the international level. These discussions are embedded in two different but overlapping issues of entrepreneurship and sustainable development and both issues point towards more active participation by universities to

[1]UM-SJTU Joint Institute, Shanghai Jiao Tong University, Shanghai, P.R. China
[2]Grameen Shakti, Mirpur-2, Dhaka, Bangladesh
[3]Department of Mechanical Engineering, Shanghai Jiao Tong University, Shanghai, P.R. China

reach out to the broader society. This, in turn, calls for changes in the nature of research, education, and administration of the higher education institutions.

In this chapter, we will first provide a literature review of the key arguments regarding the roles of the universities for sustainable development. From this review, we aim to identify the key direction for the future of higher education institutions as an active member of sustainable society. Then we will use a case of an actual application of such ideals as seen in the action-learning/research initiative taken by the Center for Entrepreneurship at the University of Michigan – Shanghai Jiao Tong University Joint Institute (JI-CFE) called Technology Entrepreneurship for Sustainable Development (TESD). This initiative started in 2018 and is an on-going effort. Through this case study, we aim at adding to the on-going discussion regarding future roles of university in responding to the global challenges of sustainable development.

1.2 Role of university for sustainable development: a literature review

In the 1990s, Etzkowitz and Leydessdorf (1995) proposed the 'triple helix model' of innovation as 'a new social contract between the university and the larger society' [2]. The model was different from the previous ivory tower model in which university maintained passive, 'linear' and arms–length relationship with industry by educating future workforce or by carrying out basic research that had potential value for the industry. By the 1990s, there had already developed a closer, more interactive, and more frequent relationship among academia, industry, and government which Etzkowitz and Leydessdorf recognized as a key component of any innovation strategy and the innovation in the context of growing international collaboration. It also meant that university, as well as, the other parties needed to adapt to the new context of institutional arrangements and for university, it meant adding a third mission, more active and integrated than traditional education and research.

This discussion coincided with the rise of a phenomenon that can be termed 'entrepreneurial universities' surrounding the issues of regional development and innovation [3–6]. Despite increasing literature on this topic, however, as Schmitz *et al.* (2017) point out that the empirical models for institutional roles of the university are very fragmented, lacking in holistic and systematic consideration. In other words, there is no dearth of arguments and experimentations but these efforts are still not being accumulated to create a systematic framework for universities to follow. As a consequence, although there is a general consensus that universities need to make an academic innovation to incorporate new teaching techniques, programmes, and curriculum, the exact nature or directions for these innovations have not been satisfactorily explored (p. 386) [6].

In the meantime, similar arguments for universities to take a more active role in collaboration with other institutions of the society were raised in relation to the issue of sustainable development. Since the publication of the *Brundtland Report (Our Common Future)* in 1987, sustainable development became an important keyword in all disciplines in academia and it also pushed universities to display leadership, taking active role as a responsible citizen of the global and local community. The *Agenda 21,* adopted by more than 178 governments at the United Nations Conference on Environment and Development in 1992, included a recognition 'that education, training, and public awareness are critical tools for the transition to sustainable development'. The UNESCO took up this call and launched the UN Decade of Education for Sustainable Development (DESD), 2005–2014 [7]. Academics and policymakers of Higher Education Institutions (HEIs) around the globe debated this issue under DED's platform and this led to a boom in both policy changes and research published on the issue of the role of university for sustainable development [8–17].

The resulting debates showed much overlap with the university's role for innovation and entrepreneurship. In fact, Etzkowitz and Ledesdorff (1995) acknowledges the need for 'environmental concerns' as one of the drivers for 'the multi-faceted relationship between organizations, to carry innovation forward and bring new products' (p. 4) [2] and sustainability cannot be achieved without systematic changes brought through collective and collaborative efforts among different institutions of the society including government, industry, and university.

Yet, the debates on sustainable university produced clearer directions for the universities to follow, which can be arranged into four areas of research, education, governance, and outreach. The final report of DESD, published in 2014, highlighted three major responsibilities of universities towards sustainability:

- to prepare students for the future;
- to seek an understanding of the causes of global challenges and find solutions;
- to demonstrate excellence in sustainable development practices through good governance, community relations, and the management of the institution's environmental footprint [7].

The first two points can be equated to education and research. The third point 'good governance' and 'the institution's environmental footprint' are related to internal management, which we summarize under the term 'governance'. The 'community relations', also contained in the third point, however, brings university beyond its boundaries and can be regarded as 'outreach', in which universities work as catalysts for the change in the local community. In fact, the last area of outreach is very much emphasized throughout the report advocating participatory approach by universities to facilitate capacity-building, empowering local enterprises with knowledge of sustainable development [7].

These four areas are clearly identified in a policy brief by Ferrer-Balas *et al.* (2010) and the International Centre for Climate Change and Development (ICCCD, 2016) [10,17]. In fact, there has long been a broad consensus on this even before *Agenda 21*. For example, in 1990, universities of the world got together to declare the *Talloires Declaration of University Leader for Sustainable Future*. This is the first of a series of similar declarations* that followed and the *Talloires Declaration* alone has more than 500 signatories over 50 countries in 2019 [18]. Ten action points of the declaration is shown in Box 1.1.

*Lozano *et al.* (2015) counted 11 such declarations by 2012 [9].

Box 1.1: Talloires Declaration (relevant areas added by the authors) [18]

1. **Increase the awareness of environmentally sustainable development (Outreach)**
   Use every opportunity to raise public, government, industry, foundation, and university awareness by openly addressing the urgent need to move toward an environmentally sustainable future.
2. **Create an institutional culture of sustainability (Education, research, governance)**
   Encourage all universities to engage in education, research, policy formation, and information exchange on population, environment, and development to move toward global sustainability.
3. **Educate for environmentally responsible citizenship (Education)**
   Establish programmes to produce expertise in environmental management, sustainable economic development, population, and related fields to ensure that all university graduates are environmentally literate and have the awareness and understanding to be ecologically responsible citizens.
4. **Foster environmental literacy for all (Education)**
   Create programmes to develop the capability of university faculty to teach environmental literacy to all undergraduate, graduate, and professional students.
5. **Practise institutional ecology (Governance)**
   Set an example of environmental responsibility by establishing institutional ecology policies and practices of resource conservation, recycling, waste reduction, and environmentally sound operations.
6. **Involve all stakeholders (Education, research, governance, outreach)**
   Encourage involvement of government, foundations, and industry in supporting interdisciplinary research, education, policy formation, and information exchange in environmentally sustainable development. Expand work with community and nongovernmental organizations to assist in finding solutions to environmental problems.
7. **Collaborate for interdisciplinary (Education, research, governance, outreach)**
   Approaches Convene university faculty and administrators with environmental practitioners to develop interdisciplinary approaches to curricula, research initiatives, operations, and outreach activities that support an environmentally sustainable future.
8. **Enhance capacity of primary and secondary schools (Outreach)**
   Establish partnerships with primary and secondary schools to help develop the capacity for interdisciplinary teaching about population, environment, and sustainable development.

9. **Broaden service and outreach (Outreach)**
   Nationally and Internationally Work with national and international organizations to promote a worldwide university effort toward a sustainable future.
10. **Maintain the movement (Governance)**
   Establish a Secretariat and a steering committee to continue this momentum, and to inform and support each other's efforts in carrying out this declaration.

Two notable characteristics of this declaration are, first, the interconnection among the four areas and, second, the needs for participatory, interdisciplinary and multi-stakeholder approaches. Research and education have been recognized as the traditional roles of the university. Yet, incorporating sustainability into these two areas are regarded as more than adding new courses or directing research towards this topic. To incorporate a new idea of sustainability into these traditional areas, the university's governance needs to be re-oriented towards sustainability. In addition, universities are expected to set standards for other institutions to follow by practicing sustainability themselves, which constitutes another area of governance that is related to the internal operation. These are regarded as systematic and holistic changes to university and beyond, key to the success is engaging multiple stakeholders inside and outside of the university. Therefore, outreach becomes an integral part of university's efforts to increase contribution to sustainability. These points are made in virtually all the literature on the university's role in sustainability as summarized in Table 1.1.

The reason outreach becomes so important is partly due to the changes in the paradigm in education and research that is necessary to integrate sustainability into them. For example, during the fourth UNESCO Chair Conference on Higher Education for Sustainable Development in 2011, participants made proposals in three interrelated aspects of campus, curriculum, and community. Of these, the Community Roundtable made a challenging proposal to transform the university into 'meeting places' and assessing the university's reputation by the quality of its interaction with local, regional, and national stakeholders while working on real-life problems relevant to the surrounding community and society at large. It also argued for treating students as 'co-creator' of knowledge and exposing them to interdisciplinary and transdisciplinary perspectives by encouraging them to engage with the real world [14].

This is a call for a paradigm change. All the authors reviewed here echoes the DESD final report and urge universities to move away from the traditional discipline-based, compartmentalized research and education, aimed at producing knowledge within the scientific community. In its place, they advocate participatory, inter-(or trans-)disciplinary, co-production of knowledge in collaboration with broader stakeholders (enterprise, NGO's and government) aimed at producing social impacts. Education and research in the traditional paradigm of the ivory

Table 1.1 Roles of the university for sustainable development as discussed by various authors

	Research	Education	Governance and operation	Outreach
Ferrer-Balas *et al.* (2010) [10]	Participatory action research; Transformation towards a more balanced; synergistic, trans-disciplinary, and holistic perspective	Emphasis on learning to learn	New course ranking and assessment methods; Participatory approach as the most effective way to change values within university members	Innovative interactions with practitioners
Sedlacek (2013) [11]	Knowledge creation and transfer	Educate and train	Internal governance	External governance at the national and regional level
Karatzoglou (2013) [12]	A new research and teaching agenda for universities as the centres of development of sustainability science	Promotion of integration, synthesis, critical reasoning, and system-thinking skills	A change in universities' own management practices	Assumption of a leading role in coordinating, promoting, and enhancing the engagement of local authorities and other societal stakeholders
Dlouhá, J. *et al.* (2013) [13]	Responsive to society; trans-disciplinary collaboration	Critical approach; Sustainability values; Implementation of participative learning strategies; Social learning that provides an opportunity for the emergence of new solutions within a given dialogue	Developing a new measure of quality based on 'sustainability impacts' (not just 'scientific impacts'); Undertake meaningful internal transformation to fulfil the new missions and roles	Greater openness and communication with all social actors; Partnership and networks; capacity building and training
Mülller-Christ *et al.* (2014) [14]	From the generation of new disciplinary knowledge to the generation of trans-disciplinary knowledge through action research	Integrating sustainability to curriculum	Develop quality criteria and enhance quality assurance; Transforming campus by engaging all members; linking university accountability with	Community: Turn university into 'meeting places' Engage students with the real world

			campus sustainability; thinking beyond the university's physical boundaries to provide a transferable model for the surrounding community	
Lozano *et al.* (2015) [9]	Centres and funding for holistic thinking	Courses, programmes, educating educators, transdisciplinary	Institutional Framework; Campus Operation; On-campus experience; Assessments and reporting	Outreach and collaboration: exchange programmes, joint degree, joint research, partnership with enterprises, NGOs, government
Lazzarini *et al.* (2018) [15]	From disciplinary, compartmentalized research to projects aimed at enhancing the competence of academics by connecting with a broader range of stakeholders in collaboration	Reorientation of educational programmes addressing and integrating sustainability; Convergence between sustainable development agenda and educational agenda; Pedagogical innovations	Reorienting management, evaluation and reward structure towards participatory, trans-disciplinary, and multi-stakeholder activities	Social outreach and collaboration

tower made an indirect contribution to the society by cultivating (future) workers in sustainability and by producing knowledge that can be adopted by others towards sustainability. In this old context, outreach was a non-essential, added activity that is disconnected from the university's main agenda – disciplinary research/teaching. This situation is akin to CSR done by corporations as a part of the public relations campaign but disconnected from their main business focus. In contrast, under the new paradigm, outreach is an integral part that can provide contextualized learning and research as well as creating opportunities for the university to take more active and direct role in bringing sustainability to the local community.

The outreach programmes envisioned in these works are therefore much more than offering university campus as 'meeting place' by convening conferences. They are much more than disseminating knowledge to the local community through public lectures. They are also much more than field trips where students are introduced to the context and the outcome is solely educational on students' side. They include, at the core of the new outreach programme, entrepreneurial activities such as commercialization of knowledge, creating spin-offs through incubators, and working with partners in regional development done by the members of the university. As Wakkee *et al.* (2019) note, 'entrepreneurial university' becomes a driver of sustainability through 'education and outreach' notably in developing countries [15]. This point seamlessly links the role of the university for sustainable development to the concept of 'entrepreneurial university' [6,19].

In sum, the characteristics of universities that are the leaders of sustainability can be summarized in the following four points:

1. Research and education in sustainable universities are action-based and context-driven, regarding students as co-producer of knowledge and inter-disciplinary by nature. These are also integrated with each other and with outreach activities.
2. Outreach activities in sustainable universities are integrated to partners in the local community through entrepreneurial, though not profit-making, activities in broad partnership with community stakeholders.
3. Governance in sustainable universities supports and leads the changes in internal management towards the above points.

These were also the points that were considered in the following example of the TESD.

1.3 Technology entrepreneurship for sustainable development

1.3.1 TESD model

TESD is an initiative by the Center for Entrepreneurship (JI-CFE) at University of Michigan – Shanghai Jiao Tong University Joint Institute (UM-SJTU JI) that aims to utilize university's strengths in human and social capital in active support of the sustainable development projects in local communities (Figure 1.1). It originated in

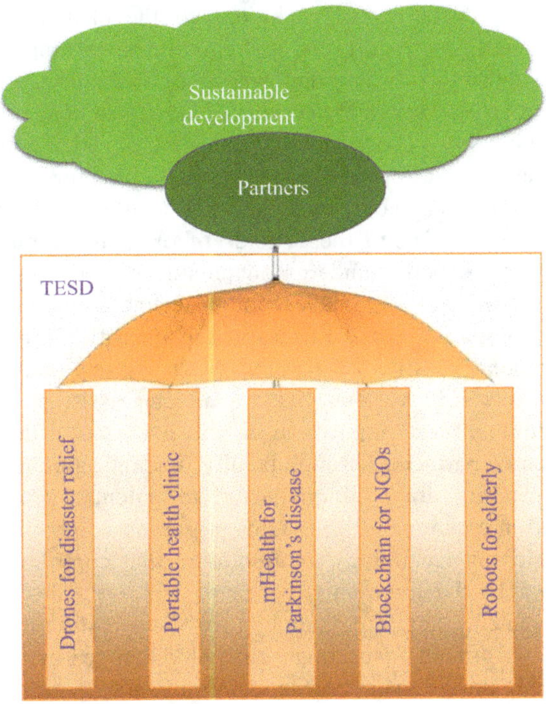

Figure 1.1 Technology entrepreneurship for sustainable development

the Entrepreneurship Week event, hosted by JI-CFE in September 2018.† This event brought together research projects in mHealth for Belt and Road which are contained in the following chapters of this book. During this conference, the participants also recognized the need to create an umbrella project that can identify possible ways to increase the social impacts by combining elements of existing projects or exploring new applications.

Then, the ensuing discussion within the JI-CFE laid down the main characteristics of the TESD project. First, as JI-CFE's main task is entrepreneurship education among undergraduate students majoring in engineering, TESD project also works in tandem with undergraduate students and carried out as an educational outreach and action learning project. Second, at the same time, students efforts will be directed towards a concrete project with visible impacts on sustainability through partnership with practitioners in the field of sustainability such as government, (social) businesses, NGOs, research institutes including other universities. Third, leveraging UM-SJTU Joint Institute's strengths in engineering, TESD

†For details, see Ro, S. *et al.* (2018). 'Entrepreneurship Week 2018'. *IEEE Leader*. (retrieved from http://www.ieee-tems.org/2018/11/25/entrepreneurship-week-2018/, August 2019)

focuses on providing technological solutions to the challenges of sustainable development by identifying, modifying, and combining existing technologies.

As such, TESD brings two abundant resources of the university – human and social capital – and employ the in the service of the global challenge of sustainable development. A university has experts in both technological and non-technological fields that can be employed to produce practical solutions for the challenges faced by partners working in sustainable development. It also has students, young people being trained competitively into these fields of expertise. Although still in the process of becoming experts, undergraduate students in engineering schools, especially in the advanced years, have enough technological awareness to work with existing technologies and make necessary modification according to specific needs of the community partners. Universities also have resources such as labs, equipment, and experts in various fields who can assist students in seeking technological solutions. More importantly, a university sits at the centre of a vast network with potential partners. Through faculty, students, alumni, and their family and friends, universities are well connected to potential community partners both domestic and international. TESD aims at putting combining these strengths together and employing technology as a solution that contributes to sustainable development efforts by the community partners.

Partner engagement, therefore, is crucial for a successful project. Partners can be divided into two groups – sustainable development partners and technology partners. Sustainable development partners are those that work in the field of sustainability. It could be a government agency, NGO, research institutes, businesses, and social businesses. The university is not institutionalized to deliver and it is not in the front of, especially localized issues such as poverty reduction, environmental protection, welfare for elderly, disabled, and underprivileged. The social network of the university makes it an ideal institution to provide a meeting place for different localized efforts to come together to create a network among themselves and create global awareness. Concrete action that contributes to the positive changes, however, necessitates in-depth knowledge of the particular situation and context and this level of intimacy cannot be retained at university because its main agenda – research and education – are different and often only allows relative short period attention to local contexts that are fast-changing and not generalizable. Therefore, for the university to become an integral part of the solution, university needs to rely on the partners, who are daily working in the particular context, to provide contextualized information and consultation based on it at every stage of the development of technology: identifying project objectives, designing engineering solution, building prototype, testing and reiterative design, implementation, and further modification. They can also grant access to the people and facilities necessary for testing prototypes and getting feedback to continuously improve technology. Many of these partners, such as Grameen Shaki, also have the ability to take the prototypes or proofs-of-concept from the university and actualize them by implementing them in real situations or even scale up to increase impacts.

Technology partners, on the other hand, are the companies and institutions that provide technology solutions that can be integrated with each other through student projects. The vast majority of these technology-based products and services are offered by private for-profit companies and are therefore available through the market. In identifying the right technology and modifying and combining them, it is necessary to build close partnership with the owners of the technology.

There are two interconnected ways in which such projects can materialize; one initiated from the field of the sustainable development project and another from sustainable technology. The first starts from the problems and challenges faced by sustainable development partners and through TESD, identifying and building the right technology solution to address this issue. The other is starting from available technologies that have potential to assist sustainable development challenges and show-case this technology with potential partners in sustainable development to generate operational model or implementation strategy built around this technology. We imagine that in reality any meaningful project will have a continuous back-and-forth cycle which is one element that TESD has to manage. Nevertheless, university's role ends at the proof of concept and showcasing to help build network and the actual implementation will be left to the partners.

In this way, TESD provides an opportunity for action-learning for students through the hands-on experience of working with partners in the field of sustainable development and in technology. This involves communicating with multiple stakeholders and such efforts are bound to be inter- or trans-disciplinary in nature. It can also lead to action-research through the partnership and it is an outreach programme that enables the university to play a more active role in the global action network for sustainable development. In essence, this project embodies the current discussion regarding the university's role for sustainable development summarized in the previous part. It is also an entrepreneurial project for the university. Both the faculty and students need to take charge and seek innovative solutions to the global challenges of sustainability. It involves putting time and resources to communicate with multiple stakeholders to identify tangible goals and work towards practical solutions. Just like any entrepreneurship project, there is also embedded risk of failure and seeking finance beyond the prearranged educational or research funding is a must to sustain such efforts. In fact, this is entrepreneurship in all its aspects except for creating a start-up company for profit. This model is being applied in multiple projects and the prominent one taking place in Bangladesh.

1.3.2 Bangladesh sustainable development challenge

From the inception in April 2017, JI-CFE sought to create action research projects through piloting suitable mHealth action research projects in a remote rural area in China with student participation. During this explorative period, undergraduate students volunteered through JI and helped in identifying local technology and development partners as well as suitable (doable and meaningful) projects. Yet a real breakthrough was made with the funding opportunity through the Global Engagement Initiative which promoted SJTU students to participate in international development projects in multidisciplinary teams. With this funding, it became possible to move TESD to overseas and Bangladesh was chosen as the first destination. It is a country along the Belt and Road Initiative, most supportive of this plan and CFE already had informal but strong linkage and collaboration with Social Businesses of Yunus Center and Grameen Groups as well as various academics of Dhaka University. 11 students were recruited in October 2018 under the project title 'Bangladesh Sustainable Development Challenge'. The team included two undergraduate students, two Ph.D. and seven masters students from eight different departments of Shanghai Jiao Tong University. It also included two media students who joined to produce multimedia reports.

The objectives of this first field trip were to make preliminary contacts with various partners and identify issues that are suitable for TESD model (Figure 1.2) to address; in other words, identifying areas where existing technologies can be combined to help local partners in bringing sustainable development for the underprivileged people in the rural and urban communities. Once the project was officially launched, the number of partners also grew and the team visited seven partners – one higher education institution, two government agents, three social businesses, and one research institute as in Table 1.2.

In January 2019, the students visited these partners and their project sites in four different municipalities in Bangladesh and identified nine projects with varying degree of feasibility. All these projects were deemed significant in terms of the social impacts, however, majority of them needed more time for students to reach a deeper understanding of the social context through more frequent visits to clarify attainable objectives so that necessary technologies can be identified and operational models can be determined. On the other hands, there were three projects with relatively clear objectives and identified interests among faculty and students and the team chose these three – list in Table 1.3 – to be carried out as the second phase of the Bangladesh Challenge project.

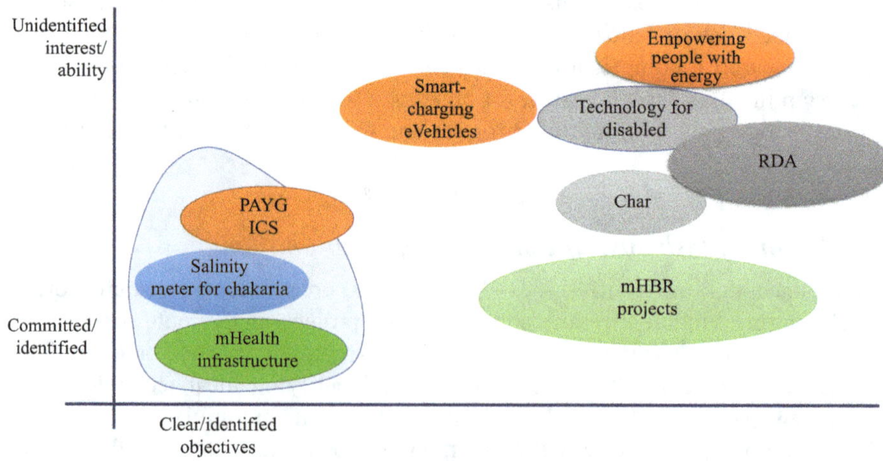

Figure 1.2 TESD model

Table 1.2 Partners of the Bangladesh Sustainable Development Challenge, 2019

Category	Partners	Projects identified
Higher education institution	• Dhaka University	• Technology for the disabled and elderly
Government institute	• A2I • Rural Development Academy	• Technology for the disabled • Education and health for the remote *Char* islands • mHealth infrastructure
Social businesses	• Grameen Shakti • Grameen Communications • Yunus Center	• Pay-as-you-go LPG cylinders • Smart-charging eVehicles • Empowering people with Energy • mHealth infrastructure
Research institute	• icddr,b	• Measuring underground water salinity

Table 1.3 Bangladesh Sustainable Development Challenge Projects, 2019

Project title	Details	Partners
mHealth infrastructure	Telemedicine infrastructure linking hospital to another hospital and mHealth infrastructure linking underserved population to hospitals or health workers in cooperation with Chinese tech companies	Renji Hospital (Shanghai, China) Shanghai Baiyulan (Shanghai, China) A2I (Dhaka, Bangladesh) SynesisIT (Dhaka, Bangladesh) Dhaka University (Dhaka, Bangladesh)
Salinity meter	Developing prototype salinity meter to measure the influence of climate change on salinity of underground drinking water on the coastal region of Chittagong	icddr,b (Dhaka, Bangladesh)
Pay-as-you-go for LPG cylinders	Developing prototype PAYG module for LPG cylinders so that rural household can afford to LPG to increase convenience and health as well as reduced greenhouse gas emission	Grameen Shakti (Dhaka, Bangladesh)

1.4 Discussion

The challenge here is motivating these stakeholders to join and continue the partnership. The immediate stakeholders for TESD (Figure 1.3) and their interests can be arranged as in Table 1.4. All institutions have a particular agenda around which the whole institutions are built. Universities are built around research and education and for-profit companies are institutionalized around short-term profit.

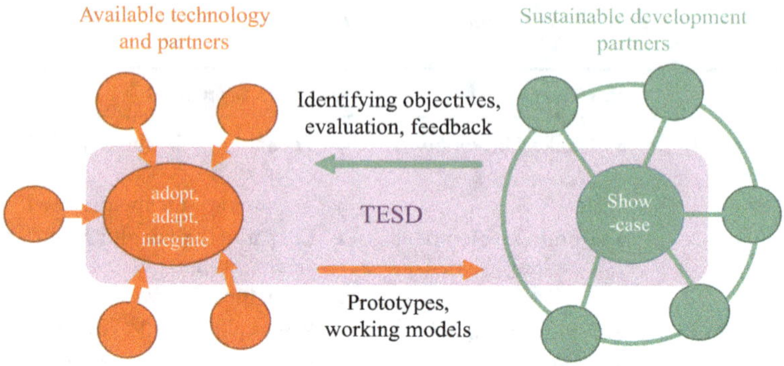

Figure 1.3 TESD stakeholders

Table 1.4 Immediate stakeholders of the TESD project

	Potential contribution to the project	**Potential gain from the project**
Sustainable development partners	Provide contextual knowledge and consultation during the project and product design; facilitate tests and implementation of the prototype;	Improvements in impact; opening new project area
Technology partners	Provide technology-based products and services; consultation during prototype building	New market, positive reputation
Students	Leading the project by identifying problems and determining designs for technological solution with partners Identifying the required technologies to modify and combine Building prototype and improving communication with partners	Entrepreneurial and innovation experience through contextual, action learning, in communication with other stakeholders
Faculty	Identify and create a network among other stakeholders Provide expert knowledge to other partners Supervise students to co-produce knowledge and social impacts Facilitate communication with other stakeholders	Innovative, action-driven educational projects; Action research

While there are welcome debates regarding necessary changes for both of the institutions in the age of sustainability, anyone who wants to see practical results need to be able to persuade stakeholders to see the value in participating in such endeavours in the language the stakeholders understand currently. Within the university, faculty members are almost solely motivated by mostly disciplinary research, students are broadly interested in education and experience but often these are expressed in terms of grades, credits or evidence of excellence that they can use in applying for jobs and graduate schools upon graduation. The structure of for-profit companies does not allow employees to divert time and resources towards projects that do not promise short-term financial gain for the company. Even CEO needs to answer to the board and shareholders for his actions. Sustainable development partners, government, NGO, research institute, social businesses all have their own unique institutional agenda and regardless of individual enthusiasm, institutional resources should not be expected for activities unrelated to their immediate goals.

After the first field trip, the Bangladesh Challenge team recognized the need to further integrate the second phase of prototype development into the educational curriculum of the university. This was necessary to motivate faculty with expertise and students who will need to put a substantial amount of time, efforts, and resources in developing and testing prototypes. Since the return of the first trip, three 'low-hanging' projects were carried out through multiple courses including senior design courses (or Capstone projects). This was possible because of the support of the faculty in charge of those courses. The leadership of the school, University of Michigan-Shanghai Jiao Tong University, also fully supported this initiative by making this experimental structure possible. And allocated financial resources to send two of the student team for additional travel to Bangladesh to confirm design requirements. In this way, outreach activities have been fully integrated into the educational structure of the institution, and this also provides motivation for students to contribute.

This, however, came at some cost. First, this meant losing the inter-departmental cooperation that characterized the first Bangladesh Challenge. Once a course structure is employed it became difficult to include students from other departments into the credit system and finding faculty members with expertise in different schools who will be interested in a project led by another school is a remaining challenge, which actually limits the kind of project that can be done as outreach to the area of expertise by volunteering faculty.

Also, most of the courses at universities are organized on the semester basis and students plan their school life accordingly. Especially with increasing number of semesters abroad, it has become difficult to get students to continue the same project over two semesters or more. This partly explains what Wakkee *et al.* (2019) noted as students' tendency to prefer low-hanging fruits type of projects but also make their hope of making these project 'serve as stepping stone toward more ambitious and ostentatious activities' [16] somewhat difficult.

This makes a long-term enduring relationship between partners and university more important. This can be achieved by non-TESD related visits and exchanges but the challenge here is the current culture based on short-term achievements. For-profit and social businesses, NGOs and government agents are all under pressure to provide evidence of short-term achievements to their investors, board, funders, and superiors. Business trips and exchanges may not be possible unless there is a reasonable chance of profit or achievement, making the long-term relationship less palatable for all concerned. Getting participation from for-profit technology partners is especially difficult because they tend to focus on market share rather than social impacts and reluctant to risk sharing their technology without matching financial prospects.

On top of this, there is the challenge of financing such an endeavour. The Internet has made international communication easy but transferring contextual information through emails, social network platforms, and video-conference is a huge challenge and it is necessary for students to travel, meet the partners and examine the local situation. In addition, building network of stakeholders needs trust which can still be best created through face-to-face interaction, especially across different cultures, but the university has been institutionalized to support disciplinary education and research which makes it difficult to justify supporting this kind of outreach activities and for the sustainable operation of TESD and funding should be created from outside the departmental box.

More challenging, however, is getting the support of the faculty. Faculty support is crucial especially since they can motivate students and also work as a link between short-term projects by students. They can also use their expert knowledge to breakdown ambitious projects and lower the branches for the students. Yet, as Lazzarini (2018) noted 'social outreach is not included as a rewarded activity of academics' [15] and it is regarded as somewhat less important than disciplinary research This, in turn, affects incentives and rewards for students who are reluctant in participating in a time-consuming projects that do not give them credits other than a line on peripheral sections of their CVs. Especially for postgraduate students, often other activities than research publications are regarded as distractions and frowned upon by their supervisors.

Wakkee *et al.* (2019) conclude that education and outreach as the first characteristics of the university through which it can be the driver of sustainable development [16]. Yet, as UNESCO reports in 2014, this necessitates the 'whole-institution approaches': transforming the curricula, pedagogy, research, and operations at the core of higher education and engaging all stakeholders [8]. As the same report laments the 'whole-institution approach' were found to 'have been the exception rather than the rule' (p. 127). The reason for this is embedded in the institutional characteristics of university. Ferrer-Balas *et al.* (2010) characterizes higher education sector with 'high resistance to change' (p. 608) [10]. As Lazzarini *et al.* (2018) observed, 'sustainable development is not yet comprehensively integrated into higher education system and the pace of change has been little and slow' (p. 238) [15]. Institutional characteristics of a university is not easy to change. Current research activities are characterized by 'over-specialization' and 'compartmentalization' through disciplinary boundaries and achieving 'business targets' of attracting such research funding has exceeded innovative teaching necessary to embed sustainability into university's education [15]. Under such circumstances, university's governance is still focused on managing disciplinary research and the outreach, as a newly highlighted area, receives least focus among the four areas mentioned above [9].

In this respect, the emergence of a new 'sustainability'-focused university ranking system is a welcome development. In the UK, Save The Student publishes 'University Sustainability Rankings' for 154 universities in the UK. Although it largely focuses on governance (operation) but it also considers education and engagement [20]. In North America, the Association for the Advancement of Sustainability in Higher Education (AASHE) uses Sustainability Tracking, Assessment & Rating System (STARS) and publishes voluntary reports by universities in North America since 2010 [21]. They classify reports into four ratings of platinum, gold, silver, and bronze. In 2019, 334 institutions submitted valid reports and 6 received platinum, 123 in gold, 141 in silver, 52 in the bronze category, and 12 elected not to publish scoring information. From 2018, the data are incorporated into Sierra and The Princeton Review's Guide to Green Colleges [22]. For a more global effort, Universitas Indonesia (UI) launched the UI GreenMetric World University Ranking in 2010 based on the online surveys. 719 universities were ranked in 2018 but the participation is still limited with many prominent universities and the UI is missing. Also, this is confined to the operational aspect of sustainability [23].

These efforts either dealt with the part of sustainability or limited in geographic scope. Then in 2018, the Times Higher Education took up the task of developing a global ranking system for Sustainable University which measures universities' impacts on the 17 SDGs [24]. The first of 'THE University Impact Ranking' was published in 2019 with more than 450 universities from 76 countries. It measures university's impacts on 11 items of 17 SDGs through carefully calibrated criteria based on data and evidence supplied by universities across three broad areas of 'research', 'outreach', and 'stewardship'. 'Education' is not mentioned in the criteria but it is measured through the professionals created by the university working to improve each item of the SDG under consideration [25]. Currently the ranking is published separately from THE's main ranking. It is there for anyone wish to look it up but whether this will become a significant source of information for the society to judge a university remains to be seen.

1.5 Concluding remarks

University has an important place in leading the world into sustainability and outreach can be the catalysis to channel university's strength to the community and in turn bring multi-stakeholder perspectives to the university leading to positive changes towards the university itself. Yet, there are many challenges. Whereas there is undeniable value in outreach programmes that integrates university's resources to actual sustainable development works through community partners and corporations, motivating stakeholders within university and among partners and getting their support remains the main challenge.

This boils down to the institutional needs that shape individual needs. Generally speaking, prevailing institutional focus on short-term achievements is a challenge for imaginative sustainable outreach programmes for the future. Beyond this, all institutions have their own unique needs and individuals in different positions within the same institution often have different institutionalized objectives. Focusing on universities, current institutional needs are dominated by disciplinary research and education. It is necessary to design a reward system for faculty and students to motivate them to participate in sustainable outreach projects within the framework of current institutional needs. Disciplinary research in itself is not a bad thing or a mere relics of the past, it will continue to generate innovation. Doing away with disciplinarily would be akin to arguing for returning to pre-industrial age to achieve sustainability. What we need is not discouraging existing institutional needs but building sustainability on them – disciplinary research will and need to continue and therefore, faculty member promoting sustainable outreach programmes should continue to find an opportunity for collaborative research while preparing long-term projects into short-term projects that can be done by students. In the same way, there have to be credits or other forms of recognition for students' time and effort for the outreach-related works. Efforts should be made to demonstrate potential or latent value – financial or relational – of participating in the project to corporate partners and the chances of increasing reach or raising social impacts for development partners. All this should be done in innovative use of new media beyond traditional written communication through publications, brochures, or even short articles in websites or social media, utilizing more multimedia to reach more people.

Sustainability is already in the to-do list of most of the institutions – although the interpretation of the word might differ little here and there, hardly anyone, in hardly any institution rejects sustainability outright. Therefore, those who are promoting changes should patiently find innovative ways to meet the current institutional needs as well as those of sustainable future. Just as profit is one of the bottom lines for the new sustainable future together with the planet and people. Incorporating current institutional needs will be the key to making sustainable university programme sustainable. This requires persistent efforts to demonstrate the value in the new programme to all partners in the way that they can willingly render support, and the TESD experience shows that support will come. Much good can be achieved by universities if we channel their resources towards sustainability: what we need is a metamorphosis of university towards a more integrated active participant of the sustainable development.

References

[1] UNDP, n.d. 'Goal 3: Good health and well-being', *Sustainable Development Goal.* [retrieved from http://undp.org/content/undp/en/home/sustainable-development-goals/goal-3-good-health-and-well-being.html, August 2019]

[2] Etzkowitz, H. and Leydesdorff L. 1995. 'The triple helix – University-Industry-Government relations: a laboratory for knowledge-based economic development'. *EASST Review* 14(1): 14–19.

[3] Clark, B. R. 1998. *Creating Entrepreneurial Universities: Organization Pathways of Transformation* Guildford: Pergamon.

[4] Schmitz, A., Urbano, D., Dandolini, G. A., de Souze, J. A. and Guerrero, M. 2017. 'Innovation and entrepreneurship in the academic setting: a systematic literature review'. *International Entrepreneurship and Management Journal* 13: 369–395.

[5] Sandström, C., Wennberg, K., Walli, M. W. and Zherlygina, Y. 2018. 'Public policy for academic entrepreneurship initiatives: a review and critical discussion'. *Journal of Technology Transformation* 43: 1232–1256.

[6] Muller, S. 2016. 'A progress review of entrepreneurship and regional development: what are the remaining gaps?'. *European Planning Studies* 24(6): 1133–1158.

[7] Leonidou, E., Christofi, M., Vrontis, D., and Thrassou, A. 2018. 'An integrative framework of stakeholder engagement for innovation management and entrepreneurship development'. *Journal of Business Research (in press)* 1–14. Retrieved from https://doi.org/10.1016/j.jbusres.2018.11.054

[8] UNESCO. 2014. 'Shaping the Future We Want: UN Decade of Education for Sustainable Development 2005-2014 (Final Report)'.

[9] Lozano, R., Ceulemans, K., Alonso-Almeida, M., *et al.* 2015. 'A review of commitment and implementation of sustainable development in higher education: results from a worldwide survey'. *Journal of Cleaner Production* 108: 1–18.

[10] Ferrer-Balas, D., Lozano, R., Huisingh, D., Buckland, H., Perre, Y. and Zilahy, G. 2010. Going beyond the rhetoric: system-wide changes in universities for sustainable societies'. *Journal of Cleaner Production* 18: 607–610.

[11] Sedlacek, S. 2013. 'The role of universities in fostering sustainable development at the regional level'. *Journal of Cleaner Production* 48: 74–84.

[12] Karatzoglou, B. 2013. 'An in-depth literature review of the evolving roles and contributions of universities to education for sustainable development'. *Journal of Cleaner Production* 49: 44–53.

[13] Dlouhá, J., Huisingh, D. and Barton, A. 2013. 'Learning networks in higher education: universities in search of making effective regional impacts'. *Journal of Cleaner Production* 49: 5–10.

[14] Müller-Christ, G., Sterling, S., van Dam-Mieras, R., Adomßent, M., Fischer, D. and Rieckmann, M. 2014. 'The role of campus, curriculum, and community in higher education for sustainable development – a conference report'. *Journal of Cleaner Production* 62: 134–137.

[15] Lazzarini, B., Pérez-Foguet, A. and Boni, A. 2018. 'Key charactiristics of academics promoting sustainable suman development within engineering studies'. *Journal of Cleaner Production* 18: 237–252.

[16] Wakkee, I., van der Sijde, P., Vaupell, C. and Ghuman, K. 2019. 'The university's role in sustainable development: activating entrepreneurial scholars as agents of change'. *Technological forecasting and Social Change* 141: 195–205.

[17] Bhowmic, J., Huq, S. and Selim, S. 2018. 'The Role of Universities in Achieving the Sustainable Development Goals'. *ICCCAD Policy Brief.* (retrieved from http://www.icccad.net/wp-content/uploads/2015/12/Policy-Brief-on-role-of-Universities-in-achieving-SDGs.pdf, August 2019)

[18] University Leaders for a Sustainable Future. n.d. *Talloire Declaration Signatories List*. (retrieved from http://ulsf.org/96-2/, August 2019)

[19] Guerrero, M., Urbano, D. and Fayolle, A. 2016. 'Entrepreneurial activity and regional competitiveness: evidence from European entrepreneurial universities'. *Journal of Technological Transfer* 41(1): 105–131.

[20] Save the Student. n.d. 'University Sustainability Rankings'. (https://savethestudent.org/extra-guides/university-sustainability-environment-league-table.html)

[21] AASHE. n.d. 'Sustainability Tacking Assessment & Rating System (STARS)'. (https://stars.aashe.org/)

[22] Sierra and The Princeton Review. n.d. 'Guide to Green Colleges'. (https://bestcolleges.com/features/greenest-universities/)

[23] Universitas Indonesia. n.d. 'UI GreenMetric World University Ranking'. (http://greenmetric.ui.ac.id)

[24] Times Higher Education. 2018. 'THE developing ranking based on Sustainable Development Goals'. (retrieved from https://timeshighereducation.com/news/developing-ranking-based-sustainable-development-goals, August 2019)

[25] Times Higher Education. n.d. 'Methodology'. (retrieved from https://timeshighereducation.com/world-university-rankings/methodology-impact-rankings-2019, August 2019)

Chapter 2

Be friends with the future – Global innovation and entrepreneurship collaboration system in the field of medical health

Zhang Zhigang[1,2]

Whether it is a scientist, entrepreneur, politician, or economist, we will find ourselves in a confusing world. Everyone tries to have a deeper understanding of the world from a certain angle. The twentieth century is a remarkably productive one for human society, especially for physics. Albert Einstein's theory of general relativity helped us view gravity not as a force but as a distortion of space [1]. Then Max Planck, Erwin Schrödinger, and Werner Heisenberg gave us quantum mechanics—and a fresh understanding of the subatomic world [2]. In the middle of the century, two new forces were discovered deep within the atom (the strong and weak nuclear forces). Finally, in the twentieth century's last decades, we got the Standard Model of particle physics—an accounting of all the particles and forces known to exist in our universe [3]. Human cognition of the micro-world has been able to meet the needs of human society.

We are full of confidence in understanding the nature of the world's operations. However, in the first 20 years of the twenty-first century, we have seen human society enter an unprecedented stage of complexity, and the prospects are not optimistic. When we put a lot of research and observations based on the experience, the world we could see is limited. We predict the future based on experience and judge the social progress with personal judgment. It may bring us to the path of retrogression. We need to see more fundamental laws of world development, and thus we can see the inevitable macroscopic trend of future development. On this basis, we will plan our resources, our time, our energy, and our way of cooperation. So we can make reasonable and correct choices relatively quickly when we take the world as a mega system. The future of this system is to be a brand new life. Understanding the future and to be friends with the future, so we could make the future of the world.

In this chapter, we will briefly describe the pyramid model for the evolution of complex systems to clarify the stage of human social development firstly. Then we

[1]Advanced Industrial Technology Research Institute (AITRI), Shanghai Jiao Tong University, Shanghai, China
[2]Shanghai neoBay Venture Capital Co., Ltd., Shanghai, China

will analyze the opportunities and future development trends of the healthcare industry at the current stage. We will also explain how to promote global cooperation in the field of the healthcare industry through the construction of an innovation and entrepreneurship ecosystem.

2.1 Folding: the basic driving force of social development

More and more researchers, economic development practitioners and policy-makers are taking human society and the economy as systems. Innovation and entrepreneurship are taken as the key to a better economy. Innovation is taken as the source of competitive advantage—for individuals, for organizations, and for society [4]. Researches are evaluating the capacity of the community to host and support an entrepreneurial ecosystem and the capacity of entrepreneurs to grow themselves and their businesses in support of community economic development [5]. During the last three decades, there has been an impressive rise in alliance research, with studies examining topics as diverse as investment patterns, organizational governance choices, network structures, trust formation, and so forth [6]. An innovation ecosystem consists of economic agents and economic relations as well as the non-economic parts such as technology, institutions, sociological interactions, and the culture [7]. Even for established companies in countless industries, they have recognized the need to access globally dispersed knowledge networks to develop and acquire innovations necessary to better serve their customers [7]. In some researchers view, innovation ecosystem is not yet a clearly defined concept, much less a theory. Moreover, the idea carries pitfalls, notably its over-emphasis on market forces, and its flawed analogy to natural ecosystems [8].

Some more exciting characteristics of systems are revealed. Some bestsellers take us to a new understanding of the world. We are trying to cultivate synthetic life. However, as we cultivate synthetic life in our artifacts, we cultivate the loss of our command. "Out of control," to be honest, is a great exaggeration of the state that our enlivened machines will take. They will remain indirectly under our influence and guidance but free of our domination [9]. Living systems, from the smallest bacteria to the largest cities and ecosystems, are quintessential complex adaptive systems operating over an enormous range of multiple spatial, temporal, energy, and mass scales [10]. The world will be different when we take the real world as systems.

The great challenge of our time is to build and nurture sustainable communities and societies, designed in such a way that our activities do not interfere with nature's inherent ability to sustain life. The first step in this endeavor is to understand the principles of organization that nature's ecosystems have evolved to sustain the web of life [11].

Finally, in the recent 100 years, the holistic perspective (systems thinking) became popular and will help us to better understanding the world. However, this not enough. The world is evolving far faster than we could imagine. After

13.8 billion years of cosmic evolution, development has accelerated dramatically here on Earth: Life 1.0 arrived about 4 billion years ago, Life 2.0 (we humans) arrived about a 100 millennia ago, and many AI researchers think that Life 3.0 may arrive during the coming century, perhaps even during our lifetime [12].

2.1.1 The basic model of a complex system

The primary goal of social development is to achieve sustainable development at all levels. Whether it is individuals, enterprises, social organizations, or countries, the most fundamental appeal of humankind is the sustainable development of the world. A fundamental feature of social development is the continuing increase in complexity at different levels above the elementary particle scale. We could take the world as a super-complex system composed of a large number of complex systems interacting at different levels. The basic laws of social evolution follow the fundamental laws of complex system evolution at all levels.

We could define a boundary for the system and abstract the system into the model shown in Figure 2.1. Complex systems consist of many interacting components. A network can be used to represent complex systems. Nodes in the network represent the components of the system, and connections between nodes represent their interactions. The interactions between the internal nodes of the system make the system as a whole to exhibit certain functions and interact with the outside world through outside connections. This system can be an enterprise, can be a social organization, can be a dog, can be a person, can be a cell, can be a country, can be humankind, can also include the entire planet.

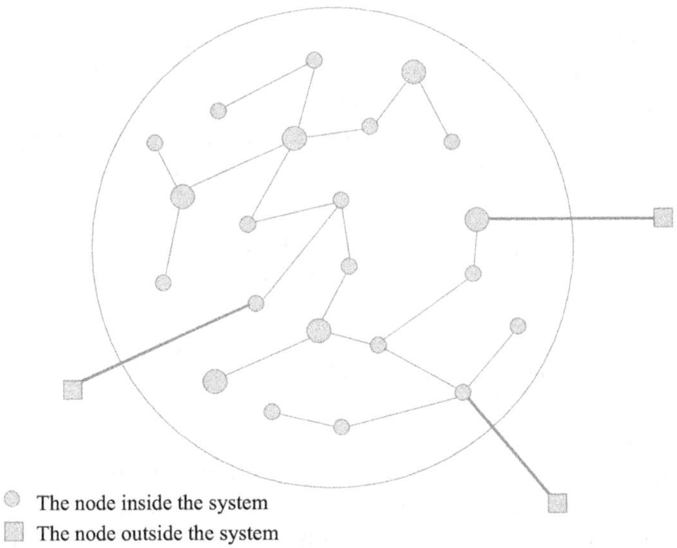

Figure 2.1 The simplified model of a system

To study a system must first define the boundary of the system, then study the interrelationship of the internal nodes of the system to ensure the optimal cooperation between the internal nodes, and study the relationship between the system and the environment to ensure the survival of the system in the environment.

If we want to solve a person's health problems, we must define the boundary between this person and the external environment and study the impact of the interrelationship between the internal nodes on the sustainable survival and development of this person. Also, to study how this person interacts with the environment to ensure the sustainability of the superior system through collaboration to obtain the support needed for this person's sustainable development as a node of the superior system. The fields about the human internal system such as medicine and life sciences. The fields about the interactions between human and external society include psychology, sociology, management science, and so on. To solve the sustainable development problem of an enterprise, we must first study the impact of the interactions between internal nodes on the sustainable survival and development of the enterprise and how could the enterprise play a role in the social economy and political system to get external resources and support needed.

The management of the enterprise and the interactions between the enterprise and society are further divided into different areas for research. All of these systems can be abstracted into a basic model of a complex system of nodes, and the fundamental driving force for the system to continue to develop and evolve is the change in connectivity between nodes.

For the evolution of complex systems, let us make a few definitions:

Node: A node is a basic unit in a system. The boundary of a node could be defined. A node should have at least one connection with other member nodes of the system.

Connection: A connection is a relationship between nodes in a system. In different systems, the connotations of connections can be completely different. There can be different types of connections between two nodes.

Distance: The distance between two nodes is a comprehensive representation of the overall effect of the connections between the two nodes.

In order to better understand the meaning of distance, we could study the "distance" relationship between nodes in a three-node system composed of three people first. We could take three cousins of mine who live in different villages of my hometown Sancha as our examples. We are about the same age. When we were young, we studied at the same school in the town. We can meet each other almost every day. After graduating from high school, the three cousins returned to their villages. The approximate location of the three villages and the road system of the town in 2000 shown in Figure 2.2.

One day in the summer of 2000, we had a family gathering at the restaurant opposite the high school at noon. Cousin A walked to the restaurant from his home. The straight-line distance from cousin A's home to the restaurant is about 2 km. There is a seasonal river between cousin A's village and the restaurant, and the water level in the river is usually high in the summer. He needed to walk upstream

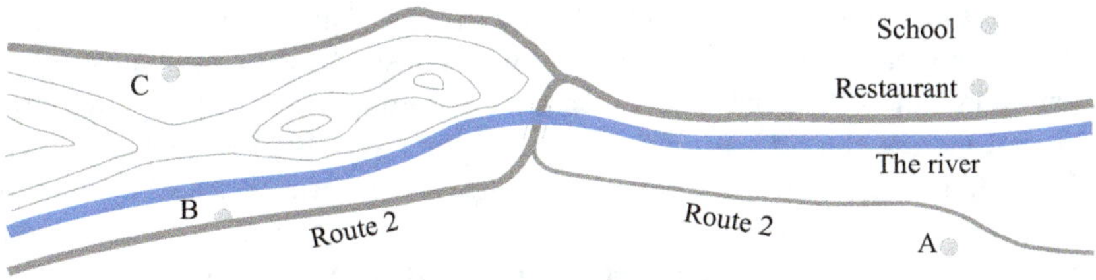

Figure 2.2 The Sancha Town and the road system in 2000

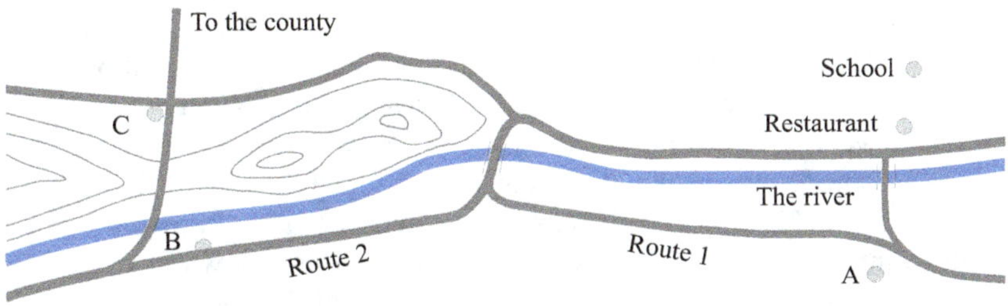

Figure 2.3 The road system of the town in 2018

along the river for about 5 km to cross the bridge (route 1). It took about 2.5 h to get to the restaurant. Cousin B lived in the upper reaches of the river and came to the restaurant by bicycle. He needed to cross the same bridge to get to the restaurant (route 2), and it took him about 30 min. Cousin C lived 8 km away from the restaurant. He came to the restaurant by motorcycle, and it takes him about 10 min.

The straight-line distance between cousin B and cousin C was less than 2 km. There is a mountain in between. In 2000, if they wanted to meet each other, they had to detour through the bridge. There was another problem that affected the communication between my cousins. At that time, they did not have phones or mobile phones. If they had to meet each other, they would ask other people to take messages for them. It usually took more than a week to set up the connections. So after graduating from high school, the three cousins rarely met. We find that when the three cousins wanted to meet in the town in 2000, the physical distance between the homes was meaningless. Their distances in time were 2.5 h (for A), 30 min (for B), and 10 min (for C), respectively, plus more than a week of lead time.

In the summer of 2018, there was another family gathering. In the past few years, a new bridge was built on the river near cousin A's house. A highway to the county was built. With a tunnel, the new road passes by both cousin C's and cousin B's house. It takes about 5 min to drive from cousin B's house to cousin C's house, so they often meet each other, drinking tea, chatting, and playing Chinese chess. We can find the road system of the town in 2018, in Figure 2.3.

Occasionally, three cousins will gather at the same restaurant in the town. Cousin A was still used to walking. It takes cousin A half an hour to walk to the restaurant. It takes about 10 min for cousin B and cousin C to drive to the hotel.

In 2018, the three cousins had mobile phones and WeChat. Although cousin B and cousin C did not have much chance to meet with cousin A. They often chat through WeChat and greet each other. They even play mahjong online in a WeChat group, and the lost money can be sent to the winner with a WeChat red packet.

In 2018, although the three cousins still need to meet in town, they can communicate with each other at any time by WeChat or by phone. Cousin A and cousin B's houses are very close, and they meet at least twice a week. From 2000 to 2018, the time cost of both the travel time and the communication time for meeting each other have changed dramatically, and they can schedule the meeting time anytime and anywhere. The lead time of meeting with each other for the three cousins are listed in Table 2.1.

When nodes collaborate in a system, the total cost of collaboration between two nodes can be considered as the distance between them. When there is no collaboration between the two nodes, the distance between them is infinite. In the social relationship between the three cousins, from 2000 to 2018, the distance between them has changed a lot, if only take the costs of travel time between each two of them into consideration, the changes that occur are shown in Figure 2.4.

From the perspective of communication, it is crucial that the cost of connection between them falls from about 7 days to negligible. When there are more types of connections, the connection cost is decreasing, and the integrated distance between nodes is getting closer and closer.

In the development process of the system, the process of making the distance between nodes smaller and smaller can be called folding. The folding at all levels is the fundamental driving force for system evolution. From the above example, we can see that from 2000 to 2018, the relationship between the three cousins has changed a lot:

1. The time cost required to meet each other was reduced, and the connection in this dimension was strengthened.
2. The time cost required for mutual communication had dropped significantly, and the connection in this dimension had been significantly enhanced.
3. The relationship between each two of them has changed. The time cost of cousin B and cousin C's meeting is much less than the time cost of cousin A meeting with either of them separately. Therefore, they meet much more

Table 2.1 The lead time of meeting with each other for the three cousins

	The lead time for meeting face to face		**The lead time for communication directly**	
	In 2000 (min)	**In 2018 (min)**	**In 2000 (days)**	**In 2018 (min)**
ABC	190	50	10	<1
AB	180	40	7	<1
AC	160	40	7	<1
BC	40	5	7	<1

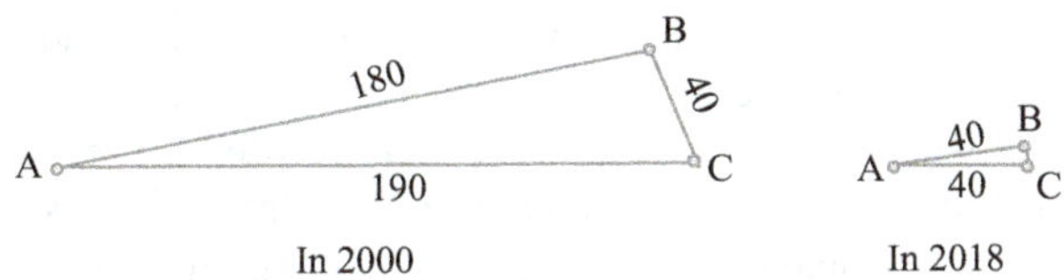

Figure 2.4 The costs of travel time been changed from 2000 to 2018

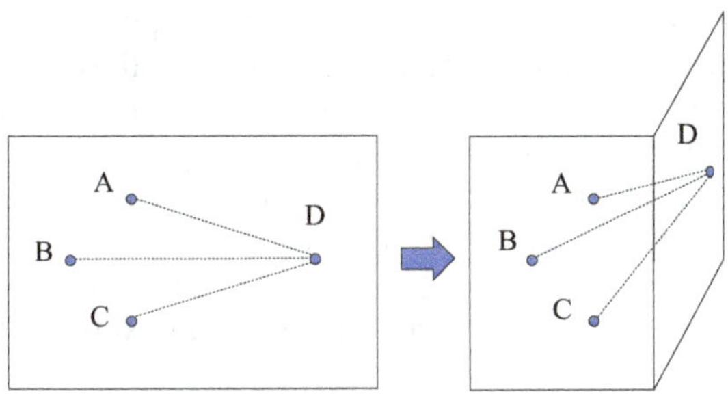

Figure 2.5 A piece of paper is folded

frequently. Moreover, their chances of meeting cousin A are still minimal. Imagine if something urgent happened, cousin B and cousin C must ask each other for help first instead of asking for help from cousin A.

4. If we take both the cost of physically meeting and the cost of communication, the distance between each of them is significantly reduced, but the distance between cousin B and cousin C is relatively small.

If we extend this model of distance variation between nodes to a system consisting of a large number of different types of nodes, we will see that for many systems, the overall trend is that the distances between nodes in the system are shrinking (direct and indirect distance). As shown in Figure 2.5, it is like the nodes on a piece of paper. After the paper is folded, the mutual positional relationship will change complexly. If the folding process continues to occur, the overall development trend of complex systems is that the "space" of the system is compressed, and the "density" is increased. The system is no longer "sparse."

As the "density" of the system increases, the relationship between the nodes also changes, and the cooperative relationship between the nodes must also be adjusted accordingly with the overall changes of the system.

2.1.2 Pyramid model for the evolution of complex systems

The process of the evolution of complex systems can be seen as the process of the interconnections and interactions of nodes in the system, that is, the process of system folding. With the folding process occurring, according to the sizes and types of nodes in the system and the types and characteristics of connections between nodes, the system can be roughly divided into four levels: individual, group, organization, and life (the "life" here is in the broad sense, a system with corresponding characteristics can be regarded as such a "life"). The hierarchy of the system is determined by the degree of coupling of nodes in the system in terms of matter, energy, information, cognition, decision making, and execution. As shown in Figure 2.6, the degree of coupling at different levels in the system at different stages.

In the process of complex system evolution, the nodes in the system are coupled and coordinated at different levels of matter, energy, information, cognition, decision-making, and execution. The whole progress follows a growing pyramid model. As shown in Figure 2.7, the collaboration of nodes higher-level system depends on the ability of the collaboration of the lower level. Only when efficient cooperation is formed at all levels can the system evolve into a perfect life system. A life system should be sustainable over some time. As the environment changes, the cooperative relationship between the internal nodes of the living system changes, and the self-consistency, self-adaptive ability and flexibility of the system also change.

This pyramid model is the essence of all life forms. In the pyramid model, matter and energy are the fundamental support for the nodes survival, and the other higher levels are the process of establishing the collaboration mechanism. When

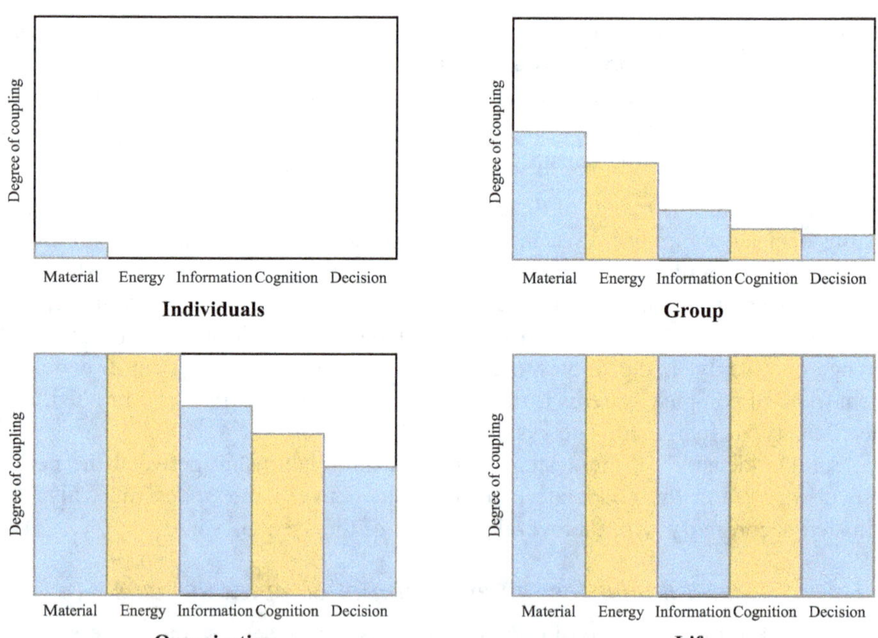

Figure 2.6 The degree of coupling

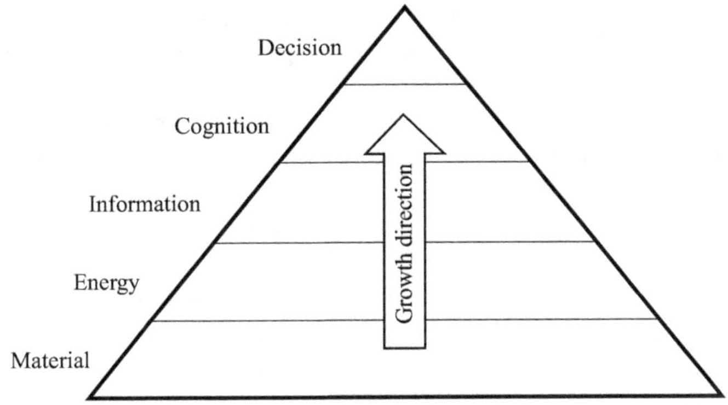

Figure 2.7 The pyramid model of complex systems evolution

the connections between a large number of nodes are enhanced, the distances between nodes are decreased, and the density of the system is increased. So the nodes in the system need to establish new ways of collaboration through competition and cooperation. "Life" is the self-consistent stage of the system. Not all systems can evolve into a self-consistent life system. Many systems will collapse in the process of resource competition because they do not form a reliable collaboration mechanism.

Skeletal and DNA evidence suggests that our species, Homo sapiens, evolved in Africa and then spread across the globe date to before 100,000 years ago. After Homo sapiens came out of Africa, they showed extraordinary ability to cooperate, won in the competition with the robust Neanderthals, and began colonizing the world [13]. From the earliest families to the tribes, to the countries, Homo sapiens evolved a large number of different types of collaboration system and social organization such as religions, enterprises, nonprofit organizations, schools, and militaries. These collaborative methods have significantly increased the scale of human beings. Through the construction of different levels of collaborative life systems, they have gradually evolved into the form of today's national. Each country is composed of a large number of different levels and different types of "life" systems.

Let us review several critical revolutions in the development of human society.

- The cognitive revolution, allowing independent individuals to establish a closer connection. In the face of the environment, human capabilities are no longer limited by individuals.
- The agricultural revolution has established a solid material foundation and, through a clear social division of labor, can achieve goals that cannot be achieved by individuals on a large scale.
- The industrial revolution, that is, the emergence of steam engines, allows human society to use large-scale natural energy that can be controlled and possessed by individuals. Human society has elemental "physical energy".

- The electrical revolution, human society has established a sophisticated, standardized, easy to be distributed energy supply system that can be precisely controlled.
- The information technology revolution represented by computer technology has enabled human beings to have, primary "neurons" and weak "neural systems," and their ability to communicate in information processing and information has been greatly enhanced. The density of the world increased dramatically.
- The revolution brought about by key innovations such as artificial intelligence is to make human society as a whole more "smart." Let human society form a unity in terms of cognition, decision-making, and execution.

After the Second World War, the establishment of a large number of international collaborative organizations and collaborative systems, the establishment of coordination mechanisms between countries in the political, military, economic, cultural, scientific, educational, environmental, medical, and health fields, so that the distances between countries are significantly decreased. Especially when the Internet emerged, the cost of communication dropped dramatically. The increase in scale and the reduction in distances make the world quickly become incredibly crowded. The global division of labor, efficiency optimization, and the formation of a global collaboration system are inevitable trends. For the first time, all human beings have the opportunity to become a new life. As with all systems transformation to life, competition, and cooperation coexist, local conflicts and the common interests of the system coexist, and the re-division of system members is inevitable.

In the process of evolution and formation of life systems without human participation, the characteristics of life emerge from systematic behavior, and could not be detected or controlled by the individual nodes within the system. Therefore, the direction of system evolution is uncertain and usually decided through the natural selection by the external environment based on the adaptability to the environment. This type of evolution is costly, slow, and not necessarily sustainable.

In the system of human society participation, in addition to the increase of system density and complexity, the passive and local responses of nodes in the system lead to new features emerging from the system, the unique cognitive ability of human society and the recognition of higher-level life can avoid system crashes. Especially in the past more than a century, many outstanding leaders of human society have formed a consensus on globalization and promoted the development of human society into the next stage. However, the current situation is not optimistic, and the forces opposing our common future are gradually strengthening. The process of the evolution of human society is a process in which super life is nurtured, born, grown, and matured. Everyone, every organization is part of the life process of this super life system. The future of human society must be the cooperation of the whole world, thus forming the most complex and most extensive life system in the universe. This is the future and the destiny of human society. We have no choice and cannot afford the consequences of a system collapse. The only thing human beings can do is to see this future, to conform to the inevitable trend of future development, to be friends with the future, and to achieve the future of humankind.

2.2 Opportunities and development trends of the medical and health industry under the background of globalization

In the process of human society development, through the collaboration between individuals and the deepening of the cognition of themselves, with the division of labor, the profession of doctor and the field of medicine have gradually emerged. In this long process, influenced by social cognition and changes in technology level, human beings have experienced different stages of cognition to their health and life system. In different countries and regions, in the process of development, plants, animals, and minerals in the natural environment have been used as medicines to treat diseases. There are also different types of psychotherapy that make humans feel healthy and safe.

2.2.1 New developments in the field of human health through the development of science and technology and globalization

Since the establishment of the human science system, medical technology has also developed rapidly. Human studies on themselves are deepening at different levels. At the forefront of medical research, there have excellent understandings and corresponding solutions for most nonsystemic diseases. Numerous research results in the nonmedical field have been widely used in the fields of medicine and health, and human cognition of environmental change has been continuously enhanced so that the overall health of human beings has been dramatically improved and life expectancy has been extended. The medical level has reached an unprecedented height. In recent years, breakthroughs in some critical areas of technology, especially the development of information technology and the application of artificial intelligence in the medical field, have not only promoted the advancement of medical technology but also improved the spread of medical technology and the efficiency of the use of medical resources. We are delighted to see that there have been rapid developments in the following areas.

1. The development of data science reshapes human cognition of itself

   Various calculation methods have begun to be widely used in drug research, as well as the development of innovative disease targets and informatics analysis systems. It plays an essential role in computer-aided design of genes and proteins, comparative genomic analysis, biological system models, cell signaling and gene regulation network research, expert databases, and biological software packages. Scientists are expected to directly decipher the genetic language in nucleic acid sequences by computational biology methods and simulate the information flow process in life, thus understanding a series of laws such as metabolism, development, and evolution.

2. The application of artificial intelligence technology in the field of medical and health has dramatically improved the efficiency of health management, diagnosis, and treatment

   The integration of artificial intelligence technology and medical health has deepened. With the gradual maturity of technologies such as voice interaction, computer vision, and cognitive computing, the application scenarios of artificial intelligence in the field of medical health are becoming more and more abundant. Artificial intelligence technology has also gradually become an essential factor affecting the development of the medical industry and improving the level of medical services. The application of artificial intelligence in the medical industry mainly includes: artificial intelligence virtual assistant based on speech recognition technology, intelligent diagnosis of medical image based on computer vision technology, analysis of massive literature information, accelerated drug development, intelligent medical robot engaged in medical or auxiliary medical treatment, intelligence analysis based on intelligent health management for personal health big data.

3. A large number of new medical devices and equipment have emerged

   Clinicians are increasingly working with medical device and equipment developers. Clinicians are involved in the entire life cycle of medical devices and equipment development and application. A new model of medical device innovation, involving doctors, scientists, entrepreneurs, and capitals, will significantly advance the development and clinical use of medical devices and equipment. The increase in the level of medical care worldwide and the extent of medical access have placed new demands on the cost and weight of medical devices and medical equipment. The emergence of new markets has brought human society into a whole new phase in terms of medical devices and therapeutic levels. Capital's focus on this area also gives this field the ability to get better and sustainable resources support.

4. Global medical basic research areas improved significantly

   The rapid development of materials science, manufacturing technology, the use of a large number of related fields of technology in the field of life sciences and medicine has enhanced human understanding of themselves and can adopt a large number of new methods to deal with traditional and emerging diseases, as well as incurable diseases with traditional methods. For example, scientists use synchrotron radiation facility to promote the development of medical technology in different directions. The synchrotron radiation facility can be used to crack the three-dimensional structure of biological macromolecules, and rapidly determine the three-dimensional crystal structure of proteins, creating excellent conditions for the life science research in the coming "post-genome era." New X-ray microscopy and tomographic imaging technologies provide direct access to subcellular structure images, giving scientists a whole new life dynamic view. The two-color subtraction angiography technique in the synchrotron radiation facility provides a quick and precise early diagnosis of cardiovascular disease.

2.2.2 The new challenges that globalization brings to the healthcare field

1. Globalization has accelerated the spread of infectious diseases and brought new challenges to disease control

   As the global "density" increases, the scale of cross-border personnel exchanges has increased significantly. The German Company IPK International Travel Consulting published the 2018 World Cross-Border Tourism Analysis and the 2019 Outlook Report during the 2019 Berlin International Tourism Trade Fair through an analysis of 90% of the global cross-border travel market [14]. According to the report, the number of cross-border tours around the world totaled 1.4 billion in 2018, an increase of 5.5% over the previous year, reaching a record high. The spread of infectious diseases is becoming more serious. Human response to acute infectious diseases is still in the emergency response mode, and only major high-risk diseases that seriously threaten the overall safety of society can attract attention and global cooperation.
2. The medical capacity is not popular enough

   In the globalization map, the gap between economically backward regions and the global economic and political centers is huge, and it is impossible to obtain proper medical resources services and support. Japan has the life expectancy of more than 84 years in 2019, while 13 countries and regions have the life expectancy of fewer than 60 years, and Central African Republic has a life expectancy of only 53.008 years [15]. Lack of medical resources remains the most important factor affecting human life expectancy.
3. Basic research in the field of healthcare is costly

   The investment in R & D companies has a long period of return on the market. The medical system is relatively conservative. As a result, the intermediate costs of medicines and medical devices remain high. Even in developed countries, it is challenging to achieve universal healthcare. In developing and underdeveloped countries, the primary healthcare system is more challenging to achieve full coverage. It is hoped that with the development of information technology, the distances within the world will shrink, the density of the world will increase, and the folding will accelerate. Ultimately, if the efficiency of medical research and development can be significantly improved, the intermediate links between medical facilities and medicines will be reduced. Cost reductions are achieved through new technologies in the field of artificial intelligence that improve the efficiency of physician diagnosis and treatment.
4. Health habits and drinking water issues

   Good hygiene practices and safe drinking water are prerequisites for ensuring health. There are still a large number of areas in the world that cannot guarantee safe drinking water or treated tap water. In the dry areas, it is not even possible to guarantee that all the tableware will be properly cleaned and that the regular bathing will not be guaranteed. These make it easier to produce and spread disease. We need to solve the daily drinking water safety problems with new technologies through economic development. Residents' health habits also seriously affect health. Toilets are also a severe problem in many places. It is necessary not only through economic development and technological means but also in cultivating people's living habits and health concepts to enhance their quality of life. At the same time, indirectly solve the health problem.

5. Pesticide residues and other harmful substances in the environment are harmful to humankind

   Although governments have strict regulations on the use of pesticides and pesticide residues, in the course of use, a large number of pesticide residues caused by repeated use have caused significant impact and harm to the environment and human beings themselves. At the same time, the accumulation of heavy metals and other chemical wastes in the soil, as well as the residues of substances that have a chronic impact on the environment and humans, have led to a significant increase in the incidence of cancer in some areas. Improper disposal of waste, as well as dioxin emissions into the environment during waste incineration, have also caused harm to humans.

6. Research and understanding of human themselves are not sufficient

   Although human beings have made significant progress in many fields, the understanding of the nature of life and the microscopic and systemic diseases is still at a relatively early stage. In most cases, it is not possible to grasp the specific information and respond promptly to the initial stages of the health problem. It is generally necessary to wait until the disease is severe before it can be discovered and intervened. This often leads to high costs and poor therapeutic results. People need to predict health problems earlier, manage their health as soon as possible, and be able to prevent problems before they are harmed. Although this topic is everyone's attention, there is no suitable solution. For the majority of ordinary people in developing and underdeveloped areas, there are no necessary conditions for solving health problems.

7. Obesity caused by the living habits

   Humans have the ability to survive in a food-poor environment during evolution, and this ability may lead to obesity in a food-sufficient environment, resulting from poor eating habits, lifestyle habits, and mental stress. The problem of obesity has become increasingly severe. The number of obese people worldwide has increased dramatically. Cardiovascular diseases, digestive diseases, endocrine diseases, joint soft tissue damage, reproductive decline and psychological disorders, heart disease, diabetes, atherosclerosis, fatty liver, gallstones, edema, gout, etc. caused by obesity not only affect the beauty of the body and bring inconvenience to life but also take a lot of people's lives.

2.2.3 Globalization has brought new opportunities for humankind to solve health problems

At the same time, we also face many new opportunities. In the context of globalization, the cost for human beings to solve medical health problems through global collaboration has fallen dramatically. Despite the significant increase in the cost of new drug development, most new drugs are likely to be available to the global market, resulting in excess returns, so the essential drivers of R & D remain. Computational biology and computational chemistry can help drug discovery organizations design and screen new drugs more efficiently, dramatically reducing the cost of drug development. The collection, analysis, processing, and application of data can help us better detect and control epidemics from a global and systematic perspective. We can get disease information in a timely manner and respond quickly.

The 2013–2016 Ebola virus disease (EVD) epidemic in West Africa was the largest in history and resulted in a huge public health burden and significant social and economic impact in those countries most affected. Its size, duration, and geographical spread present important opportunities for research that might help national and global health and social care systems to better prepare for and respond to future outbreaks. Fighting the Ebola virus is a meaningful collaboration for all humanity to work together to solve medical health problems. The large-scale investment in basic medical research and the enhancement of scientific research has accelerated drug development and our understanding of human beings and diseases. The application of technologies from different fields in healthcare gives us more ways to deal with medical health issues. The development of science and technology not only allows us to understand people from the perspective of reductionism but also allows us to recognize the human life system from the perspective of systematics and the perspective of holism. The collaborative system of human society can help us better solve medical health problems from different angles.

Medical health issues are problems for all human beings and require all human beings to solve these problems through a more efficient collaborative system. We do not just have to solve local problems. We have to solve systemic problems. This is the future of medicine. Be friends with the future and achieve a healthy future for humanity.

2.3 Building a global innovation and entrepreneurship ecosystem to promote global collaboration in the field of healthcare

Science and technology play an increasingly important role in the process of globalization [16]. We need to improve the production efficiency of materials and energy needed to support the sustainable development of human society through the development of science and technology. New technologies are also needed to help us build connections and consensus at all levels of information, cognition, and decision making. The university carries the essential functions of knowledge production and talent cultivation in human society. In the current development context, it is the hard work of the whole world to transform the innovations formed by universities and institutions into the fundamental driving force of social development through innovation and entrepreneurship.

Nowadays, the Central Government of China regards mass innovation and entrepreneurship as new engines for the sustainable development of our country. In this innovation-driven era, the roles of Chinese universities have changed profoundly. One of the essential responsibilities of Chinese universities is to serve society and the industry. It becomes essential for universities to release the innovation power into related industries, create more business entities and foster new industrial trends by connecting industrial enterprises with research teams closely.

2.3.1 A global innovation and entrepreneurship community as an application layer for the university

Shanghai Jiao Tong University (SJTU) is a comprehensive, research-oriented, and internationalized top university in China. SJTU enjoys an increasingly high scientific research level and technology innovation level. Like other universities, SJTU has implemented the technology transfer model for many years and devoted itself to transforming research achievements into industries.

However, the services and the resources on the campus alone are not enough to support an ongoing development of the startups and the entrepreneurs. Hence, a vast gap does exist here. Why is it so hard to realize the technology transfer? The difficulty results from the complexity of the mechanism of a university. Within this system, the trajectories for individual research and its access to the industry are even more complicated. Therefore, it is no simple matter to have an efficient result through a centralized organization within a closed or semi-closed structure. What's more, there is a metaphor for the startups at the first stage of their business: the newly born babies. Psychologically, it is tough to let them get away from home and make a living alone. Thus, an open ecosystem should be built providing all kinds of resources and services for them based on their lifestyles. So here comes the conception of the neoBay.

neoBay Global Entrepreneurship and Innovation Community (neoBay), was co-founded on April 11, 2015, by SJTU, People's Government of Minhang district, and Shanghai Land Group (SL). With its focus on incubating technology-based startups within the ecosystem of innovation and entrepreneurship, neoBay aims at attracting and converging global resources relevant to innovation and entrepreneurship in favor of SJTU's technology transfer as well as a hub for innovation and entrepreneurship resources communication.

If we take the university as a smartphone with compelling hardware system and a high-quality and stable software operating system, but it has limited functions for industrial users. Through the improvement of industrial service capabilities, neoBay has cooperated with the industrialization service office (AITRI, Advanced industrial technology research institute) and the School of Innovation and Entrepreneurship in Shanghai Jiao Tong University to establish the "application layer" of the university, as shown in Figure 2.8. while the neoBay ecosystem is like an App store for smartphones. Through collaboration with various developers (incubators and service organizations), neoBay has cultivated a large number of outstanding entrepreneurial teams. These entrepreneurial teams are industry-oriented Apps of the university.

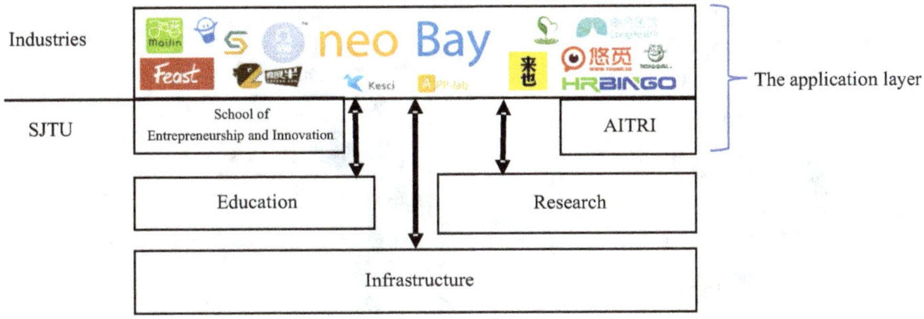

Figure 2.8 The neoBay ecosystem as the application layer of SJTU

So we call it the "application layer" of the university. In this way, more people can play their greatest strengths and capabilities in this innovative and entrepreneurial ecosystem.

2.3.2 From technology transfer model to collaborative innovation model

From the researcher's perspective, traditional industrialization process of science and technology mainly depends on limited resources from their own. Moreover, they have to finish all the transfer work to realize the idea. For most researches had to finish all the necessary tasks which took up over 80 percent of the whole process. While now, most of the work is done by doctoral candidates and postgraduates. This often leads to the mismatch between research findings and industry's demands. As a result, only some great research achievements can be industrialized through AITRI, while some other technical breakthroughs are not able to be industrialized. The situation becomes more challenging when some of the accomplishments can only be approved after a long time, due to the complicated research and development cycle. When the products are finally introduced to the market, they have already lost competitiveness.

By providing services from AITRI and neoBay together, we connect research teams with industries more efficiently. In this way, we can build up a superior university-industry cooperation model with an effective incentive mechanism. From the beginning of an idea, all the researches, developments, and technologies are tied up with industries and achieved gradually. During this process, more and more resources can be attracted and obtained to strengthen the relationship between scientific research and industries. As shown in Figure 2.9, the cooperation model changed from technology transfer model to collaborative Innovation Model.

2.3.3 The ecosystem approach in developing healthcare inside the boundary

Transferring from the technology transfer model to collaborative innovation model, Building up new connections between the most essential internal nodes of an

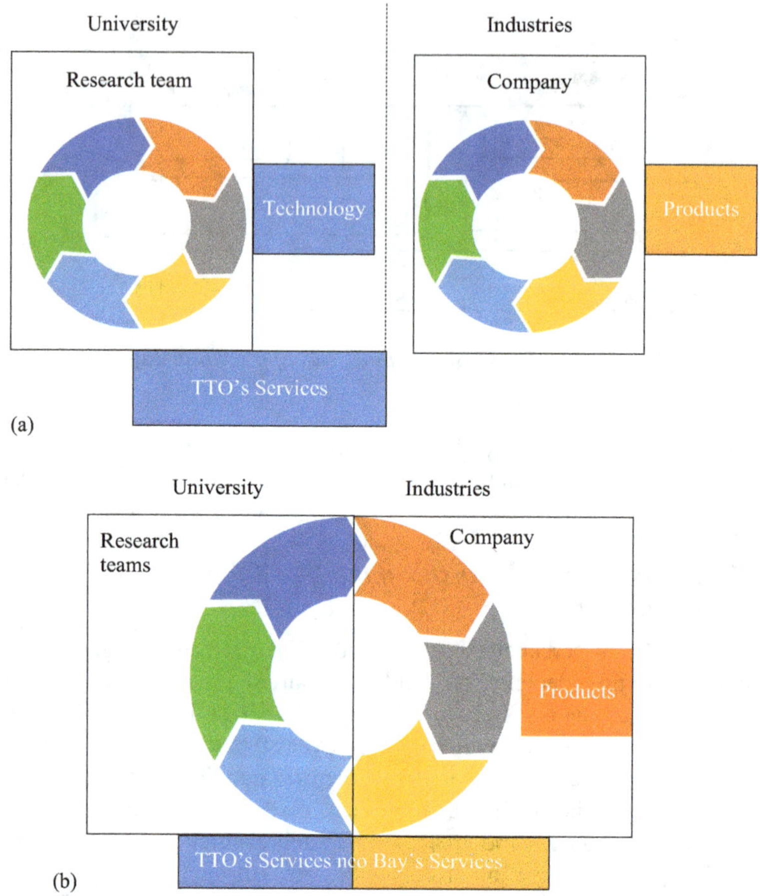

Figure 2.9 From technology transfer model to collaborative innovation model: (a) the technology transfer model and (b) the collaborative innovation model

ecosystem inside the boundary for innovation, scientific research and industries, here occurs the ecosystem approach in developing healthcare. Based on the general services and infrastructure of neoBay, we have established the Intelligence Medical Incubator of neoBay which is a key incubator for the neoBay ecosystem, focusing on attracting and incubating intelligent hospital system design and medical upgrading applications as well as the application of information technology and artificial intelligence technology in the medical field and the development of medical equipment, advancing SJTU to be the first in clinical medicine among Chinese universities.

The development of the intelligent hospital system can realize the collection, storage, processing, extraction, and data exchange of patient medical information and administrative management information.

Medical upgrading applications include the application of remote image transmission, big data processing technologies in the construction of digital hospitals, and the improvement of medical service level.

Supported by the Intelligence Medical Data Center, the intelligence medical innovation and entrepreneurship system established by neoBay is shown in Figure 2.10.

The Intelligence Medical Data Center can solve the difficulties of the self-built data platform of the entrepreneurial team in related fields, and will also serve the construction of the data platform for SJTU's medical disciplines and affiliated hospitals. The Intelligent Medical Data Center provides data storage, data processing capabilities for various types of hospitals, especially for SJTU's affiliated hospitals. The de-private medical data can be opened to relevant research teams of SJTU through the Data Open Application Agreement. Research teams can use these data and data storage and processing capabilities provided by data centers to do research work. The achievements of the research teams could be transferred to the market with the support of the industrialization department of SJTU (AITRI) and the services from neoBay entrepreneurship ecosystem. The startup teams in neoBay can work with the research teams in SJTU to propose new research topics and work together on R & D. The new achievements can be quickly iterated through cooperation with hospitals to realize the industrialization of technology and enhance the hospital's diagnosis and treatment capabilities. Entrepreneur teams in neoBay also can enjoy the low-cost data storage and processing service from the data center.

The following are brief Introductions to some entrepreneurship teams fostered by the neoBay Intelligent Medical Incubator.

1. AccuMed

   This company focuses on the efficient navigation system at a low cost for pulmonary surgery, which is based on double needle methodology and

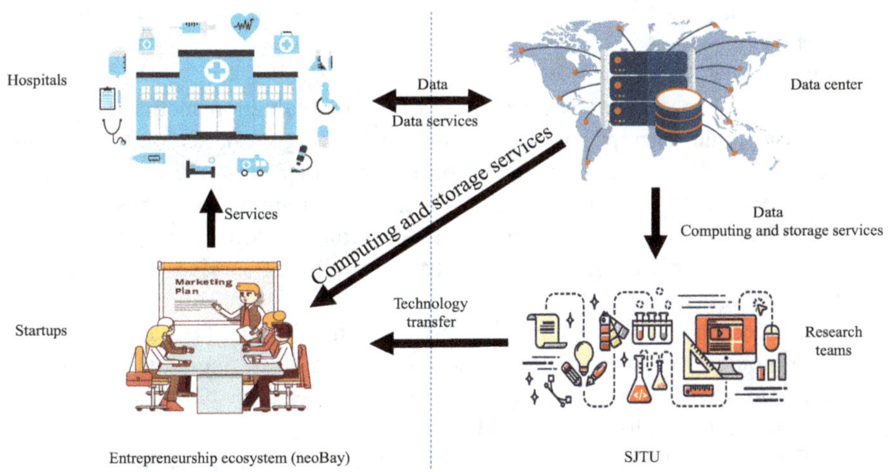

Figure 2.10 The intelligence medical innovation and entrepreneurship system

statistical model. This surgical navigation system can accurately locate the lesions and solve the problem of the movement of the lesion caused by lung respiration. In this way, the system can reduce the difficulty of lung puncture and provide effective early diagnosis and treatment of lung cancer.

2. AI Diagnostic Platform on pediatrics (Yitu Tech)

   This project concerns the pediatric diagnostics, consultation, and health education by artificial intelligence. Through the database on medical record provided by the hospitals reputed for their services in pediatric diagnosis, the team of this project takes advantage of AI and deep learning together with the clinical research to develop AI algorithm models for dozens of common pediatric diseases and realize intelligent diagnostic products.

3. Shanghai Qiyuan Biomedical Technology Co., Ltd.

   This company is a technology service company aiming at big data analysis on high-throughput gene sequencing as well as the gene diagnosis products and new medicines.

4. Lunghealth

   Lunghealth is a high-tech enterprise specialized in the early-stage diagnosis and treatment of lung cancer. They have claimed lots of Chinese patents on their accurate diagnosis technology. Some of their innovative diagnostic and interventional therapies are unique healthcare all over the world.

5. Remote Intelligent Rehabilitation Aid System

   Based on internet technology, intelligent machine vision technology, and human biomechanics research, this project enables patients to realize the rehabilitation training process at home through robotic observation of rehabilitation process, analysis on rehabilitation process by cloud computing and the remote monitoring by the medical staff of the cycle rehabilitation cycle.

6. Pulse Medical Imaging Technology (Shanghai) Co. LTD

   This startup focuses on the development of the medical instruments for clinical diagnosis and assessment for retreatment on cardiac, cerebral, and nephric diseases.

7. Shanghai NZJ Medical Device

   Based on insomnia treatment detection and evaluation methodology such as transcranial current stimulation therapy, intelligent hardware, cloud computing, big data, and other technologies, combined with the clinical experience and actual needs of a number of comprehensive hospitals and community health service centers, this startup explores a complete set of feasible insomnia diagnosis and treatment intelligent service technologies.

8. BRBIO biotechnology

   This company focuses on the research and development of the critical technologies in terms of dyeing series, stained film automatic microscopy series and whole blood platelet analysis series.

9. Weiyin Biotechnology (Shanghai) Co., Ltd

   Their project using the high-throughput sequencing technology (also known as the second generation sequencing technology, the next-generation sequencing, NGS) to detect the free DNA in the peripheral blood released from tumors (Circulating tumor DNA, ctDNA) to determine the existence of the tumor, which helps to conduct the personalized medication.

10. Analysis and interpretation of big data of genomics

    Their goal is to set up a data analysis team which provides high-quality data analysis services for universities and research institutions that study on life sciences as well as interpretation services for hospitals and consumers.

11. "Pomegranate Medicine" Clinical Research Statistics Service Platform

    It is an open service platform based on WeChat contact number. Through the business model of "S2b2c" and the assembly of the best statisticians on the epidemic disease in China, it provides the doctors with the analytical services and consultation, solving the problems related to the statistics in clinical research.

12. Human phenotype prediction based on artificial intelligence and advanced chromatin structure

    Through the application of the latest academic discovery, they predict the various physical phenotypes of the population accurately, contributing to the personalized medical care as well as the orientation on talent cultivation.

13. Hualiang smart logistics management system for hospitals

    By detecting accurately the personnel, the facilities, and the vehicles, this management system collects an enormous amount of data, analyses, and digs out the value of data, coordinating the task analysis, artificial intelligence, quantitative analysis of staff KPI and equipment usage, and improving the efficiency of the workforce and the material.

2.3.4 The collaboration with the nodes outside the boundary

The interactions between the internal nodes inside the boundary of a system alone is not enough. In order to ensure the substantial development of an ecosystem in favor of health intervention, it is quite critical that a mechanism of the collaboration with the nodes outside the boundary should be set up.

By collaborating with SJTU Medical Robot Institute and neoBay's public services, Intelligence Medical Incubator of neoBay breaks the barrier between the various industries, interconnecting the basic research and its industrialization by accelerating the transfer from the new discovery of the laboratory to the products.

SJTU Medical Robot Institute is a multidisciplinary platform studying on the subjects such as biology, medicine, machinery, materials, information, controlling, computer science, devoting itself to integrating research, education, transfer, and service. The main research includes micro–nano systems, perception and cognition, and biomimetic systems, advanced intelligent materials, surgical robots, rehabilitation robots, image navigation interventions, artificial intelligence and human–computer interaction, bio-optics and precision electromechanical systems. By researching on these domains, the institute combines the clinical research and the robotic one.

2.3.5 New model of "research and incubation in the field"

The new model of "research and incubation in the field" means scientific and technological innovation by the Shanghai Jiao Tong University, SJTU Medical Robot Institute together with the R & D funding support from neoBay public services, supporting the initial research and pushing the project from the "theoretical principle" to the "application mechanism," from the "principle prototype" to the "engineering prototype."

On the campus of SJTU, the professors, the alumni, and the entrepreneur students enjoy multidisciplinary support for their project. Outside the campus, they enjoy the convenient space and vertical resources provided by neoBay as a global innovation and entrepreneurship ecosystem around the university.

2.3.6 Case study on AccuMed

Let us take an example of AccuMed. This company focuses on the development of low-cost and high-precision surgical navigation systems and clinical solutions for surgical and interventional treatment, relying on the scientific research achievements of the School of Biomedical Engineering of SJTU. Along with its incubation and acceleration, this high-tech company, as a node in a system, has been progressively interconnected with other nodes, in other words, various resources favoring its growth. It was pre-incubated by neoBay to gain some necessary supports, such as space, public services, legal advisory on the first phase of its business, then fostered by Intelligence Medical Incubator of neoBay for its acceleration and afterwards headquartered at SJTU Medical Robot Industrial Park to acquire the vertical resources brought about by other domains. Significantly, it has gone beyond the boundary of the ecosystem by allocating its mass production in Chongchuan District, Nantong city, Jiangsu Province. The case of AccuMed is a perfect reflection of the model of a system mentioned previously. One node interconnected with others inside an original system intends to go beyond the boundary to get access to the nodes outside. For that reason, we witness the expansion of an ecosystem which contains more and more nodes outside, from a regional, a national ecosystem to a global one.

2.3.7 Create a healthy future for humankind through global collaboration

The problems in healthcare we are obliged to face up with are relevant to the destiny of mankind. In view of that, new knowledge, innovative methodology, and revolutionary patterns serving the medical advancement should be acquired through a closer and more sophisticated collaboration worldwide, assembling all the nodes inside or outside a defined ecosystem with its expanding boundary as well as interconnecting all the outcomes or efforts to solve problems in healthcare and develop endlessly the chain combining research and industry.

neoBay, Global Innovation, and Entrepreneurship Community, around the university and the research institutions, is forging a global network through the nodes for connections and collaborations. With the help of this network, we can gradually change the healthcare of humankind through the following ways.

1. By nurturing new forces in the healthcare area and building access to healthcare for them;
2. Through this network, global cooperation will be provided to provide resources and transfer new healthcare technologies to the clinic;
3. Ensuring that technological innovations in the healthcare area can spread rapidly to the world;
4. Reduce the cost of healthcare globally;
5. Improve the response capability in the medical and healthcare field.

Let us work together to create a healthy future for humankind.

References

[1] Tsujikawa, S. 'Possibility of realizing weak gravity in redshift space distortion measurements'. Physical Review, 2015; D 92, 044029

[2] Griffiths D.J. and Schroeter, D.F. Introduction to Quantum Mechanics. 3rd edn. Cambridge, UK: Cambridge University Press; 2018. p. 11–13

[3] Cottingham, W.N. and Greenwood, D.A. An introduction to the standard model of particle physics. 2nd edn. Cambridge, UK: Cambridge University Press; 2007. p. 89

[4] Smith, K.R. 'Building an innovation ecosystem: process, culture and competencies'. Industry and Higher Education, 2006; 20(4) p. 219–224

[5] Markley, D.M., Lyons, T.S. and Macke, D.W. 'Creating entrepreneurial communities: building community capacity for ecosystem development'. Community Development, 2015; 46, p. 580–598

[6] Alvarez, S., Ireland, R. and Reuer, J. 'Entrepreneurship and strategic alliances'. Journal of Business Venturing, 2006; 21(4): p. 401–404

[7] Mercan, B. and Goktas, D. 'Components of innovation ecosystems: a cross-country study'. International Research Journal of Finance and Economics, 2011; No. 76. p. 102–112

[8] Oh, D.-S., Phillips, F., Park, S. and Lee, E. 'Innovation ecosystems: a critical examination', Technovation, 2016. p. 1–6

[9] Kelly, K. Out of Control: The New Biology of Machines, Social Systems, & the Economic World. New York: Basic Books; 1994. p. 328–329

[10] West, G. Scale: The Universal Laws of Life and Death in Organisms, Cities and Companies. London UK: W&N; 2017. p. 79–81

[11] Capra, F. and Luisi, P.L. The Systems View of Life, A Unifying Vision. Cambridge, UK: Cambridge University Press; 2014. p. 362–399

[12] Tegmark, M. Life 3.0: Being Human in the Age of Artificial Intelligence. New York: Alfred A. Knopt; 2017. p. 40–45

[13] Harari, Y.N. Sapiens: A Brief History of Humankind. New York: Harper, 2015

[14] https://ipkinternational.com/en/world-travel-monitor/
[15] http://worldpopulationreview.com/countries/life-expectancy-by-country/
[16] Zahra, S. and Nambisan, S. 'Entrepreneurship in global innovation ecosystems,' Academy of Marketing Science Review, 2011; 1(1), p. 4–17

Chapter 3

Use of mobile health application to support belt and road initiatives: a cross-sectional study in China and Bangladesh

Md. Rakibul Hoque[1,2] and Shahidul Islam[3,4]

3.1 Background

Under the Belt and Road Initiative (BRI), China has introduced a new model of economic development of cross-continental connectivity. The project is envisaged to connect Asia, Europe and Africa through a network of multiple corridors and seaports. Over all, BRI will connect 65 countries, covering one-third of global output, 40% of global trade and 62% of the world population [1]. The BRI is aimed at promoting more in-depth regional cooperation among Asia, Europe and Africa as well as their adjacent areas.

Under the BRI, the Chinese government has promised to finance multi-billion infrastructure projects in Bangladesh and also committed to invest in a number of sectors, including telecoms, agriculture, power and energy in Bangladesh (beltandroad.hktdc.com). Moreover, Bangladesh is also an official partner of the proposed Bangladesh–China–India–Myanmar corridor (BCIM), one of the six corridors of BRI in 2016 when the two countries (Bangladesh-China) signed a number of deals having value of $21.5 billion [2]. Bangladesh can greatly benefit from BCIM initiative. For example, Bangladesh imports goods worth more than $12 billion from China, and exports worth a little above $1.5 billion while exports opportunities worth around $2,000 billion yearly [3].

To tap the opportunities initiated in Bangladesh and China because of BRI project, Bangladesh needs not only to develop the logistical integration by roads and transport facilities but also to enlarge the person-to-person contacts for gaining more benefits from the initiatives of BRI [3]. In this process, lots of citizens from both countries visit each other's country for business and official works and stay for a long time as expatriate.

[1]Department of Management Information Systems, University of Dhaka, Dhaka, Bangladesh
[2]School of Business, Emporia State University, Emporia, KS, USA
[3]UBD School of Business and Economics, Universiti Brunei Darussalam, Jalan Tungku Link, Brunei
[4]Department of Marketing, Comilla University, Cumilla, Bangladesh

Because of ever-increasing cross-border business and study programs between Bangladesh and China over the last two decades, the Chinese and Bangladeshi outbound travellers and expatriates in each other's countries have increased gradually but widely. However, due to the difference in weather and inadequate availability of health facilities for the foreigners in both countries, the travellers and expatriates from both countries show concerns when return to their respective countries. Under such situation, health education intervention for addressing the most commonly occurred health issues faced by them can be proven to be an effective strategy to reduce their health concerns.

The travellers and expatriates from Bangladesh and China often express for a need of an easy access to information on health issues and healthcare service available in their locality in their native language. In most of the cases, they show keenness in knowing what actions other travellers and expatriates from their respective countries take to address similar health issues. As a result, many of the common health and communication issues that are significantly associated with the travellers and expatriates' daily life and interaction are required to be explored in support of BRI between the countries.

3.2 Research problem

Due to urban crowding, environmental changes, altered sexual relations, intensified food production, and increased mobility and trade, health policy makers are facing a new height of challenges to manage many contagious diseases (e.g. tuberculosis, malaria, dengue, influenza, AIDS and Ebola viral disease) and chronic diseases (e.g. blood pressure and arthritis). This study assumes that these health issues affect not only local people but also foreign travellers and traders face various types of the above-mentioned health issues when they visit and stay in another country.

The fact of facing various health issues by foreign citizens (e.g. Chinese in Bangladesh and Bangladeshis in China) can impede the development and regular business activities because of BRI. Hence, assurance of addressing such health challenges as well as provision of continuous health services for both contagious and chronic diseases for foreign citizens should be one of the top priorities to facilitate the trading and business relationships related to BRI. In the Bangladeshi and Chinese context, not preventing and managing the above-mentioned common health issues faced by foreign citizens can negatively affect the BRI and thereby impede the sustainable regional economic growth.

3.3 Research objective

The main objective of this study is to conduct a survey for finding the needs of Chinese citizens in Bangladesh and Bangladeshi citizens in China when they face health issues. Based on the findings, a mobile health application will be developed to track and case study the common health issues they face. This mobile health application will methodically help the travelling citizens from each country to take essential and timely steps to address their health issues. It will connect citizens travelling from both countries in their local languages to get instant access: (a) to information on the nearest healthcare facilities, which can provide personalized care and (b) find information on how previous citizens from their own respective countries had acted and solved the most common and similar issues that they already had faced.

Ultimately the mobile health application will let the citizens from the two countries to share their own experiences in similar health conditions on online posts. The posts will be in their local languages arranged in different categories. The user generated posts will also contain information on which hospitals and health clinics they went and what steps they took to address any specific health issue.

3.4 Methodology

We conducted a study based on judgemental sampling which is a type of non-probability sampling that allows a researcher to include a wide range of variation or homogeneity in the population sample based on certain selection criteria. The sample selection criteria were set carefully to avail the benefits of judgemental sampling, for example, finding the best representative expatriates that the authors are interested in. Choosing other sampling method might not serve the researchers best, e.g. to use a random sampling that may include the participants who stayed in either China or Bangladesh for a brief period of time and have not had any health issues. The selection criteria were:

(i) The participants have to stay in China or Bangladesh for at least six month,
(ii) The participants who have faced any health issues and felt the need for easy access to health service information.

In the sampling process, a sample of 20 participants from Bangladesh and 30 participants from China were physically approached for face to face interview. The participants where either students or businessman by profession who the authors believe represent the best as expatriates from the respective countries. The age range of the participants were between 25 and 55 years. The participants were from different cities as shown in Table 3.1. This study was conducted on the citizens

Table 3.1 Number of the participants by cities and countries

Chinese citizens staying in Bangladesh		**Bangladeshi citizens staying in China**	
City	**Respondents**	**City**	**Respondents**
Dhaka	20	Beijing	5
		Shanghai	5
		Wuhan	15
		Guangzhou	5

staying either in China or Bangladesh for at least six months. The participants were asked about following five questions while interviewing.

(i) What health issues do you commonly face when you are travelling in China/ Bangladesh?
(ii) Where do you go or what actions do you take when you face any health problem?
(iii) Do you search on the internet and look for any mobile app to solve your health problem when travelling in this country?
(iv) What kinds of problems do you face while taking service for your health problem?
(v) If you were to use a mobile health application, which features would you like to have in that mobile health application?

3.5 Data analysis

The survey results are discussed against the five questions asked to the participants. According to Table 3.2, Chinese citizens residing in Bangladesh stated that commonly they suffer from fever (60%), influenza (i.e. flue) (45%), dengue (60%), gastroenteritis (infectious diarrhoea) (55%) and dysentery (35%). On the other hand, Bangladeshi citizens residing in China stated that the most common health issues they suffer from are muscle pain in legs (70%), skin disease (47%), itching (10%), common cold cough (57%) and sleep disorder (53%).

When asked about where the participants go or what actions they take when they have any health issue, according to Table 3.3, Chinese citizens staying in Bangladesh said that they mostly visit Chinese websites (70%). Secondly, they apply their own previous experience regarding similar health issues (80%). Then, if they do not get adequate information, they prefer to consult with their friends in China. Finally, if they feel that their previous initiatives are not enough to address any specific health issue, they visit local hospitals (mostly United Hospital Limited in Dhaka). In contrast, Bangladeshi citizens staying in China informed that they mostly use their own medicines that they brought with them from Bangladesh when

Table 3.2 The most common health issues mentioned by the number of participants

Chinese citizens travelling in Bangladesh		**Bangladeshi citizens travelling in China**	
Common disease	**Percentage**	**Common disease**	**Percentage**
Fever	60	Muscle pain in legs	70
Influenza	45	Skin disease	47
Dengue	60	Itching	10
Gastroenteritis	55	Common cold cough	57
Dysentery	35	Sleep Disorder	53

Table 3.3 Actions taken by the participants when faced by any health issue

Chinese citizens travelling in Bangladesh		Bangladeshi citizens travelling in China	
Actions taken	**Percentage**	**Actions taken**	**Percentage**
Visit the Chinese website	70	Medicine taken from Bangladesh	80
Own experience	80	Consult Bangladeshi doctors	67
Consult with friends	65	Visit Chinese doctor	53
Local hospital	55		

Table 3.4 The number of participants who would like to search internet or use mobile apps for health problems

Chinese citizens travelling in Bangladesh		Bangladeshi citizens travelling in China	
Searching online or mobile app	**Percentage**	**Searching online or mobile app**	**Percentage**
Search online	85	Search online	43
Use mobile health application	62	Use mobile health application	47

they went to China (80%). Secondly, they prefer to consult Bangladeshi doctors over phone or online on their health issues (67%). Thirdly, they visit Chinese doctors as a last resort to solve their health problems.

The survey participants were also asked whether they use internet or any mobile health application as a way to address their health problems. With this regard, Chinese participants informed that they only prefer to search for Chinese websites, forums and mobile health applications. In contrast to the Chinese participants, Bangladeshi participants informed that they hardly look for online contents or information to find solutions for their health issues, but they opined that they would like to use a mobile health application to initially search information for their health problems. Table 3.4 provides details above.

The participants reported that they face several problems when looking for options to take service for health problems. Chinese participants mainly face language barriers and they prefer not to take blood from foreigners (i.e. only take blood from other Chinese people). Similarly, Bangladeshi participants said that besides reluctance, language barrier is also a great reason for them not to visit the Chinese doctors. Table 3.5 shows the reasons informed by the participants.

Finally, the participants were asked whether they would like to use mobile health applications. Surprisingly, almost all of the participants opined that they would like to use a mobile health application initially to start addressing their health problems. When they were asked about what features they wanted to have in such mobile health applications, the Chinese participants opined that they wanted a feature where other Chinese citizens staying in Bangladesh could share their previous experiences and tips on how they acted to solve a certain but similar health

Table 3.5 Types of problems in seeking health service

Chinese citizens travelling in Bangladesh		Bangladeshi citizens travelling in China	
Problem faced while taking service	**Percentage**	**Problem faced while taking service**	**Percentage**
Language barrier	52	Language barrier	97
Prefer not to take blood from non-Chinese persons	80	Feeling reluctance in taking service from Chinese doctors	70

Table 3.6 Suggested mobile health application features

Chinese citizens travelling in Bangladesh		Bangladeshi citizens travelling in China	
Opted features in a mobile app	**Percentage**	**Opted features in a mobile app**	**Percentage**
Chinese language version	100	Bangla language version	63
English version	25	English version	77
Reading and posting about previous and new experience in similar situation	70	Scope of experience share and learning from others experience in the same situation	73
Customized health alerts and tips	57	Customized health alerts and tips	65
Audio/Video call to doctor	85	Audio/Video call to doctor	90
Review/Comments	78	Review/Comments	95

problems. They also suggested to provide information on the mobile health application regarding in which hospital or clinic they could receive special service, such as Chinese doctors for Chinese citizens. Furthermore, they informed that they wanted a Chinese language version of mobile health application that they could use for making appointments with the doctors where previously other Chinese citizens had visited or where there were special services available for foreign citizens. In contrast, the Bangladeshi participants also suggested for the Bangla language version for their convenience. They were also interested to get information on what health issues other Bangladeshis had come across while staying in China and how they coped with those health problems. They were also interested to obtain health tips and alerts customized for meeting their needs. Table 3.6 shows the common features that participants want in a mobile health application.

3.6 Discussions

This study aims to develop mHealth initiatives between Bangladesh and China by considering a standardized questionnaire based on frequently suffering health issues, first aid health seeking behaviour, and desired health application features in mobile while travelling to other countries. This study evaluates the participants' preferences for mobile health applications, finding evidence that the demand exists among Chinese participants as well as Bangladeshi participants. The finding reflects that mHealth tools can help by providing round-the-clock real-time solution [4] and address not only chronic medical situation [5] but also commonly faced health challenges. Hence, the borderless accessibility to mHealth application may create ubiquitous opportunities for citizens of Bangladesh and China to learn about the health status and to manage suddenly inflicted health problems and symptoms.

This study also shows promise to develop and use of customized mHealth apps. For instance, this study identifies that the participants from both counties (i.e. Chinese citizens in Bangladesh and Bangladeshi citizens in China) expect to learn about frequently sought health information using a mobile app or having a mobile app platform to share their health treatment experience that they have to already addressed in specific but frequently occurred health situations. In general, the major implication of this study is that it reveals about the most solicited healthcare supports that the participants need through mobile health intervention. Also, this study specifically supports previous findings on the impact of users' responsiveness towards mobile health app features, e.g. interactive service features, personalized health information, receiving quick response to patients' request, information regarding respondents' online access frequency for healthcare services [6].

The study also advances further credence to the view that citizens from both countries are recommending features like audio/video call to doctor (e.g. 'Active Call') and review/comments functions to be present in the app. This study implies that the lack of a definitive service design may hinder the users' motivation for use and interaction with the mobile health applications. Hence, healthcare providers need to broaden their concepts of health applications development process, design and use in smartphones, mobile devices, personal digital assistance and laptop to improve service features that integrate global citizens, i.e. Chinese and Bangladeshis. In the next section, this study will propose a mobile health application that may allow decision-makers to consider global health needs as well as personalized healthcare services for its users.

3.7 Proposing a mobile health application

The literature on mobile health shows that mobile health applications are widely adopted in the process of taking healthcare services today. The rapid pace of mobile phone adoption and its promise of universal connectivity also support such technology adoption globally. For example, WeChat mobile app's official account was found to be useful, sustainable, feasible for improving the health literacy on malaria of Chinese expatriates in the malaria-prone Niger [7]. On the other hand, Lindlar, Mika and Gerzer studied the usefulness of teleconsultation and second opinion services support for travellers and expatriates and concluded telemedicine as a the most cost-effective tool [8]. Moreover, study shows that peer interaction in online forum can effectively provide advice, interactive support, and information on how to prevent HIV and other sexually transmissible diseases among the expatriates and travellers [9]. Such scope of using mobile apps has led agencies and foundations to design and develop various mobile health applications to meet various health needs. Therefore, based on the suggestions that the authors have obtained from the survey, development of a mobile health application is proposed to meet the needs of Chinese and Bangladeshi citizens staying in each other's countries. With the cooperation between mobile health service providers and partner institutions from Bangladesh and China, this mobile application will monitor and help in tracking the health status, health behaviour and health care action status of its users.

According to the suggestions provided by the participants discussed in the previous section, the proposed features and the screenshots of the user's interface (UI) of the mobile application are given below. Figure 3.1 shows the UI of the proposed mobile application with three icons which imply the integration of three main features which would enable its users to avail the service they need specifically.

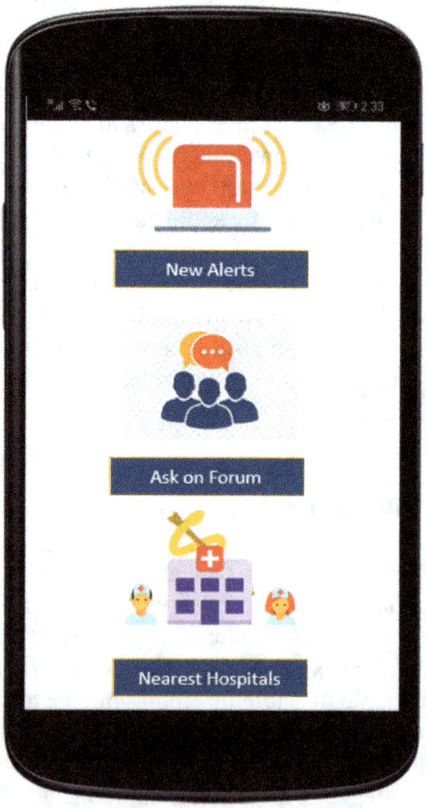

Figure 3.1 UI design of the proposed mobile application

Feature 1 (icon 1: New Alerts) would provide alerts and tips regularly about the most recent and frequent health issues that Chinese and Bangladeshi expatriates face in Bangladesh and China, respectively. The alerts and tips will be customized in Chinese and Bangla language accordingly. Feature 2 (icon 2) would enable its Chinese and Bangladeshi users to post and share their experiences in addressing their specific health problems during their stay in Bangladesh and China correspondingly. This second main feature is also known as 'Ask on Forum' where the users will read, ask and share their previous experiences like on social media. Finally, the third feature (icon 3) would allow its users to make appointments with doctors who have experience of treating the most common health problems that Chinese and Bangladeshi expatriates face.

Figure 3.2 shows how the UI would look like in Chinese language. Figure 3.3 shows how besides reading about previous experiences of other users, the users will also be enabled to ask about their health problems against which the other users will also reply with their suggestions. On the other hand, Figure 3.4 shows the option to make appointment with local doctors in the nearest hospital.

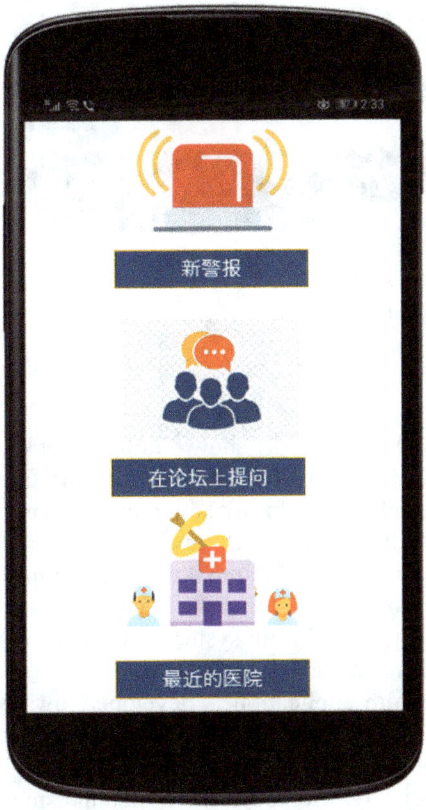

Figure 3.2 UI design in Chinese language of the proposed mobile application

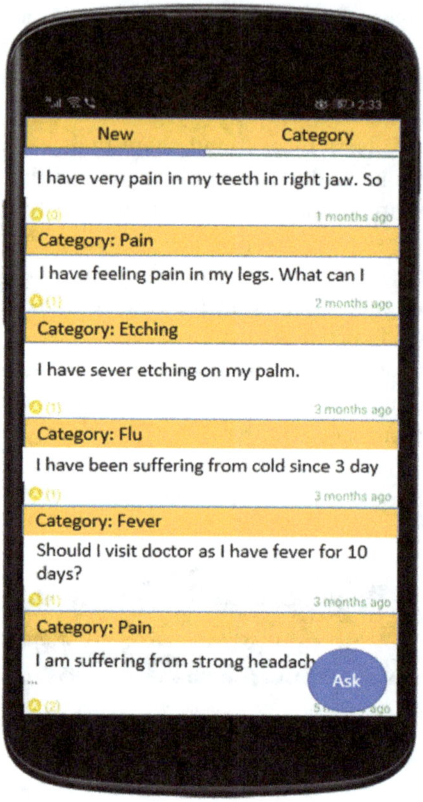

Figure 3.3 Asking questions about health issues to get reply from experienced users

Figure 3.5 (technical framework) shows how the back end (i.e. the database, programming code like PHP or Python and other media files stored in the cloud) interacts with the front end (i.e. UI for making appointment, asking other users and reading health alerts and tips). The development of such user specific (expatriates) mobile health application would help to make new relationships between hospitals in respective local areas to facilitate the diffusion of beneficial ICT innovations and ensure that the overall pattern of health system development meets the needs of the foreign citizens staying in Bangladesh and China.

Once the mobile health application is developed, awareness about the application will be created. Awareness about new innovation and technology is essential for wide-range quick adoption. In future versions, the bugs in the mobile application will be fixed periodically. Moreover, a longitudinal study will be conducted in both countries to increase the users' acceptance of the mobile application by identifying the factors that act as barriers to the application adoption.

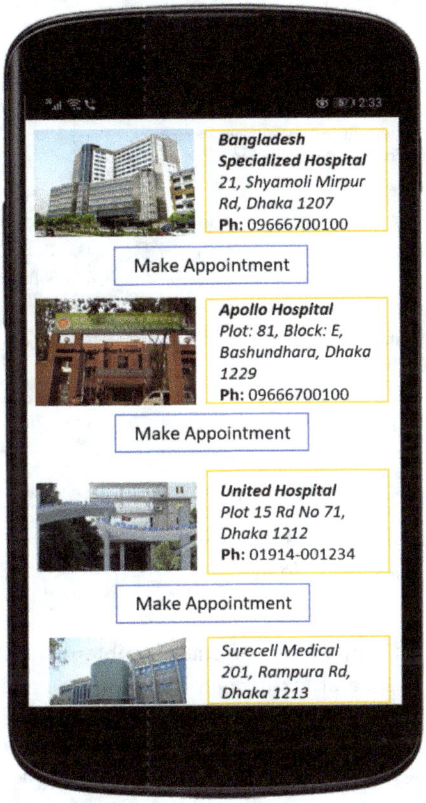

Figure 3.4 List of nearest hospitals for making appointment

Continuous improvement of the mobile application will make it easier for Chinese and Bangladeshi expatriates to get medical treatment not only easily but also timely. In this process, methodological and intermittent usability test of the mobile application is significant. Otherwise, the purpose of the mobile application will not be served aptly. In future, artificial intelligence can be used to incorporate a digital assistance to direct the users for taking appropriate and optimized actions to solve their health issues.

3.8 Conclusion

Because of the dissimilarities found in the regional, environmental, healthcare provision and cultural contexts in both countries, Chinese and Bangladeshi expatriates generally face health problems related to food variation, seasonal variation and communication, which can lead to various health issues and barriers in seeking healthcare services in foreign countries. With this regard, this simple but significant study shows that language barrier between health service providers and

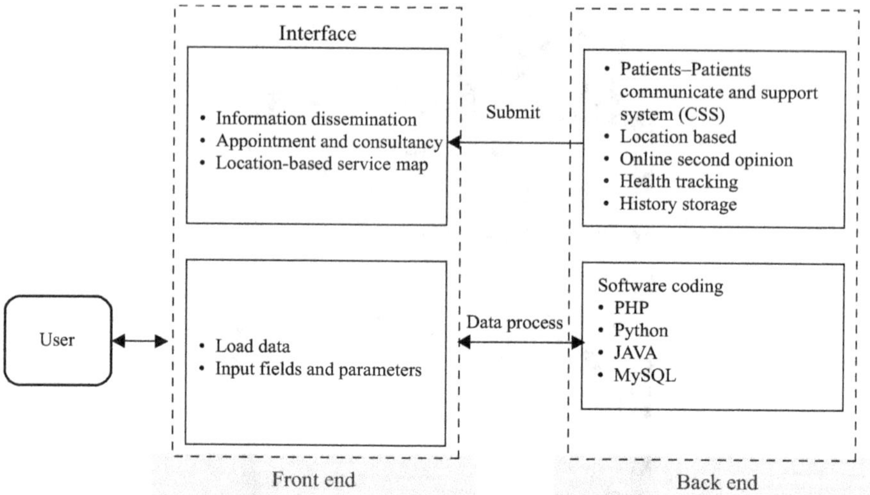

Figure 3.5 A technical framework to understand how the front end (i.e. UI) and back end work (i.e. cloud)

Chinese and Bangladeshi patients is the main problem that the participants often face. Besides, the lack of special facilities for the Chinese and Bangladeshi patients also is an important issue which needs to be addressed. Similarly, the participants also think that timely health alerts and tips can prevent their health issues. Therefore, based on these significant findings, the authors have proposed a mobile health application to fulfil the needs of Chinese and Bangladeshi expatriates who often face health issues that ultimately impede their regular work activities.

Another note-worthy implication of this study is that the findings of the study show us how information technology (IT), e.g. mobile health app as a health service information sharing platform, can be contextually utilized by the Chinese and Bangladeshi travellers and expatriates according to their individual health knowledge capacity and fulfil the custom health needs. Subsequently, such custom-built use of mobile app can be an effective strategy for disease prevention and minimization of the Chinese and Bangladeshi citizens staying in each other's country which would ultimately facilitate the process of grasping and availing the immense economic possibilities that have emerged because of the BRI.

After developing and piloting the proposed mobile app, the success of this small initiative will be followed by large scale mHealth applications to help Bangladesh to meet its 'Vision 2041' and to help China to meet its 'Healthy China 2030' vision. China already has made a huge stride in terms of its public health. Eventually, this cooperative effort of mobile health application will be a useful solution for about 1 million Chinese tourists who travel to Bangladesh every year [10]. Similarly, Bangladeshi citizens travelling in China (e.g. diplomats, scholars, students, traders and freelance visitors) will also be benefited from this mobile health application.

In the end, this study argues that the proposed mobile health (mHealth) application and its features will allow the Chinese and Bangladeshis in each other's country to circumvent many possible health problems. The resultant effect of the proposed mobile application will help us to understand and fulfil the demands of cross-country health services, and then to serve for the successful materialization and growth of the BRI.

References

[1] ESCAP. China's "One Belt, One Road" Initiative: An ESCAP Report. Vol. 43, Population and Development Review. John Wiley & Sons, Ltd (10.1111); 2017 September.

[2] Saimum R. What One Belt One Road means for Bangladesh. Dhaka Tribune. 2017 October.

[3] Daily Star. One Belt, One Road a golden opportunity: analysts. The Daily Star. 2017 Jun.

[4] Kumar S, Nilsen W, Pavel M and Srivastava M. Mobile health: revolutionizing healthcare through transdisciplinary research. Computer (Long Beach Calif). 2013;46(1): 28–35.

[5] Hilliard ME, Hahn A, Ridge AK, Eakin MN and Riekert KA. User preferences and design recommendations for an mHealth app to promote cystic fibrosis self-management. JMIR mHealth uHealth. 2014;2(4): e44.

[6] Islam S, Hoque R and Jamil A. Predictors of users' preferences for online health services. J Consum Mark. 2019 (conditionally accepted).

[7] Li W, Han LQ, Guo YJ and Sun J. Using WeChat official accounts to improve malaria health literacy among Chinese expatriates in Niger: an intervention study. Malar J. 2016;15(1): 567.

[8] Lindlar M, Mika C and Gerzer R. TEMOS–Telemedicine for the Mobile Society Telemedical Support for Travellers and Expatriates. In: Space Technologies for the Benefit of Human Society and Earth. Springer; 2009. p. 179–200.

[9] Crawford G, Maycock B, Tobin R, Brown G and Lobo R. Prevention of HIV and other sexually transmissible infections in expatriates and traveler networks: qualitative study of peer interaction in an online forum. J Med Internet Res. 2018; 20(9): e10787.

[10] Xinhua. Bangladesh expects 1 million Chinese tourists next year: PM. China Daily. 2015 September.

Chapter 4

Behind the popularity of "online mutual aid": how does the Chinese one-child policy generation appraise and control cancer risk of their aging parents?

Ying Shen[1] and Da'an Huang[1]

> "I am the only child and caregiver. I do not dare to die because my parents and my grandparents rely on me...... My family cannot afford a serious disease like cancer. Online mutual aid is an economical choice for me."
>
> ——female, 22, university student
>
> "Cancer is catastrophic. I bought cancer online mutual aid for my parents, but I did not explain what it is to them. My parents would not understand or trust this new product. I believe it will do some help when we need it. Even though we won't need it, it is great that I can help others."
>
> ——male, 27, editor

Those were reasons given for joining in the online mutual aid in a previous study [1]. The popularity of "online mutual aid" (also named crowdfund medical aid), an innovation in China, manifests the deep worries of the one-child policy (OCP) generation about their parents' cancer risk. *

4.1 Introduction

Ant Financial launched a mutual aid plan focused on cancer treatment of senior citizens (60–70 years old) on May 8, 2019. In 4 months, 3.4 million of this product had been bought by children for their parents. Meanwhile, Waterdrop, a Tencent-backed online mutual aid platform, have recruited 13.4 million users for the senior cancer mutual aid plan (51–65 years old). Those plans allow seniors to get medical

[1]Guangxi University

*The one-child policy in China was conducted from 1979 to 2016. In this study, one-child policy generation only refers to children (both only-children and children with siblings) who were born between 1979 to 1999 (20–40 years old), because they are more likely to do cancer control for their aging parents (42–70 years old) than those born after 1999.

aid of up to RMB 100,000 if they are diagnosed with cancer by contributing less than RMB 3 ($ 0.44) per month. The founder of Waterdrop Mutual, Shen Peng, once told the media that people born in the 1980s and 1990s are the target consumers for these products [2]. The popularity of these senior cancer mutual aid products reflects the deep concern of the generation about the cancer risk of their aging parents.

Cancer is the leading cause of death in China [3]. The polluted air, increasing obesity and drinking rate, high smoking prevalence, and low physical activity [4], make cancer a severe public health concern. For low- and some middle-income Chinese people, cancer equals "unaffordable medical expense and a high probability of a terminal illness" [1]. Mean expenditure per cancer patient exceeded the annual household income in China, and 77.6% of families with a newly diagnosed cancer patient reported that out-of-pocket expenditure is an unmanageable financial burden [5].

By the end of 2018, there were 250 million people aged over 60 in China, accounting for 17.9% of the whole population [6]. Additionally, filial piety, a virtue of respect for one's parents, elders, and ancestors, implies the obligation that the young generation should look after their parents when they are old and provide them with proper treatment when they become ill. Therefore, getting cancer and seeking treatment is not an individual, but a family issue.

Unfortunately, the OCP (1979–2016) results in a dramatic demographic transition in China: a shrinking working population and an enlarging aged population. With the increasing cancer incidence with the aging population, the "4 (parents) – 2 (only-children couple) – 1 (child)" family configuration is very fragile [7]. In the next 20–30 years, this tendency will continue or become even worse. In 1985, experts already warned that the OCP undermines the family's ability to provide security for its elders [8]. Meanwhile, the deficiency of public health services and low public medical insurance reimbursement rate pose significant challenges to the only-children caregivers [9]. Thus, identifying the Chinese OCP generation's parents cancer risk assessment and risk management strategies is imperative and urgent.

Cancer control continuum has stages from cancer etiology, prevention, early detection, diagnosis, treatment, survivorship, to the end of life (see Figure 4.1). Scholars have used this concept to conduct research on health education or intervention [10]. According to cancer control continuum, individuals could control cancer risk through cancer prevention, early detection (secondary prevention), and treatment. Between 30% and 50% of all cancer cases are preventable, and

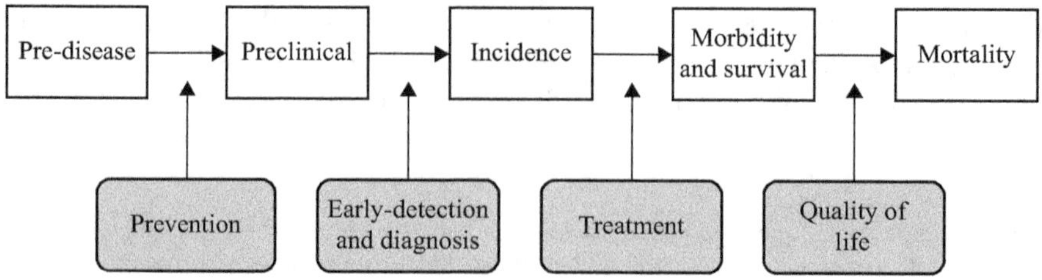

Figure 4.1 Types of interventions along the cancer continuum [10]

prevention is the most cost-effective long-term strategy for cancer control [11]. According to the American National Cancer Institute, cancer prevention includes tobacco control, diet, physical activity, sun protection, HPV vaccine, limited alcohol use, and chemoprevention [12]. Screening and early detection will help improve cancer outcomes by providing care at the earliest stage or reducing the risk of developing cancer [13], such as bowel cancer, breast cancer, cervical cancer [14]. In China, cancer medical expense is catastrophic for most families with cancer patients [4]. The main public medical insurances only cover certain portions of the total expense. Therefore, private medical insurance is a key factor of treatment quality and health outcomes. Previous researches show that uninsured cancer patients have a higher risk of death than privately insured patients [15–19]. The same health difference was also found in China [20].

Protection motivation theory (PMT), founded by R.W. Rogers in 1975, has been frequently used in cancer researches (e.g., individual and community cancer prevention or health interventions) [21]. According to PMT model [22], protection motivation (see Figure 4.2) is developed from both the threat appraisal process and the coping appraisal process. Threat appraisal process comprises vulnerability and severity, which are the factors of perceptions of threat. Another aspect of threat appraisal is maladaptive response rewards, including intrinsic and extrinsic rewards. Rewards refer to the positive perspective of starting or continuing unhealthy behavior. It decreases the probability of adaptive response. Coping appraisal, the ability to deal with and averting the threat, consists of response efficacy, self-efficacy, and response costs. Response efficacy refers to the belief that protective action will work. Self-efficacy means the belief of the ability that one can take positive action. Response costs are any costs related to the recommended behavior.

PMT model has been applied to cancer health education or intervention studies, focusing on cancer prevention and early detection/screening, such as exercise, sun protection, Pap test, mammography [23–30]. PMT have been proved to be a

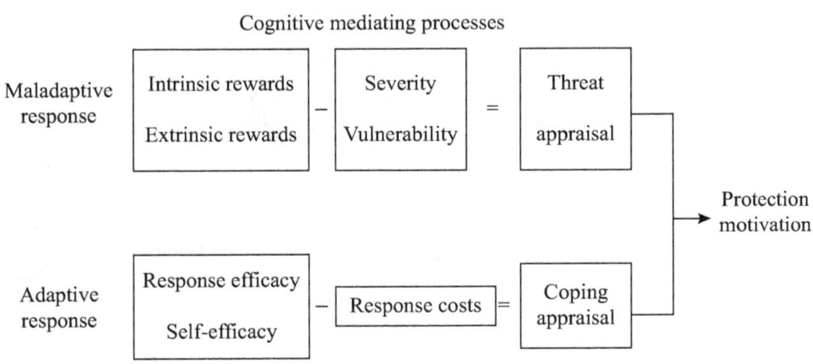

Figure 4.2 Cognitive mediating process of PMT (adapted from [22])

viable model for understanding the social-psychological process of health behavior adoption to conduct health intervention.

In this study, we combined the cancer control continuum with PMT model to answer questions as follows:

1. How does the OCP generation appraise the cancer risk of their aging parents?
2. What kind of coping strategies did they adopt to manage the cancer risk of their aging parents?
3. Are there differences between only-children and children with siblings on cancer risk appraisal and risk control of their aging parents?
4. What caused the differences (if any) between only-children and children with siblings on cancer risk appraisal and risk control of their aging parents?

4.2 Methods

4.2.1 Measures

A self-administrated questionnaire was designed by the authors according to the PMT model and the cancer control continuum (see Figure 4.3). Firstly, cancer control behavior and cancer control motivation (CCM) modules includes five questions each, including cancer prevention, early detection/screening, public medical insurance, private medical insurance, and online mutual aid. Five-level Likert scale was used to rate protection motivation, and dichotomous answers (yes/no) are used to measure their protection behavior. The five questions for measuring respondents cancer control behavior (CCB) are: "In the past one year, did you ever try to convince or help your parents to do cancer prevention/do early detection/get public medical insurance/get private medical insurance/get online mutual aid?" (yes = 1, no = 0). CCM module consists of five similar questions: "In the next

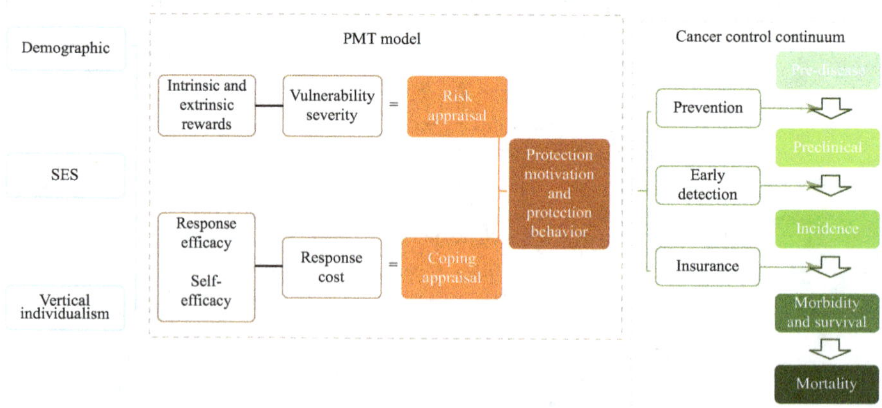

Figure 4.3 Theoretical framework of the questionnaire

year, will you try to convince or help your parents do cancer prevention/do early detection/get public medical insurance/get private medical insurance/get online mutual aid?" (not at all likely = 1, extremely likely = 5). The score of CCB and CCM is the sum of five questions in each module.

Secondly, the risk appraisal and coping appraisal process consisted of three modules each. Cancer risk appraisal process have the severity of cancer (3 items), the vulnerability of cancer (3 items) and intrinsic and extrinsic rewards (3 items). These are followed by coping appraisal process, including response efficacy (5 items), self-efficacy (3 items) and response costs (3 items, and each item has 4–5 elements). Above 6 modules are rated at a typical 5 level Likert scale from "strongly disagree" to "strongly agree."

Moreover, another cultural variable named vertical collectivism (VC) (4 items) is designed to measure the difference of the belief of Chinese core family values such as filial piety between only-children and children with siblings. According to Triandis and Gelfand, individualism and collectivism are the importance of attitudes and norms as determinants of social behavior. VC is related to family integrity [31]. Scholars have conducted researches on family values and individualism of Chinese one-child generation [32,33]. Previous studies in the 1980s and 1990s indicate that only-children are more likely to be individualistic, compared with children with siblings [34,35]. The researches of Feng indicate that there is no significant difference in the socialization process and personality between only-children and children with siblings [36]. Another research shows that the core Chinese traditional values of family, such as filial piety and harmonious family, are still welcomed among the young generation [37]. In this study, VC has four items: (1) Children, no matter how busy they are, should often go home to visit their parents. (2) Parents and children should live together as much as possible. (3) I have to take care of my parents, even if I have to sacrifice my personal needs. (4) Family happiness comes prior to personal interests/future. Four items are measured by a 5 level Likert scale from "strongly disagree" to "strongly agree." The score of VC is the sum of four questions.

Demographic and social-economic status (SES) comprise gender, education, occupation, monthly income, marriage, only-child or not and age. Meanwhile, the occupation and insurance coverage of their parents are also investigated to examine their parents' SES.

4.2.2 Respondents and statistics

The OCP started from 1979 and ended by 2016 in China. Therefore, we recruited participants who were born during 1979 to 1999, including only-children and children with siblings. Questionnaires are self-administrated and distributed on the most popular Chinese questionnaire website: wjx.cn. At the same time, the authors also distribute the questionnaire on social media. The data collected on the website was transferred to IBM SPSS Statistics for Macintosh, Version 25.0 (NY: IBM Corp.). In the process of analysis, descriptive statistics, *t*-test and ANOVA were used. The reliability of each module in the questionnaire was measured by Cronbach's coefficient. The Cronbach's coefficient of most modules is higher than 0.7, which shows the reliability of the questionnaire. The significance level was set at $p < 0.05$.

4.3 Results

A total of 307 questionnaires were collected in September 2019. Questionnaires completed in less than 100 seconds or with more than ten consecutive identical answers were deleted for the sake of validity. Questionnaires of respondents who were not aged 20–40 were removed. In total, 274 questionnaires were valid.

Table 4.1 shows the difference between CCB, CCM and VC by demographic variables. There was no significant difference in CCB, but a significant difference in CCM and VC between men and women ($p = 0.044$). That is to say, male respondents had a stronger sense of family integrity and belief of core Chinese family values. However, their CCM for parents was not as strong as that of women.

Among different monthly income groups, the CCB of the income group below 3,000 yuan was significantly lower than that of other income groups ($p = 0.004$). However, there was no significant difference in CCM and VC among different income groups. The VC of married respondents was significantly higher than VC of unmarried respondents ($p = 0.001$), indicating that married ones are more likely to agree with the Chinese traditional family values. There was a significant difference in CCM among different age groups, and the groups aged 24–31 had a higher CCM score than other groups. There were no significant differences in CCB, CCM, and VC among the respondents with different educational levels and occupations.

The average scores of PMT modules of all respondents are shown in Table 4.2 Modules with a high average score were severity (88.5%), response efficacy (88.3%), and CCM (82.5%). CCB (47.4%) and vulnerability (60%) had the least average scores. In CCB and CCM modules, private medical insurance and online mutual aid had the least average scores. Although there was no significant difference in total CCB and CCM scores between only-children and children with siblings, the latter was more active in convincing/helping parents to get public insurance ($p = 0.004$).

The average score of only-children on intrinsic and extrinsic rewards was lower than that of children with siblings ($p = 0.005$). However, no significant difference was found between these two groups in VC. The item with the highest average score was "Children, no matter how busy they are, should often go home to visit their parents" (87%), and the lowest was "Parents and children should live together as much as possible" (66.8%).

The first item of vulnerability was "the trend of cancer incidence in the past ten years" (sharply decreased = 1, slightly decreased = 2, stable = 3, slightly increased = 4, sharply increased = 5), and the average score of all respondents was 4.02 (80.4%). The second item was "what is the current cancer incidence in China?" (1/1,000 = 1, 1/800 = 2, 1/500 = 3, 1/200 = 4, 1/100 = 5) (The age-standardized cancer incidence in China was 201.7/100,000 in 2018 [2].), and the average score of all respondents was 2.61 (52.2%). The third item was the

Table 4.1 Characteristics of respondents (n = 274)

Variables		Frequency (Percent)	CCB		CCM		VC	
			Mean (SD)	*p* value	Mean (SD)	*p* value	Mean (SD)	*p* value
Gender	Male	85(31%)	2.21(1.54)	0.255	19.86(4.31)	0.048	15.58(2.88)	0.044
	Female	189(69%)	2.44(1.47)		20.96(4.24)		14.78(3.08)	
Education	High school and below	9(3.3%)	2.11(1.54)	0.608	20.67(3.04)	0.197	17.22(2.64)	0.050
	2–3 years college	20(7.3%)	2.60(1.98)		19.95(4.57)		15.75(2.20)	
	Bachelor	132(48.2%)	2.45(1.55)		21.19(4.06)		15.10(3.19)	
	Masters and above	113(41.2%)	2.24(1.42)		20.07(4.53)		14.64(2.94)	
Occupation	Students	115(42%)	2.06(1.46)	0.116	20.47(4.17)	0.320	14.97(3.03)	0.544
	Private company staff	48(17.5%)	2.67(1.55)		21.04(4.52)		14.92(2.68)	
	Self-employed	14(5.1%)	2.64(1.34)		20.50(3.05)		16.36(2.47)	
	Staff of state-owned company/government affiliated institution	63(23%)	2.52(1.53)		20.08(4.92)		14.89(3.27)	
	Public servants	12(4.4%)	2.83(1.64)		23.17(2.33)		15.83(3.04)	
	Others	22(8%)	2.45(1.68)		20.73(3.67)		14.68(3.47)	
Monthly income	3,000 and below	125(45.6%)	2.01(1.42)	0.004	20.54(4.09)	0.333	15.06(3.13)	0.666
	3,000–5,000	42(15.3%)	2.79(1.62)		21.60(3.86)		15.38(3.08)	
	5,001–8,000	50(18.2%)	2.56(1.57)		19.96(5.11)		14.60(2.82)	
	Above 8,000	57(20.8%)	2.68(1.51)		20.67(4.19)		15.05(3.01)	
Marriage	Single	191(69.7%)	2.27(1.54)	0.113	20.59(4.25)	0.842	14.64(3.02)	0.001
	Married	83(30.3%)	2.59(1.47)		20.70(4.40)		15.92(2.91)	
Only-child or not	Yes	125(45.6%)	2.33(1.55)	0.687	20.34(4.62)(4.62)	0.335	14.74(3.43)	0.158
	No	149(54.4%)	2.40(1.51)		20.85(3.98)		15.27(2.65)	
Age	20–23	89(32.5%)	2.07(1.59)	0.149	20.20(4.21)	0.012	14.88(3.09)	0.855
	24–27	82(29.9%)	2.44(1.48)		21.27(3.62)		14.88(2.63)	
	28–31	45(16.4%)	2.69(1.31)		21.87(3.37)		15.38(2.93)	
	32–35	17(6.2%)	2.76(1.79)		20.12(5.22)		14.94(3.94)	
	36–40	40(14.6%)	2.35(1.55)		18.98(5.59)		15.30(3.50)	
	Missing	1(0.4%)						

Table 4.2 The difference of PMT constructs between only-children and people who have siblings

Items	Only-children ($N = 125$)	Children with siblings ($N = 149$)		All	
	Mean (SD)	Mean (SD)	*p* value	Mean (SD)	Percent
***CCB* (*α* = 0.650)**	***2.33(1.55)***	***2.40(1.51)***	***0.687***	***2.37(1.53)***	***47.4%***
Cancer prevention	0.72(0.45)	0.69(0.46)	0.605	0.70(0.46)	70.4%
Early detection	0.55(0.50)	0.50(0.50)	0.424	0.53(0.50)	52.6%
Private medical insurance	0.35(0.48)	0.30(0.46)	0.319	0.32(0.47)	32.1%
Public medical insurance	0.46(0.50)	0.64(0.48)	0.004	0.56(0.50)	55.8%
Online mutual aid	0.24(0.43)	0.28(0.45)	0.510	0.26(0.44)	25.9%
***CCM* (*α* = 0.850)**	***20.34(4.62)***	***20.85(3.98)***	***0.335***	***20.62(4.29)***	***82.5%***
Cancer prevention	4.52(0.85)	4.42(0.84)	0.343	4.47(0.84)	89.4%
Early detection	4.51(0.85)	4.37(0.87)	0.171	4.43(0.86)	88.6%
Private medical insurance	3.94(1.21)	3.98(1.08)	0.796	3.96(1.14)	79.2%
Public medical insurance	3.77(1.42)	4.30(0.96)	0.000	4.06(1.22)	81.2%
Online mutual aid	3.60(1.37)	3.78(1.20)	0.257	3.70(1.28)	74.0%
***VC* (*α* = 0.775)**	***14.74(3.43)***	***15.27(2.65)***	***0.158***	***15.03(3.04)***	***75.2%***
Children, no matter how busy they are, should often go home to visit their parents	4.34(0.82)	4.36(0.69)	0.898	4.35(0.75)	87.0%
Parents and children should live together as much as possible	3.21(1.25)	3.45(1.07)	0.086	3.34(1.16)	66.8%
I have to take care of my parents, even if I have to sacrifice my personal needs	3.65(1.06)	3.80(0.87)	0.204	3.73(0.96)	74.6%
Family happiness is prior to personal interests/ future	3.54(1.10)	3.66(0.93)	0.303	3.61(1.01)	72.2%
Intrinsic and extrinsic rewards (negative) (α=0.869)	***8.50(3.58)***	***9.60(2.70)***	***0.005***	***9.09(3.17)***	***60.6%***
Cancer is severe, and I feel calm when I don't think about it	2.85(1.30)	3.10(1.10)	0.087	2.99(1.20)	59.8%
I avoid talking about cancer with my family because we can't afford it	2.69(1.26)	3.17(1.05)	0.001	2.95(1.18)	59.0%
Talking about death and cancer would make my parents uncomfortable	2.96(1.39)	3.32(0.97)	0.015	3.16(1.19)	63.2%
Vulnerability (α = 0.659)	***9.25(2.35)***	***8.80(2.09)***	***0.095***	***9.00(2.22)***	***60.0%***
What is the trend of cancer incidence in China in the last ten years?	3.98(1.01)	4.05(0.91)	0.505	4.02(0.96)	80.4%

(Continues)

What is the current cancer incidence in China?	2.85(1.44)	2.41(1.36)	0.010	2.61(1.41)	52.2%
What is the probability of your parents getting cancer?	2.42(0.97)	2.34(0.96)	0.449	2.38(0.96)	47.6%
***Severity* (α = *0.748*)**	***13.33(1.75)***	***13.21(1.77)***	***0.57***	***13.27(1.75)***	***88.5%***
Physical pain and possible death	4.54(0.65)	4.48(0.65)	0.395	4.51(0.65)	90.2%
Psychological worries and sadness about bereavement	4.59(0.65)	4.50(0.63)	0.255	4.54(0.64)	90.8%
Financial pressure and the risk of returning to poverty	4.20(0.87)	4.23(0.82)	0.733	4.22(0.84)	84.4%
***Response efficacy* (α = *0.829*)**	***21.06(3.20)***	***20.64(2.72)***	***0.242***	***20.83(2.95)***	***83.3%***
Some cancers could be prevented if improving lifestyle scientifically	4.23(0.74)	4.19(0.64)	0.656	4.21(0.69)	84.2%
Screening and early detection are useful and helpful to get early diagnosis and treatment	4.56(0.63)	4.38(0.58)	0.015	4.46(0.61)	89.2%
Public medical insurance can relieve financial pressure and provide better treatment for cancer patients	4.27(0.81)	4.22(0.71)	0.585	4.24(0.75)	84.8%
Private medical insurance can relieve financial pressure and provide better treatment for cancer patients	4.17(0.91)	4.10(0.70)	0.500	4.13(0.80)	82.6%
Online mutual aid can relieve financial pressure and provide better treatment for cancer patients	3.82(0.98)	3.74(0.90)	0.451	3.78(0.94)	75.6%
***Self-efficacy* (α = *0.475*)**	***9.46(2.08)***	***9.36(1.96)***	***0.678***	***9.41(2.01)***	***62.7%***
I have the ability to help my parents prevent cancer and mitigate its consequences	3.47(0.95)	3.50(0.91)	0.827	3.49(0.93)	69.8%
I believe I can successfully help my parents prevent cancer and mitigate its consequences	3.42(0.95)	3.41(0.90)	0.896	3.42(0.92)	68.4%
With my current living conditions and family relationships, what I can do is very limited (reversed)	2.57(1.05)	2.45(1.00)	0.370	2.50(1.02)	50.0%
***Response costs* (α = *0.849*)**	***42.34(8.74)***	***43.77(7.70)***	***0.154***	***43.12(8.20)***	***66.3%***
The cost of helping parents prevent cancer	13.07(2.89)	13.40(2.55)	0.315	13.3(2.71)	66.5%
The cost of helping parents do early detection	12.84(3.09)	13.17(2.77)	0.356	13.0(2.92)	65%
The cost of helping parents get private medical insurance	16.43(3.79)	17.19(3.50)	0.085	16.85(3.65)	67.4%

Italic and bold texts are modules, and others followed are items in each module.

probability of parents getting cancer (much lower than average = 1, slightly lower than average = 2, same as average = 3, slightly higher than average = 4, much higher than average = 5). The average score of all respondents was 2.38 (47.6%). A significant difference was found between only-children and children with siblings in the second item ($p = 0.01$).

The average severity score of all respondents was 88.5% of the total score, which means that the perception of cancer severity is very high. The highest score of response efficacy items was early detection (89.2%), and the lowest was online mutual aid (75.6%). The average score of only-children on early detection efficacy was significantly higher than children with siblings ($p = 0.015$). No significant difference was found in the self-efficacy and response costs modules between only-children and children with siblings.

In addition to examining the differences in PMT structure between only-children and children with siblings, the medical insurance coverage of their parents was also investigated (see Table 4.3). There are three main public medical insurance schemes in China: urban employee-based basic medical insurance scheme (UEBMI, an institutional medical insurance), urban resident-based basic medical insurance scheme (URBMI) and new rural cooperative medical scheme (NRCMS) [38]. Public servants, staff of state-owned companies/government affiliated institutions and staff of private companies with employee medical insurance are covered by UEBMI, which provides more benefits and a higher reimbursement rate than URBMI and NRCMS.

From the data we collected, 68.8% of fathers and 56.8% of mothers of only-children have UEBMI, while only 29.5% of fathers and 15.4% of mothers of children with siblings have UEBMI. After adding up the score of UEBMI of fathers and mothers (yes = 1, no = 0), the average score of only-children parents was 1.26, and that of the children with siblings' parents was about 0.45 (p = 0.000) (see Table 4.4).

The proportion of both parents with private medical insurance in only-children families was 31.2%, while that in more than one children families was only 19.5%. There was a significant difference in the scores of both parents covered with private medical insurance between two kinds of families ($p = 0.026$). Furthermore, there was also a significant difference in the average score of online mutual aid coverage between the two groups ($p = 0.032$). It shows that only-children parents are more likely to have online mutual aid products (see Tables 4.5 and 4.6).

Table 4.7 shows the response costs of cancer control behavior. Lacking reliable information was the biggest obstacle to help parents prevent cancer and do early detection. Unfamiliarity with private insurance products, poor financial condition, and difficulty in making a claim were three top obstacles to get parents private medical insurance for the OCP generation.

4.4 Discussion

Understanding the cancer risk appraisal and risk control of parents among the OCP generation will help us understand: (1) the role that the OCP generation plays in

Table 4.3 The occupation of OCP generation parents

Only-child	Occupation	Father		Mother	
		Frequency (Percent)	Cumulative Percent	Frequency (Percent)	Cumulative Percent
Yes	Public servants	27(21.6%)	68.8%	11(8.8%)	56.8%
	Staff of state-owned company/government affiliated institution	46(36.8%)		45(36.0%)	
	Staff of private company (including employee medical insurance)	13(10.4%)		15(12.0%)	
	Staff of private company (no employee medical insurance)	4(3.2%)	31.2%	3(2.4%)	43.2%
	Self-employed	24(19.2%)		28(22.4%)	
	Farmer/immigrant workers	5(4.0%)		5(4.0%)	
	Unemployed	6(4.8%)		18(14.4%)	
	Total	125	100.0%	125	100.0%
No	Public servants	8(5.4%)	29.5%	2(1.3%)	15.4%
	Staff of state-owned company/government affiliated institution	26(17.4%)		18(12.1%)	
	Staff of private company (including employee medical insurance)	10(6.7%)		3(2.0%)	
	Staff of private company (no employee medical insurance)	2(1.3%)	70.5%	1(0.7%)	84.6%
	Self-employed	29(19.5%)		31(20.8%)	
	Farmer/immigrant workers	66(44.3%)		62(41.6%)	
	Unemployed	8(5.4%)		32(21.5%)	
	Total	149	100.0%	149	100.0%

Table 4.4 The average score of UEBMI coverage of parents

Only-child	*N*	Mean	Std. deviation	*p* value
Yes	125	1.2560	0.85103	0.000
No	149	0.4497	0.72070	

cancer control in Chinese families; (2) the strategies and obstacles of cancer control in Chinese families; (3) the potential health impact of the OCP on parents of OCP generation.

First of all, the average CCM score was 20.62 (82.5%), and the average CCB score of all respondents was only 2.37 (47.4%). That shows that CCM of the OCP generation is strong, but they are not doing well enough in cancer control behavior.

Table 4.5 The insurances coverage of OCP generation parents

Only-child		Public medical insurance (UEBMI, URBMI, and NRCMS) Frequency (Percent)	Private medical insurance Frequency (Percent)	Online mutual aid Frequency (Percent)
Yes	Both have	103(82.4%)	39(31.2%)	19(15.2%)
	Only one has	6(4.8%)	11(8.8%)	2(1.6%)
	None	2(1.6%)	48(38.4%)	83(66.4%)
	I don't know	14(11.2%)	27(21.6%)	21(16.8%)
	Total	125(100%)	125(100%)	125(100%)
No	Both have	124(83.2%)	29(19.5%)	9(6%)
	Only one has	16(10.7%)	13(8.7%)	5(3.4%)
	None	2(1.3%)	81(54.4%)	119(79.9%)
	I don't know	7(4.7%)	26(17.4%)	16(10.7%)
	Total	149(100%)	149(100%)	149(100%)

Table 4.6 The average scores of insurance coverage of OCP generation parents

	Only-children Mean (SD)	Children with siblings Mean (SD)	*p* value
Private medical insurance	0.71(0.91)	0.48(0.80)	0.026
Public medical insurance	1.70(0.69)	1.77(0.55)	0.320
Online mutual aid	0.32(0.73)	0.15(0.50)	0.032

Response costs results could provide with some clues of the reasons for the gap between CCM and CCB: not enough reliable information is the main barrier to help parents do cancer prevention and early detection. Unfamiliarity with private medical insurance, poor financial condition, and the difficulty in making a claim are the main costs of getting private medical insurance for parents. Therefore, the government and relevant health promotion institutions should enhance the work on the dissemination of cancer prevention and early detection information.

Surprisingly, there was no significant difference in CCM and CCB between only-children and children with siblings. From the data analysis, three potential reasons could explain this phenomenon: Firstly, the institutional medical insurance coverage of only-children parents is higher than parents with more than one child. Therefore, only-children are under less pressure. The regulation of the OCP in China could support this explanation: the parents who have more than one child will lose their institutional jobs. Thus, parents who are civil servants, staff of state-owned companies and government affiliated institutions are more likely to comply with the policy requirement and have only one child. On the contrary, children with

Table 4.7 Response costs of cancer control behavior

Response costs		**Only-children Mean (SD)**	**Children with siblings Mean (SD)**	***p* value**
Cancer prevention	Total	13.07(2.89)	13.40(2.55)	0.315
	Time	3.20(1.09)	3.26(0.98)	0.061
	Financial condition	3.46(1.04)	3.51(0.94)	0.701
	Lacking reliable prevention information	3.53(0.97)	3.61(0.94)	0.474
	Difficulty in communication with parents	2.88(1.15)	3.03(1.01)	0.267
Early detection	Total	12.84(3.09)	13.17(2.77)	0.356
	Time	3.22(1.01)	3.25(0.97)	0.839
	Financial condition	3.34(1.08)	3.45(0.97)	0.359
	Lacking reliable information	3.43(1.04)	3.49(1.02)	0.664
	Difficulty in communication with parents	2.85(1.10)	2.98(1.05)	0.312
Private medical insurance	Total	16.43(3.79)	17.19(3.50)	0.085
	Time	3.05(1.05)	3.10(0.99)	0.671
	Financial condition	3.35(1.09)	3.50(0.95)	0.242
	Difficulty in finding a suitable insurance	3.71(0.99)	3.72(0.94)	0.913
	Difficulty in making a claim	3.48(0.99)	3.58(0.97)	0.415
	Difficulty in communication with parents	2.84(1.10)	3.30(1.04)	0.001

siblings in this study are more active in persuading/helping parents to get other public insurance plans (URBMI and NRCMS). Secondly, parents of only-children have stronger cancer risk awareness and are more likely to do cancer risk control by themselves. Even though no difference of private medical insurance CCM and CCB between only-children and children with siblings was found, but there is a significant difference in the coverage of private medical insurance between parents of only-children and parents with more than one child. It indicates that parents of only-children are more likely to get private medical insurance by themselves to control cancer risks. Besides, children with siblings tend to think that it is difficult to convince parents to get private medical insurance, while only-children are less likely to regard it as a problem ($p = 0.001$). Thirdly, in the intrinsic and extrinsic rewards module, the average score of children with siblings was higher than only-children. This indicates that children with siblings are more likely to have uncertainty avoidance, while only-children are more positive to face cancer risks of their parents.

Moreover, the average score of severity of cancer of all respondents was high, the average score of vulnerability of their parents was relatively low. For instance, although the average score of cancer incidence in China is close to "slightly increased," the average score of cancer incidence rate and the likelihood of their parents getting a cancer is below average. This contradictory result indicates that respondents' vulnerability appraisal of their parents is not very objective.

In our hypothesis, the VC score of only-children and children with siblings would be different, further influencing CCM and CBC. However, the research results negated this hypothesis. It suggests that the traditional core family values, such as filial piety and care-giving obligations, are still accepted by both only-children and children with siblings. In addition, no significant difference in VC between different age groups, and it echoes conclusions of previous researches.

Additionally, the low coverage of private medical insurance suggests that families of OCP generation is fragile in the risk of cancer. Even though the coverage of Chinese only-children parents is 31.2%, it is still much lower than the average 70.2% (2015, 18–64 years old) private medical insurance coverage in the USA [39].

However, online mutual aid is becoming prevalent among OCP generation, especially among only-child families. The online mutual aid coverage of both only-children parents was 15.2%, while that of parents with more than one child was only 6%. It indeed provides the OCP generation with an affordable and complementary option to mitigate the risk of cancer. At the same time, online mutual aid is improving cancer risk awareness and cancer prevention education by introducing users to cancer patients that they helped every month. Nevertheless, the relatively low average response efficacy score of online mutual aid suggests that OCP generation doubt its reliability and efficacy.

4.5 Limitations

The educational level of respondents in this study is relatively high. 96.7% of respondents have at least 2–3 years of college education. Therefore, the results in this study are only applicable to 20%–30% of the whole population, according to the *China's 2010 Population Census Data* [40]. In our previous qualitative research on online mutual aid, we found that personal life experience and health information resources also influence their cancer risk appraisal and risk control motivation. Due to the limitation of the length of the questionnaire, we did not include these variables. Besides, the correlation analysis and regression analysis are recommended to identify the predictors of OCP generation's CCM and CCB in future researches.

References

[1] Shen Y., Wu H. and Ray P. K. 'Why is crowdfunded medical aid so popular and successful in China?' *Asian Hospital and Healthcare Management*. 2018, vol. 40, pp. 30–33

[2] Anonymous. '水滴互助沈鹏：做80后90后心中互助保障第一品牌 (Waterdrop Mutual Shen Peng: we strive to be the top choice of mutual aid among people born in the 1980s and 1990s)' [online]. 2016. Available from http://qlwb.com.cn/2016/0812/696734.shtml [Accessed 28 Aug 2019](In Chinese)

[3] Feng R. M., Zong Y. N., Cao S. M. and Xu R. H. 'Current cancer situation in China: good or bad news from the 2018 Global Cancer Statistics?' *Cancer Communications*. 2019, vol. 39(1), 22

[4] Center for Health Statistics and Information. An analysis report of national health services survey in China, 2013 [online]. 2016. Available from http://nhfpc.gov.cn/ewebeditor/uploadfile/2016/10/20161026163512679.pdf (In Chinese)

[5] Huang H. Y., Shi J. F., Guo L. W., *et al.* 'Expenditure and financial burden for common cancers in China: a hospital-based multicentre cross-sectional study'. *The Lancet.* 2016, vol. 388, S10

[6] National Bureau of Statistics. Statistical Bulletin on National Economic and Social Development, 2018 [online]. 2019. Available from http://stats.gov.cn/tjsj/zxfb/201902/t20190228_1651265.html [Accessed 28 Aug 2019](In Chinese)

[7] Flaherty J. H., Liu M. L., Ding L., *et al.* 'China: the aging giant'. *Journal of the American Geriatrics Society*. 2007, vol. 55(8), pp. 1295–300

[8] Bongaarts J. and Greenhalgh S. 'An alternative to the one-child policy in China'. *Population and Development Review*. 1985, vol. 11(4), pp. 585–617

[9] Li X., Zhou Q., Wang X., *et al.* 'The effect of low insurance reimbursement on quality of care for non-small cell lung cancer in China: a comprehensive study covering diagnosis, treatment, and outcomes'. *BMC Cancer.* 2018, vol. 18(1), pp. 683–683

[10] Hiatt R. A. and Breen N. 'The social determinants of cancer – a challenge for transdisciplinary science'. *American Journal of Preventive Medicine.* 2008, vol. 35(2), pp. S141–S150

[11] WHO. Cancer prevention [online]. Available from https://who.int/cancer/prevention/en/ [Accessed 28 Aug 2019]

[12] National Cancer Institute, Division of Cancer Control and Population. Cancer Control Continuum [online]. 2017. Available from https://cancercontrol.cancer.gov/od/continuum.html [Accessed 28 Aug 2019]

[13] WHO. Cancer-Early diagnosis and screening [online]. Available from https://who.int/cancer/prevention/diagnosis-screening/en/ [Accessed 28 Aug 2019]

[14] WHO. International Agency for Research on Cancer. European Code Against Cancer [online]. Available from http://cancer-code-europe.iarc.fr/index.php/en/ [Accessed 29 Aug 2019]

[15] Niu X., Roche L. M., Pawlish K. S. and Henry K. A. 'Cancer survival disparities by health insurance status'. *Cancer Med.* 2013, vol. 2(3), pp. 403–11

[16] Fedewa S. A., Lerro C., Chase D. and Ward E. M. 'Insurance status and racial differences in uterine cancer survival: a study of patients in the national cancer database'. *Gynecologic Oncology.* 2011, vol. 122(1), pp. 63–68

[17] Slatore C. G., Au D. H. and Gould M. K. 'An official American Thoracic Society systematic review: insurance status and disparities in lung cancer practices and outcomes'. *American Journal of Respiratory and Critical Care Medicine*. 2010, vol. 182(9), pp. 1195–1205

[18] Ward E., Halpern M., Schrag N., *et al.* 'Association of insurance with cancer care utilization and outcomes'. *CA: A Cancer Journal for Clinicians*. 2008, vol. 58(1), pp. 9–31

[19] Brookfield K. F., Cheung M. C., Lucci J., Fleming L. E. and Koniaris L. G. 'Disparities in survival among women with invasive cervical cancer'. *Cancer.* 2009, vol. 115(1), pp. 166–178

[20] 黄枫 (Huang F.), 吴纯杰 (Wu C. J.). '城镇不同社会医疗保险待遇人群死亡率交叉现象研究 (A study on mortality of city residents with different social medical insurance)'. 人口研究. 2010, vol. 34(01), pp. 95–105

[21] Floyd D. L., Prentice-Dunn S. and Rogers R. W. 'A meta-analysis of research on protection motivation theory'. *Journal of Applied Social Psychology*. 2000, vol. 30(2), pp. 407–429

[22] Rogers R.W. 'Cognitive and physiological processes in fear appeals and attitude change: a revised theory of protection motivation' in: Cacioppo J. and Petty R. (eds). *Social Psychophysiology* (New York, Guilford Press, 1983), pp. 153–77

[23] Courneya K. S. and Hellsten L. A. M. 'Cancer prevention as a source of exercise motivation: an experimental test using protection motivation theory'. *Psychology, Health & Medicine.* 2001, vol. 6(1), pp. 59–64

[24] McClendon B. T. and Prentice-Dunn S. 'Reducing skin cancer risk: an intervention based on protection motivation theory'. *Journal of Health Psychology*. 2001, vol. 6(3), pp. 321–28

[25] Babazadeh T., Nadrian H., Banayejeddi M. and Rezapour B. 'Determinants of skin cancer preventive behaviors among rural farmers in Iran: an application of protection motivation theory'. *Journal of Cancer Education*. 2017, vol. 32(3), pp. 604–612

[26] Prentice-Dunn S., Jones J. L. and Floyd D. L. 'Persuasive appeals and the reduction of skin cancer risk: the roles of appearance concern, perceived benefits of a tan, and efficacy information'. *Journal of Applied Social Psychology*. 1997, vol. 27(12), pp. 1041–1047

[27] Rahaei Z., Ghofranipour F., Morowatisharifabad M. A. and Mohammadi E., 'Determinants of cancer early detection behaviors: application of protection motivation theory'. *Health promotion perspectives*. 2015, vol. 5(2), pp. 138–146

[28] Bai Y., Liu Q., Chen X., *et al.* 'Protection motivation theory in predicting intention to receive cervical cancer screening in rural Chinese women'. *Psycho-Oncology*. 2018, vol. 27(2), pp. 442–449

[29] Seyde E., Taal E. and Wiegman O. 'Risk-appraisal, outcome and self-efficacy expectancies: cognitive factors in preventive behaviour related to cancer'. *Psychology & Health*. 1990, vol. 4(2), pp. 99–109

[30] Helmes A. W. 'Application of the protection motivation theory to genetic testing for breast cancer risk'. *Preventive Medicine.* 2002, vol. 35(5), pp. 453–462

[31] Triandis, H. C. and Gelfand, M. J. 'Converging measurement of horizontal and vertical individualism and collectivism'. *Journal of Personality and Social Psychology*. 1998, vol. 74(1), pp. 118–128

[32] Chen R. 'Weaving individualism into collectivism: Chinese adults' evolving relationship and family values'. *Journal of Comparative Family Studies*. 2015, vol. 46(2), pp. 167–179

[33] Moore R. L. 'Generation Ku: individualism and China's millennial youth'. *Ethnology.* 2005, vol. 44(4), pp. 357–376

[34] Poston D. L. and Falbo, T. 'Effects of the one-child policy on the children of China' in: Poston D.L., Yaukey D. (eds.). *The Population of Modern China* (Boston, Springer, 1992)

[35] 陈科文 (Chen K. W.). '关于独生子女合群性的初步研究 (A study on the gregariousness of Chinese only-children)'. 心理学报. 1985, vol. 3, pp. 264–270

[36] 风笑天 (Feng X. T.). '独生子女青少年的社会化过程及其结果 (The process and results of socialization of Chinese only-children teenagers)'. 中国社会科学. 2000, vol. 6, pp. 118–131+208

[37] 徐安琪 (Xu A. Q.). '家庭价值观变迁:去传统化?去集体主义化? (The change of Chinese core family values: detraditionalization? de-collectivism?)'.中国研究. 2012, vol. 2, pp. 171–199+245

[38] Meng Q., Fang H., Liu X., Yuan B. and Xu J. 'Consolidating the social health insurance schemes in China: towards an equitable and efficient health system'. *The Lancet.* 2015, vol. 386(10002), pp. 1484–92

[39] Anonymous. Lack of health insurance coverage and type of coverage [online]. Available from https://cdc.gov/nchs/data/nhis/earlyrelease/Early release201609_01.pdf [Accessed 30 Aug 2019]

[40] National Bureau of Statistics of the People's Republic of China. The Sixth National Population Census of the People's Republic of China [online]. Available from http://stats.gov.cn/tjsj/pcsj/rkpc/6rp/indexch.htm [Accessed 2 Sep 2019] (In Chinese)

Chapter 5

Understanding health professionals' perspective on delivering health information on social media: a case study in Bangladesh

Rashadul Hasan[1], Mahfuz Ashraf[2] and Numa Sarkar[3]

5.1 Introduction

Human health is considered as a social matter, not just a matter of an individual [1]. In modern times, by enabling the creation of support systems for health matters, social media platforms are providing a space to share health information. In the healthcare setting, using social media platforms health professionals (HPs) can impact on how information on health issues are generated, shared and discussed [2,3]. Today, the patients use social media to seek advice from HPs more than any time before [4].

Social media have gained access to all of our lives, in general, individual and professional states of affairs [5]. Many social media platforms are available to HPs, such as social networking sites, blogs, microblogs, wikis, discussion forums and mobile applications. They use these platforms to enhance professional networking, health-information sharing and public health programmes. In contrast, the general people (users) also seek for health information on social media-based interactive platforms. These platforms are important place for them to search for health information, discuss their experiences with health issues, and information management – an important component of coping with health-related issues [6].

Although, users use social media to educate themselves better, the quality and accuracy of the available information on social media are the matters of concern. Therefore, HPs' participation on social media platforms is important to reduce the influence of misinformation, while their participation also increases their reputation by elevating their own content in search results [7]. In this way, these social media platforms are fundamentally reshaping the way of commutation by HPs [8,9]. The other significant outcomes of using social media platforms for health information sharing by the HPs are reengineering the way of user engagement [10] and

[1]Research Division, Bhalo Achi Healthcare and Research Ltd., Dhaka, Bangladesh
[2]Entrepreneurship and Innovation, Crown Institute of Higher Education, North Sydney, Australia
[3]Division of Education and Innovation, Ashraf Begum, Sydney, Australia

repurposing online information (using something for a new or different purpose) [11]. Yet, there is a lack of study of statutory regulations on health information sharing on social media, which is important to establish rules and expectations around health information sharing on social media. Besides, in the healthcare setting, policy issues are significant to consider when using social media [5].

While HPs are contributing and sharing health information on a global scale on social media and educating the users and communities, until today, most of the studies have investigated the users' perspectives and the quality of available information. For example, according to a systematic review on social media for health communication, the most common studies were on the quality and reliability of available information, and the users' engagement, confidentiality, privacy and barriers such as socioeconomic and gender factors [12]. On the other hand, many studies also investigated the HPs' perspectives. These studies have explored: how HPs contribute on social media by ensuring that available information is correct [13]; what barriers HPs face while using social media (e.g. skills) [2]; how HPs can undertake online educational courses for health information and health care delivery [14]; and what guidelines HPs might follow to prevent the distribution of poor-quality information [15]. Besides, study reports that the issues of privacy, patient consent, HPs' credentials and license, safety and security are critical for HPs when using social media for healthcare activities [5]. However, no studies have theoretically investigated which factors motivate the HPs in health-information sharing on social media.

The healthcare systems are always evolving that recognise the social elements, for example social relationship, social inclusion, culture, community, lifestyle and education, as influencing factors in health quality difference [16]. In the context of healthcare systems, the interactions between these elements influence health and lead to considerable variances in health quality conditions among various groups of people. For example, because of various differences in social elements, often a considerable health quality discrepancy between the indigenous and non-indigenous population in Australia is reported [17]. However, to lower such health quality discrepancy, the presence of HPs on social media for healthcare activities can be very useful. In this regard, a common and pertinent question is whether HPs should be encouraged to participate on social media for healthcare activities [18].

The connection between healthcare and social media-based communities is a significant and promising area of study in information system (IS) research [18]. In addition, it is also important to know what conditions influence the HPs for participating in the social media-based communities for healthcare activities. Therefore, in this chapter, the authors aim for a case study and a theoretical review to understand which factors motivate the HPs in health-information sharing on the social media. This case study-based study will be useful for statutory regulations and policy formation regarding engaging the HPs' for health-information sharing on social media.

The following sections in the study proceeds as follows: (1) first, a case study on a mobile app-based social media platform used for disseminating health information among the underserved communities in Bangladesh; (2) second, literature review on the facts and findings on the health-information sharing on the social media; (3) third, an overview of the theoretical background and perspective to explain the underlying the reasons that can motivate the HPs' health-information sharing on the social media; (4) fourth, proposing a theory-based conceptual framework for future study and policy-making and (5) fifth, the conclusion, recommendations and contribution of this study.

5.2 Case study: Good Health app

Bangladesh has full coverage of mobile network with very high demand for social media. The country has a total population of more than 160 million; there are only approximately 96,000 registered general practitioners (GP/doctors) available. According to the WHO, approximately 44% of member states (countries) have less than 1 physician for every 1,000 of population [19]. In Bangladesh, there is only one GP for every 1,700 patients. However, according to Millennium Development Goal, at least 2.5 physicians per 1,000 people needed to provide adequate coverage with primary care interventions. Although 70% of total population live in rural areas, only 25% of total qualified GPs are practicing in rural areas [19]. Besides, the rural citizens in Bangladesh have been suffering from 'digital divide'. However, there is an increase of social media usage across the country. By using this advantage, the dissemination of health knowledge and information can be reached to the Bangladeshi rural citizens conveniently, the people who do not have adequate access to healthcare support in general practice.

Although mobile apps technologies have successfully addressed many healthcare issues related to clinical decision support such as for field health workers' information assistance, for cardiovascular disease, incorporating patient data streams, and offering epidemiological support for managing infectious disease, few apps have focused on a social media features-based platform where the HPs can share health information. For this reason, Good Health app was developed as a social media-based platform where the HPs can share health knowledge with the app users (Figure 5.1).

The people in rural and remote areas may receive poor or inadequate treatment due to the lack of effective medical diagnostic facilities and expertise. They may not even get appropriate consultation, precaution, awareness and education on food, nutrition and lifestyle that could assist them to prevent and manage health complications. To address this gap, Good Health app was developed by a private IT firm in the capital city of Bangladesh for providing general healthcare decision support and medical information dissemination. It took more than 15 months of users and intervention design study to start the pilot by engaging rural users before the large-scale lunching for everyone across the country. As a result, using design science research (DSR) guidelines [19] the IT team developed the solution artefact to address user demand for general practice services.

Primarily, Good Health app system provides a healthcare information dissemination platform where HPs can share health information and contribute to the

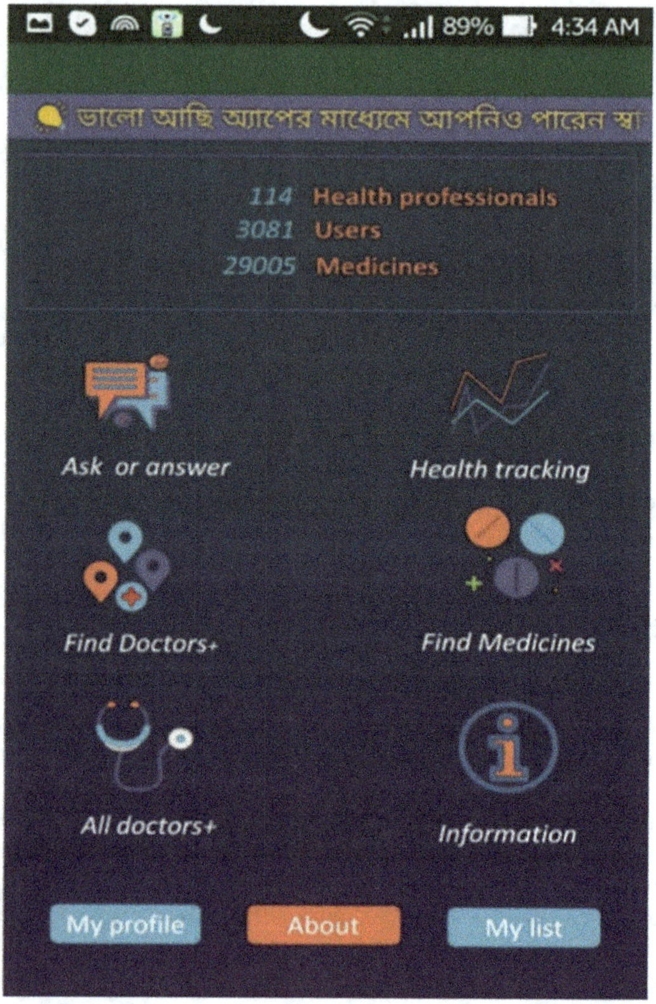

Figure 5.1 Main menu/theme of Good Health app mobile app (screenshot taken on 10th November 2018)

healthcare process. It connects the HPs socially and let them increase their social branding by contributing to the society (i.e. by sharing health information and answering to users' queries on the app that has all the social media functions). Using Good Health app, the HPs can provide free advice to the people, and get liked by the people. The likes inspire the HPs more to contribute voluntarily and eventually bring free health service to the people. By using the app, the available HPs can also evaluate a patient's condition and comment on regarding diagnosis or treatment. In the solution, a doctor-rating technique is used which 'incentivises' doctors and HPs to provide expert support and disseminate medical knowledge using the app.

The pilot test of this apps shows that the practical usefulness of the decision support: through the means of HPs health information sharing or answering and commenting against users' questions. Currently, there are 1.5 new MBBS doctors and 12 new users on average who are downloading this app weekly. Mostly, the young doctors and users are showing more keenness to use the app to seek information. Ultimately, using the app and the user-based rating system, the HPs become familiar to social media users which encourage them to asynchronously participate in providing free health information more. In this way, through the participation in health information sharing using the social media-based app, they can increase awareness about their profile.

5.3 Literature review

Social media platforms function as a two-way communication system that permits information sharing between multiple parties. From the point of scope of scholarly communication, these platforms provide convenient environments for health information sharing and exchange [20]. Everyday millions of social media users globally seek information for understanding disease aetiology, treatment options, second opinion, patient or doctor insights, and self-management knowledge [21]. Today, the HPs are increasingly using social media to support, promote and increase the spread of information in order to improve their both personal and community health practices [15]. By realising the power of sharing information, the HPs are more interested to join online physician communities [22].

Social media as a low-cost, powerful, and effective platforms have been proven to be effective in health information sharing [23]. The use of social media tools can be a way of more democratic and, in many cases, effective communication in healthcare [9]. According to Google, 5% of all searches are health related [24], while as per another report, more than 80% of individuals ages 18–24 would be likely to share health information through social media platforms [22]. In a study, more than 40% of respondents reported that information found via social media would affect the way they coped with a chronic condition or their approach to diet and exercise [22]. Therefore, understanding this scope, a survey shows that 81% of hospitals expressed an interest in participating in the hospital's social media strategy [25]. As it is reported by Google, the YouTube traffic to hospital sites has increased year-over-year which was 119% in 2012 [26]. On the other hand, majority of HPs are flexible for integrating social media platform for educating, however, their perceived barriers and potential benefits significantly influence their use of social media for educating [26].

In a study report, it is found that there are at least 967 hospitals on Twitter and around 3,000 hospitals have a company page on LinkedIn [27]. Another study shows that 53% of physician practices in the United States have a Facebook page, and users are 60% more likely to trust those HPs who have presence on social media platforms unlike who are not [28]. The social media platforms may include a wide range of PC and mobile applications, however the essential features of them are: (1) services are internet based, (2) contents are user-generated and (3) profiles are user-specific [29]. For example, social networking sites (Facebook), micro-blogging sites (Twitter), wikis, online forums, and online blogs and social media platform-based mobile applications. However, in social media platforms, when the concern is health information sharing, the most studied topic is the quality and reliability of information [12]. Therefore, it is important to validate accuracy of available information found through participation of HPs. Similarly, as the users are increasingly interested to acquire health knowledge from these platforms, understanding the motivational factors for health information sharing by HPs in the context of social media platforms is important.

5.4 Theoretical perspective

Motivation for the HPs in health-information sharing on social media can be influenced by the socio-psychological factors. The socio-psychological factors deal with how an individual and society are interlinked. The importance of socio-psychological factors in health has been increasingly recognised [30]. These factors are the combination of both the social and the psychological factors that influence the personality of an individual. Theories such as Social Penetration Theory and Social Exchange Theory consist of socio-psychological factors.

The perspective of Social Penetration Theory has been found to be important in the context of relationship building between HPs and patients [31]. For example, Social Penetration Theory can explain how interpersonal communication between family caregivers of elders with dementia moves from relatively non-intimate levels to more intimate ones. On the other hand, the perspective of Social Exchange Theory has been found to be important in the context of resources exchanged between HPs and patients [32]. For example, Social Exchange Theory can explain how the client-nurse interaction depends on the mutual exchange of resources. Therefore, it is important to find the scopes of Social Penetration Theory and Social Exchange Theory to understand what socio-psychological factors motivate HPs in health-information sharing on social media.

There is study from the users' perspective based on Social Exchange Theory which explains that socio-psychological factors such as 'sense of self-worth' and 'reputation enhancement' motivate the users to share health information on online health communities (OHC) [33]. Previous study on information sharing on social media has highlighted that socio-psychological factors such as 'perceived online relationship commitment' and 'altruism' factors have influence on knowledge-sharing behaviour and motivation [34]. Likewise, 'personal benefits' and 'community-related benefits' factors have influence on the motivation for information sharing on social media [35]. Currently, no theory-based study is found in the literature that helps us to conceptually understand what socio-psychological factors motivate the HPs to share health information on social media platforms [33].

For this reason, the Social Penetration Theory and Social Exchange Theory are conceptually discussed below to propose a theory-based conceptual framework that can explain which factors motivate the HPs in health-information sharing on the social media.

5.4.1 Social penetration theory

Social Penetration Theory was proposed by Altman and Taylor in 1987 [36]. Its proposition is that, individuals (in our case both HPs and general people) extend their relationship from comparatively shallow relationship to intimate relationship through the means of interpersonal communication and reciprocity [36]. According to Social Penetration Theory, as the relationship become deeper and more trustful, individuals dynamically self-disclose each other as if their layers of personality are revelled over time. For this reason, it is also called 'onion theory' of personality [37]. Moreover, this self-disclosure process makes stronger relationship if individuals feel positive.

Based on the perspectives Social Penetration Theory, the self-disclosure involves three factors: (1) personal characteristics, (2) reward and (3) context/situation [37]. While the personal characteristics factor is influenced by the specific aspects of socio-psychological factors (e.g. beliefs, such as political, religious, cultural), more intimacy and disclosure happen if the reward (e.g. recognition) is perceived greater than the cost. Finally, the moral consideration, satisfaction level, commitment and effort influence the context/situation and shape the responses in self-disclosure process [37].

5.4.2 Social exchange theory

Social Exchange Theory can explain the behavioural causes of exchanging knowledge, views, opinions in social media [38]. According to Social Exchange Theory, individual persons support and assist each other as a norm of reciprocity [39]. Improvement of knowledge management through exchanging knowledge in social media is important and as well as helpful and beneficial. In OHC knowledge sharing is a kind of exchange behaviour which can be explained well by Social Exchange Theory [33].

Based on the perspectives Social Exchange Theory, previous studies have developed three main factors related to the concept of knowledge sharing. These are: (1) reciprocity, (2) reputation and (3) altruism [40]. According to Social Exchange Theory, a series of interactions between two individuals leads to an obligation of reciprocity. It is standardly believed that in a bidirectional transaction, if something has given, something has to be returned as well as a part of mutual and complementary arrangement. Social Exchange Theory suggests that various types of resource can be exchanged in the process of reciprocity, such as exchanging love, information, money, goods, services, etc. Ultimately such exchange of resource in form of interdependent transactions develop the relationship between two individuals – the fundamental notion of Social Exchange Theory [41].

5.5 Proposing a theory-based conceptual framework

As health-information sharing on social media has two-way benefits [42], understanding the socio-psychological factors that motivate the HPs for health-information sharing on the social media would ultimately increase the following benefits: (1) dissemination of quality health information, (2) the reduction of misinformation on health issues, (3) widen the access to health information, (4) access to more tailored information, (5) more social and emotional supports from the HPs, (6) more public health surveillance, (7) meeting the socio-psychological needs of the HPs and (8) improved health outcomes using social media platforms [12]. Therefore, there is a need for developing a conceptual framework based on theories to understand how the socio-psychological factors motivate HPs for health-information sharing on the social media platforms.

Based on the discussion form the theoretical perspective above, the Social Penetration Theory explains the more specific reasons that why HPs are motivated for their online self-disclosure to build deeper relationship with users based on three factors: (1) Personal Characteristics, (2) Reward and (3) Context/Situation. On the other hand, the Social Exchange Theory explains why HPs are motivated to share health information based on the three knowledge-sharing factors: (1) Reciprocity, (2) Reputation and (3) Altruism. Therefore, a theory-based conceptual framework would bring the socio-psychological outlook to understand how these abovementioned factors motivate HPs for health-information sharing on the social media platforms. In addition, a conceptual framework would generate new interpretations of motivation for health-information sharing by HPs, particularly on social media platforms. Figure 5.2 shows the conceptual framework.

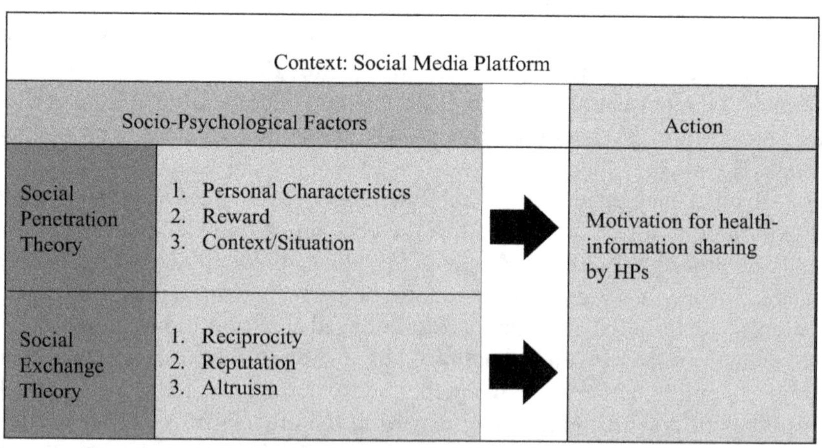

Figure 5.2 A conceptual framework to understand how socio-psychological factors motivate HPs for health-information sharing on the social media platforms

5.6 Conclusion

The main objective of this research was to understand which factors motivate the HPs in health-information sharing on the social media. In this process, a theory-based conceptual framework is proposed based on Social Penetration Theory and Social Exchange Theory after analysis a case study in Bangladesh. The framework can be useful to identify and understand the nature of influences that the socio-psychological factors have on the motivation for health-related information sharing by HPs on social media platforms. The understanding of socio-psychological factors that motivate the HPs for health-information sharing on the social media would ultimately increase the following benefits such as: (1) dissemination of quality health information, (2) the reduction of misinformation on health issues on social media, (3) widen the access to health information, (4) access to more tailored information, (5) more social and emotional supports from the HPs, (6) contribute in more public health surveillance, (7) meeting the socio-psychological needs of the HPs and (8) improved health outcomes using social media platforms.

5.7 Recommendations

The future research needs to test the proposed conceptual framework using a quantitative study, which will help the healthcare policy makers to engage HPs on social media for healthcare contribution. The authors suggest another empirical study in another context to test if the proposed six motivational factors (Figure 5.2) can motivate the HPs to disseminate authentic health information on mobile app. In that way, social media as a cheap but effective medium will contribute in healthcare better and can contribute to improve the mHealth intervention strategy and usefulness. For instance, social media-based Good Health app provides a platform to HPs to help its users in decision support and more reliable primary care advice. This social media-based mobile app is also a low-cost approach to reduce digital divide in Bangladesh beside delivering health information easily to a large population who are underserved.

5.8 Contribution

The beneficiaries of this study can be classified into three categories:

1. The HPs:

   The understanding what socio-psychological factors influence the HPs would benefit the HPs by meeting their socio-psychological needs (e.g. social recognition, social rewards satisfaction from useful feedback). This will ultimately help the HPs to gain more benefits resulted from knowledge sharing by them.
2. The users:

   They would learn about the ways they should follow for feedback and engaging with HPs to motivate them for more health information sharing. This will ultimately increase their access to quality and correct health information on social media platforms.

3. The social media platform researchers:

   They would learn about the new perspectives on how socio-psychological factors influence HPs for health information sharing on the social media platforms and help them to integrate important evidence-based functionalities (e.g. rating system, feedback system, recognition system, reward system) on social media platforms that would further motivate HPs for health information sharing.

References

[1] Bandura, A. Health promotion by social cognitive means. Heal. Educ. Behav. 31, 143–164 (2004).

[2] Antheunis, M. L., Tates, K., and Nieboer, T. E. Patients' and health professionals' use of social media in health care: motives, barriers and expectations. Patient Educ. Couns. 92, 426–431 (2013).

[3] Alsobayel, H. Use of social media for professional development by health care professionals: a cross-sectional web-based survey. JMIR Med. Educ. 2, 1–8 (2016).

[4] Chretien, K. C. and Kind, T. Social media and clinical care: ethical, professional, and social implications. Circulation 127, 1413–1421 (2013).

[5] Lambert, K. M., Barry, P. and Stokes, G. Risk management and legal issues with the use of social media in the healthcare setting. J. Healthc. Risk Manag. 31, 41–47 (2012).

[6] Brashers, D. E., Goldsmith, D. J. and Hsteh, E. Information seeking and avoiding in health contexts. Hum. Commun. Res. 28, 258–271 (2002).

[7] Dosemagen, S. and Aase, L. How Social Media Is Shaking Up Public Health and Healthcare. huffingtonpost (2016).

[8] Dutta-Bergman, M. J. Health communication on the web: the roles of web use motivation and information completeness. J. Commun. 54, 253–269 (2004).

[9] Hawn, C. Report from the field: take two aspirin and tweet me in the morning: how twitter, facebook, and other social media are reshaping health care. Health Aff. 28, 361–368 (2009).

[10] Sama, P. R., Eapen, Z. J., Weinfurt, K. P., Shah, B. R. and Schulman, K. A. An evaluation of mobile health application tools. JMIR mHealth uHealth 2, 6 (2014).

[11] Boulos, M. N. K. and Wheeler, S. The emerging Web 2.0 social software: an enabling suite of sociable technologies in health and health care education. Health Info. Libr. J. 24, 2–23 (2007).

[12] Moorhead, S. A., Hazlett, D. E., Harrison, L., Carroll, J. K., Irwin, A. and Hoving, C. A new dimension of health care: systematic review of the uses, benefits, and limitations of social media for health communication. J. Med. Internet Res. 15, (2013).

[13] McNab, C. What social media offers to health professionals and citizens. Bull. World Health Organ. 87, 566 (2009).
[14] Usher, W. T. Australian health professionals' social media (Web 2.0) adoption trends: early 21st century health care delivery and practice promotion. Aust. J. Prim. Health 18, 31–41 (2012).
[15] Ventola, C. L. Social media and health care professionals: benefits, risks, and best practices. P T 39, 491–520 (2014).
[16] Hurowitz, J. C. Toward a social policy for health. N. Engl. J. Med. 130 (1993).
[17] Bowes, J. and Grace, R. Review of early childhood parenting, education and health intervention programs for Indigenous children and families in Australia (2014).
[18] Fichman, R. G., Kohli, R. and Krishnan, R. The role of information systems in healthcare: current research and future trends. Inf. Syst. Res. 22, 419–428 (2011).
[19] Miah, S. J., Hasan, N., Hasan, R. and Gammack, J. Healthcare support for underserved communities using a mobile social media platform. Inf. Syst. 66, 1–12 (2017).
[20] Gu, F. and Widén-Wulff, G. Scholarly communication and possible changes in the context of social media. Electron. Libr. 29, 762–776 (2011).
[21] Susannah Fox. Health Topics. (2011).
[22] PWC. Social media "likes" healthcare From marketing to social business. (2012).
[23] Sharma, P. and Kaur, P. D. Effectiveness of web-based social sensing in health information dissemination – a review. Telemat. Informatics 34, 194–219 (2017).
[24] Google. A remedy for your health-related questions: health info in the Knowledge Graph (2015).
[25] Afiah. The Increasing Importance of Social Media in Healthcare (2014).
[26] Google. The Digital Journey to Wellness: Hospital Selection (2012).
[27] Dyrda, L. 10 things to know about social media in healthcare: Who's using it? Does it make a difference? (2016).
[28] CDW Healthcare. The Healthcare Social Media Shakeup (2013).
[29] Obar, J. A. and Wildman, S. S. Social media definition and the governance challenge: an introduction to the special issue. Telecomm. Policy 39, 745–750 (2015).
[30] Prentice-Dunn, S. and Rogers, R. W. Protection motivation theory and preventive health: beyond the health belief model. Health Educ. Res. 1, 163–161 (1986).
[31] Bylund, C. L., Peterson, E. B. and Cameron, K. A. A practitioner's guide to interpersonal communication theory: an overview and exploration of selected theories. Patient Educ. Couns. 87, 261–267 (2012).
[32] Byrd, M. E. Social exchange as a framework for ClientNurse interaction during public health nursing maternal-child home visits. Public Health Nurs. 23, 271–276 (2006).

[33] Yan, Z., Wang, T., Chen, Y. and Zhang, H. Knowledge sharing in online health communities: a social exchange theory perspective. Inf. Manag. 53, (2016).
[34] Ma, W. W. K. and Chan, A. Knowledge sharing and social media: altruism, perceived online attachment motivation, and perceived online relationship commitment. Comput. Human Behav. 39, 51–58 (2014).
[35] Munar, A. M. and Jacobsen, J. K. S. Motivations for sharing tourism experiences through social media. Tour. Manag. 43, 46–54 (2014).
[36] Carpenter, A. and Greene, K. Social Penetration Theory. Int. Encycl. Interpers. Commun. (2016).
[37] Baack, D., Fogliasso, C. and Harris, J. The personal impact of ethical decisions: a social penetration theory. J. Bus. Ethics 24, 39–49 (2000).
[38] Hamoud, M. W., Tarhini, A., Akour, M. A. and Al-Salti, Z. Developing the main knowledge management process via social media in the IT organisations: a conceptual perspective. Int. J. Bus. Adm. 7, 49 (2016).
[39] Gouldner, A. W. The norm of reciprocity: a preliminary statement. Am. Sociol. Rev. 25, 161–178 (1960).
[40] Shiau, W. L. and Luo, M. M. Factors affecting online group buying intention and satisfaction: a social exchange theory perspective. Comput. Human Behav. 28, 2431–2444 (2012).
[41] Cropanzano, R. and Mitchell, M. S. Social exchange theory: an interdisciplinary review social exchange theory: an interdisciplinary review. J. Manage. 31, 874–900 (2005).
[42] Torabi, S. Towards understanding users' motivation to share health information on Facebook (2016).

Section II

Portable health clinic

Chapter 6

Mapping the need for preventive healthcare services in remote South Asian communities

Faiz Shah[1], *Rowena Alcoba*[1], *Seema Medhe*[1] *and Sajid Omar Farook*[1]

6.1 Overview of healthcare access in the SAARC and ASEAN nations along the belt and road region

The most intrinsic factor of life is health. People free from disease, illness, and injury are more capable of enjoying life. Healthy populations also exhibit a greater capacity of work and thus productivity. Health therefore is a key determinant of the overall development of a country, and a significant factor in achieving all other development targets. In addition to its pragmatic implications for development and wellbeing, the importance of innovation in primary healthcare provision is underscored when understanding healthcare provision as a fundamental human right. The concept of the right to health is enshrined universally in various contemporary frameworks. Article 25 of the United Nations Universal Declaration of Human Rights (1948), for example, states that "everyone has the right to a standard of living adequate for the health and well-being of himself and of his family, including food, clothing, housing and medical care and necessary social service." The International Covenant on Economic, Social and Cultural Rights (1966), also recognizes the "right of everyone to the enjoyment of the highest attainable standard of physical and mental health." Specifically, the UN (2019) refers to the right to the provision of resources necessary to realize a minimum standard of healthcare to which all individuals are entitled. This can be outlined more clearly when examining four criteria adopted by the Committee on Economic, Social and Cultural Rights by which to evaluate the right to health. These include Availability – that healthcare services are available in a sufficient quantity, Accessibility – that they are physically accessible and affordable, Acceptability – that they are gender-sensitive and culturally acceptable), and Quality – that healthcare is of good quality, such as trained professionals, safe drugs, etc. Against these criteria, SARC and ASEAN countries along the Belt and Road Region demonstrate a general lack of healthcare. This serves not only as a major impediment to development, poverty

[1]Yunus Center, Asian Institute of Technology, Bangkok, Thailand

alleviation, and the wellbeing of people in these communities, it amounts to a violation of a basic human right. There are various reasons for the lack of healthcare provision in these regions, apart from gaps in state policy, service delivery systems.

Firstly, and perhaps most obviously, many individuals lack the financial means to pay for basic healthcare services. Impoverished people living in underdeveloped communities quite simply cannot afford treatment in clinics and hospitals. Even if they did, however, the lack of means to reach said services, such as transportation to hospitals, are also insufficient [1]. Hence, not only is healthcare inaccessible in rural regions along the Belt and Road axis, it is often unaffordable. When coupled with the relatively high prevalence of disease in rural regions, this spells a clear need to compensate for the significant unmet health-related needs in underdeveloped regions. Countries such as Bangladesh, Cambodia, India, Pakistan, and Sri Lanka, all represent this healthcare dilemma in various ways, and are examined in this chapter.

The documented lack of primary healthcare in unreached communities requires solutions that do not create further expectations from already stretched primary healthcare services. Achieving the goal of a healthy population requires well planned public health services and systems, backed up by effective community health education, and efficient public health professionals. More importantly, public health research confirms that improvement in general health indicators are more directly the outcome of innovative prevention strategies. In the digital age, this can be achieved by applications that boost primary healthcare coverage and affordability for those who otherwise lack access to it. The premise of implementing mobile healthcare technologies such as the Portable Health Clinic lies in doing precisely this.

A more compelling case for mobile technologies in the delivery of health care emerges from the Healthcare Access report (2019), which identifies a general shortage of numbers, typically in rural areas, for remote healthcare facilities, diagnostic and clinical technologies, or medical professionals, in proportion to the target populations. PHC aims to overcome this triple-impediment by redefining the role of the typical healthcare delivery professional, using ubiquitous and affordable technology to overcome a costly, time-consuming, and inefficient approaches [2]. This redefined role means professionals typically located in static units such as hospitals, clinics, laboratories, or other institutions, with no incentive to travel for serving in remote regions, do not have to move from their base.

Instead, PHC creates employment opportunities for local health workers already resident in unreached communities, equipping them with basic PHC operating skills to simply link the patient wherever they are, to a doctor or healthcare provider using video call technology. To improve access for home-based women and children in addition to creating female employment in underdeveloped regions, local women are given a priority as PHC health workers. They own and operate a portable kit comprising diagnostic equipment and sensors linked with a remote data server managed by Grameen Health. All PHC patient records are archived in a software system, “GramHealth,” which can be accessed in real time by doctors deployed at a static call-center, who can then provide e-prescriptions and referrals for diagnosis or expert consultation with the video conferencing tool included in the PHC briefcase [3]. The PHC re-imagines the traditional, static service unit model where patients see doctors, by having a local health worker become the bridge between patient and doctor, thus creating access without in any way compromising the integrity of healthcare quality.

This chapter will discuss the use of the Portable Health Clinic as a practical answer to the high burden of health in underdeveloped and developing member nations of the South Asian Association for Regional Cooperation (SAARC), comprising Afghanistan, Bangladesh, Bhutan, India, Maldives, Nepal, Pakistan, and Sri Lanka, and The Association of Southeast Asian Nations (ASEAN), formed by Brunei, Cambodia, Indonesia, Lao, Malaysia, Myanmar, the Philippines, Singapore, Thailand and Vietnam. The following section will examine data on the current state of health services availability for rural populations in the aforementioned nations.

6.2 State of health services availability for rural populations in the ASEAN and SAARC regions

6.2.1 *Baseline demographics of population distribution*

Information on sociodemographic factors of the SAARC and ASEAN countries are exhibited in Table 6.1. Singapore and Brunei fall under high-income group nations as per their GNI index. Few of the countries in this geographic region are upper-

Table 6.1 Socio-demographic factors of the SAARC and ASEAN nations

Country	% rural population	% urban population	GINI index	% Poverty
Afghanistan	75	25	NA	38.3
Bangladesh	64	36	32.4	31.5
Bhutan	60	40	37.4	12
Brunei	23	77	NA	NA
Cambodia	77	23	NA	17.7
India	66	34	35.7	21.9
Indonesia	23	77	38.1	11.2
Lao	66	34	36.4	23.4
Malaysia	25	75	41	0.4
Maldives	61	39	38.4	NA
Myanmar	70	30	38.1	32.1
Nepal	81	19	32.8	25.2
Pakistan	64	36	33.5	24.3
The Philippines	64	36	40.1	21.6
Singapore	0	100	NA	NA
Sri Lanka	82	18	39.8	6.7
Thailand	51	49	36.5	7.2
Vietnam	65	35	35.5	13.5

NA—not available

middle-income countries, such as Maldives, Thailand, and Malaysia. Excluding Nepal and Afghanistan, the rest of the countries comprise under the group, as Nepal and Afghanistan are lower-income countries. This categorization illustrates the level of development in this geographic area.

Sociodemographic factors are important in the regimentation of health status (Hutchison *et al.*, 2010). Afghanistan has the highest proportion of the population living in poverty, at 38.3%, followed by Myanmar at 32.1% and Bangladesh at 31.5%. This large group of people is, in the majority of cases, incapable of accessing healthcare, in spite of the fact that they are mostly dependent on the public healthcare services for any health issues. Malaysia has the lowest proportion of the population in poverty (0.4%), most of whom live in rural areas. Out of the total population residing these nations, 60.41% of the population live in rural areas, while only 39.51% live in urban areas. Sri Lanka has the highest rural population (82%), followed by Nepal (81%), and Cambodia (77%). Singapore is the only nation with a 100% urban population, followed by Brunei (77%), Indonesia (77%), and Malaysia (75%). The GINI index of all these nations is from 32.4 to 41, although no data for GINI index are available for Afghanistan, Cambodia, Singapore, and Brunei.

6.2.2 State of health

State of health for populations of each of these countries are stated according to six determinants recorded from World Bank data. They include maternal mortality rate (MMR), infant mortality rate (IMR), life expectancy, prevalence of diabetes (PVD), prevalence of HIV (PVHIV), and health access index. The highest rate of maternal mortality per 1,000 live births was found in Afghanistan (17.7%), followed by Pakistan (10.9%) and Lao (10.3%) (Figure 6.1). An upper-middle-income country, Thailand, was noted with the lowest rate of maternal mortality (0.6%), followed by Singapore (0.8%) and Sri Lanka (1.9%). Pregnancy intricacy and complications in offspring birth are could be the causes of death as well as infirmity to expectant women in developing countries (WHO). This determinant is vital to

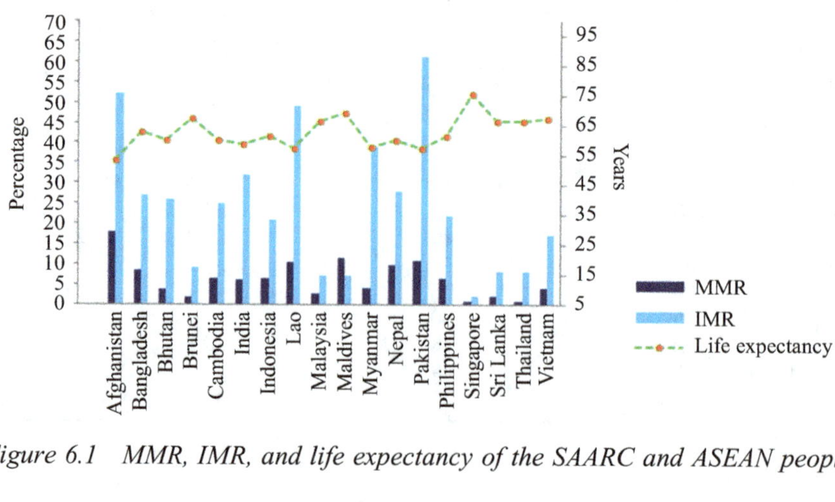

Figure 6.1 MMR, IMR, and life expectancy of the SAARC and ASEAN people

depict pregnancy-related risks. The reasons for the highest rate of maternal mortality in Pakistan could be post-partum hemorrhage, sepsis, eclampsia, and anemia. Postpartum hemorrhage could lead to the death of the mother if blood transfusion facility is not available on time. Sepsis and eclampsia, on the other hand, are complications associated with childbirth and due to improper pre and postnatal treatments. The causative factors for the highest MMR in Afghanistan are different than Pakistan. The remote rural and mountainous areas in which most of the population resides lack transport facilities delays the access to required healthcare services. Unmet need of transits to healthcare units causes the obstructive childbirth which was reported as the most prominent cause for increased MMR in Afghanistan (Lee and Eckhardt, 2017). Lack of midwives and skilled birth attendance could also be the causative factors for high MMR.

IMR was found to be the highest in Pakistan (61%) followed by Afghanistan (52%) and Lao (49%) (Figure 6.2). Obstructed childbirth, lack of skilled healthcare workers (SAB), infections, pneumonia, and diarrhea are some causes for higher IMR according to WHO. Singapore (2%) has the lowest IMR, followed by Malaysia, Maldives (7% each) and Sri Lanka and Thailand (8% each).

Life expectancy was recorded highest in Singapore (75.9 years), followed by Maldives (69.4 years) and Brunei (67.7 years), while the lowest life expectancy was recorded in Afghanistan (53.2 years). This data is an indication of the availability and quality of healthcare services in each respective country. Health access quality index data was obtained from a report presented by GBD Healthcare Access and Quality Collaborators, 2016. High-income countries like Singapore (91) and Brunei (76) was recorded to have the highest healthcare access and quality index (HAQ), followed by Sri Lanka (71). The economic sufficiency of the country enables them to not only provide advanced healthcare services but to allow access to such healthcare services to a larger number of people. This is likely the primary reason for which Singapore, as the most economically developed and urbanized country,

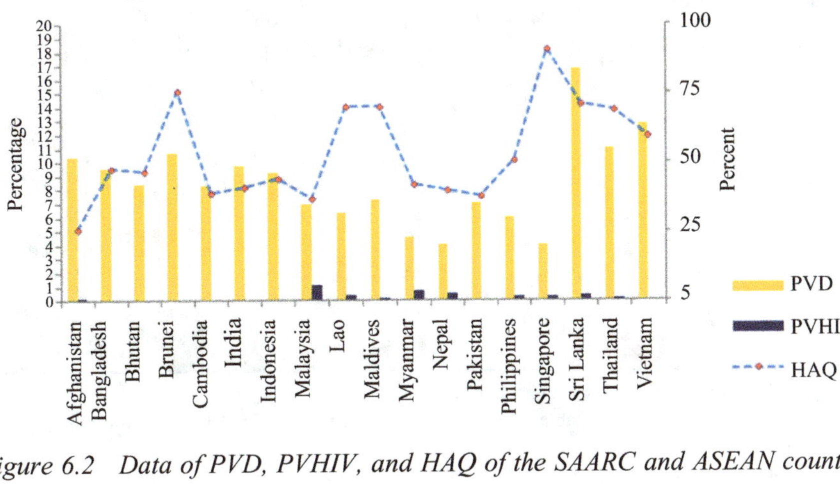

Figure 6.2 Data of PVD, PVHIV, and HAQ of the SAARC and ASEAN countries

has the highest HAQ index. Brunei was recorded to have the second-lowest rural population (23%). Because of this urbanization, healthcare services can easily reach people in need.

6.2.3 Burden of health

Noncommunicable diseases (NCDs) caused 71% of deaths globally (WHO, 2016). Table 6.2 demonstrates that the preeminent originator for death in high-income nations was NCDs, with Brunei at 85%, followed by upper-middle-income country Maldives (84%) and Sri Lanka (83%). NCDs include ischemic heart disease, stroke, coronary obstructive pulmonary disease, trachea, bronchus and lung cancer, liver cirrhosis, and diabetes mellitus. Afghanistan was reported to have highest death records, with 36%, mostly due to communicable diseases, maternal prenatal, and nutrition conditions, followed by Pakistan (35%) and Lao (31%). From this table, it can be determined that the lower-income and lower-middle-income countries are recorded to have the most deaths due to CD, MP, NC. Communicable diseases include lower respiratory tract infections, diarrheal diseases, tuberculosis, HIV/AIDS, preterm birth complications, and malaria. Death by communicable diseases was reported highest in Afghanistan (20%), followed by India (11%),

Table 6.2 Estimates of death by different causes in the SAARC and ASEAN countries

Country	**Death by NCD (% of total)**	**Death by injury (% of total)**	**CD,MP,NC (% of total)**	**PU %**	**CDR %**	**UNC (% of women age 15–49)**
India	63	11	26	15	11	13
Afghanistan	44	20	36	30	20	25
Bangladesh	67	8	26	15	8	12
Sri Lanka	83	10	8	11	10	8
Pakistan	58	7	35	21	7	20
Bhutan	69	11	21	NA	11	12
Maldives	84	8	8	11	8	29
Thailand	74	11	16	9	10	6
Indonesia	73	6	21	8	6	15
Nepal	66	9	25	10	9	24
Myanmar	68	9	24	11	9	16
Cambodia	64	10	26	19	10	13
The Philippines	67	8	25	14	8	18
Vietnam	77	10	12	11	11	6
Lao	60	9	31	17	9	20
Malaysia	74	9	18	3	9	NA
Singapore	74	10	23	NA	4	NA
Brunei	85	7	8	3	7	NA

Death by NCD—Death by noncommunicable diseases

CD, MP, NC—Death by communicable diseases, maternal prenatal, and nutritional condition

PU—Prevalence of malnourishment % of population

UNC—Un-mate need of contraception (% of married women ages 15–49)

Bhutan (11%) and Thailand (11%). Assessing the number of people dying and understanding the reason for their deaths could be a vital aid to study the efficiency of nationals health systems and consequently implement more efficient healthcare strategies. High-income countries were observed to have a paramount number of deaths due to degenerative diseases like diabetes, cardiovascular diseases. This could be due to the modest lifestyle and lack of preventive care plans. Malnutrition is one of the most important issues in regards to health and should not be neglected, particularly because the nutritional health of children will contribute to the socio-economic development of that country in the long term. The data obtained by WHO reveals that Afghanistan is counting a 30% undernourishment prevalence, which may be due to causes such as the rural and remote residence of the bulk of the population, poverty, unavailability of primary healthcare facilities, a limited health workforce, and poor quality of healthcare services. Lower-middle-income countries like Pakistan (21%) and Cambodia (10%) was noted to have the second most undernourished prevalence.

The unmet need for contraceptives prevents women from avoiding pregnancy. Planned pregnancy can also slow the rapid population growth in lower-income countries by limiting child births, which could be a contributor to the development of the country. Furthermore, a lack of knowledge about contraceptive methods, misconceptions about use, fear, rituals and cultural barriers, and gender inequality further diminish access to contraceptive aids. The Maldives was reported to have the highest percentage (29%) of unmet need for contraception, followed by Afghanistan (25%) and Nepal (24%).

6.2.4 Availability of healthcare workforce

Health workforce denotes the personnel employed to facilitate healthcare. Trained healthcare professionals are imperative assets in the healthcare structure. A better health workforce would contribute to raising the standard and accessibility of healthcare programs. Healthcare workers are comprised of nurses, midwives, community health workers, pharmacists, dentists, physiotherapists, laboratory experts, and doctors, along with other experts who serve the health sector, such as economists, administration staff, auditors, and information technologists. Many of the SAARC and ASEAN countries do not have data on the availability of health worker professionals. Data presented in Table 6.3 gives an idea about the availability of skilled health workers per 100,000 people in each country in the study. Specifically, the availability of physicians, nurses, midwives, surgical specialty workforce, and community health workers were observed. The number of physicians per 100,000 people ranged from 0.2 to 3.6 only. The number of nurses and midwives ranged from 0.3 to 7.1. Community health workers ranged from 0.1 to 1.4. Data on surgical specialty workers are not available for the majority of the countries; Singapore was reported to have 31 specialty surgical workers followed by Thailand (13) and Malaysia (11). High-income countries like Singapore, Brunei and the upper country Thailand were reported to have a skilled attendant present at birth for 100% of births, followed by Malaysia and Sri Lanka (99).

Table 6.3 Availability of healthcare professionals per 100,000 people in the SAARC and ASEAN countries

Country	Physicians	Nurses and midwives	Community health workers	Surgical specialty work force	SAB (% births)
Afghanistan	0.3	0.4	NA	0	55
Bangladesh	0.5	0.3	0.5	3	44
Bhutan	0.4	1.5	0.1	3	90
Brunei	1.7	NA	NA	NA	100
Cambodia	0.1	1	0.1	NA	86
India	0.8	NA	0.6	NA	60
Indonesia	0.2	1.3	0	NA	91
Lao	0.5	NA	NA	NA	48
Malaysia	1.5	NA	1.4	11	99
Maldives	3.6	4.1	1.4	NA	89
Myanmar	0.6	0.9	0.2	2	77
Nepal	0.6	NA	0.7	NA	53
Pakistan	1	0.5	0.1	6	55
The Philippines	1.1	NA	NA	NA	72
Singapore	2.3	7.1	0.5	31	100
Sri Lanka	0.9	NA	NA	NA	99
Thailand	0.5	2.3	0.1	13	100
Vietnam	0.8	NA	NA	NA	95

NA—not available
SAB—skilled attendant at birth

Lower-middle-income nations like Bangladesh and Lao, on the other hand, were noted to have SAB for less than 50% of births.

Lack of trained healthcare professionals is thus a large threat for developed as well as developing countries in the SAARC and ASEAN countries. The availability of specialists and trained healthcare workers should be increased to achieve the healthy population goals and consequently, overall development.

6.3 Effectiveness of PHC to rectify the high burden of health in the underdeveloped and developing countries

The above narratives outlined the clear lack of primary healthcare provision in underdeveloped regions of the SAARC and ASEAN countries along the Belt and Road Initiative to illustrate the evident need for innovation in the field of healthcare provision. The remainder of this chapter examines the effectiveness of the Portable Health Clinic as a means of rectifying this disparity and providing much-needed healthcare to needy populations who are unreached by traditional healthcare facilities that are already in place.

The main reason for which people lack access to primary healthcare is not only financial but also due to the inaccessibility and unreached nature of the rural regions in which they live. As an effort to innovate and patch the deficiencies of traditional healthcare systems, the PHC aims to eliminate the challenges posed by the latter. The fundamental premise of PHC thus lies in bringing healthcare services to the poor to improve upon its accessibility through mobilizing healthcare facilities [3].

To understand how this is done, it is important to first examine the challenges in a traditional healthcare system. Brick and mortar healthcare involve doctors operating out of hospitals and clinics. This is typically effective for a demographic capable of both affording and frequently traveling to medical institutions to carry out primary preventative healthcare. The limitations of this model begin to show, however, when examining rural, poor communities as a stakeholder, to whom these healthcare facilities are quite inaccessible. This dilemma of inaccessibility associated with brick and mortar systems, however, is not necessarily new, and neither is the concept of mobilizing facilities to improve accessibility. The move of branchless banking, for example, is a prime example of a situation in which being restricted to conventional banking branches is a limitation on the ease of access to financial services. This necessitated technology and third party retail agents to bring these services to those who are otherwise unreached [4]. The same concept is retained with the PHC. Rather than the poor needing to commute to expensive medical facilities, essential diagnostic equipment are instead brought to these communities and are operated by local health workers to provide cheap preventative healthcare at their own doorsteps.

PHC addresses not only the problem of accessibility associated with conventional healthcare provision systems but also that of affordability. While the operation of hospitals and clinics remain costly, to operate the PHC is relatively very cheap. The data below illustrate the government spending and third-party funding availability in developing countries as percentage of GDP and fiscal outlay to demonstrate the financial efficiency of PHC.

Although values for domestic general government health expenditure range vastly from 5% in Afghanistan to 95% in Brunei, the general trend clearly suggests that countries spend a sizable percentage of GDP and CHE on public health services (Table 6.4). One PHC briefcase, enough to cover checkups for an entire village or community, on the contrary, approximately costs less than $300, which is an amount an entrepreneur can borrow from micro-finance institutions such as Grameen Bank in Bangladesh [5]. Numbers are similarly relatively high for out-of-pocket healthcare expenditure and external healthcare expenditure. Compare this to the PHC, which, per service, costs patients the equivalent of about $2–5 [2]. It is evident from comparing data from the status quo to that from tested examples of the implementation of PHC that the financial problem associated with attempting to provide healthcare to underdeveloped and unreached communities is rectified by the relatively cheap portable health clinic.

A third advantage of PHC is its focus on preventative care [6]. The premise of preventative care lies in identifying health problems before they become critical

Table 6.4 Health service expenditure % of GDP and CHE

Countries	(GGHE-D) as % (GDP)	(GGHE-D) as % (CHE)	(PVT-D) as % (CHE)	(OOPS) as % (CHE)	(EXT) as % of (CHE)	(CHE) as % of (GDP)	GDP (USD)	Current Health Expenditure per capita (USD)
Afghanistan	1	5	77	77	17	10	19,543.98	57.25
Pakistan	1	68	28	65	4	3	304,951.82	39.58
Bangladesh	0	18	74	72	8	2	249,723.86	34.22
Bhutan	3	74	21	20	5	3	2,528.01	91.34
India	1	25	74	65	1	4	2,650,725.34	62.77
Indonesia	1	45	55	37	0	3	1,015,420.59	111.55
Maldives	8	73	27	19	0	11	314,710.26	1,047.84
Myanmar	1	20	74	74	6	5	67,068.75	62.11
Nepal	1	19	70	55	12	6	24,880.27	45.45
Sri Lanka	2	43	56	50	1	4	87,357.21	153.10
Thailand	3	78	22	12	0	4	455,302.68	221.92
Brunei Darussalam	2	95	5	5	0	2	12,128.09	630.63
Cambodia	1	22	59	59	19	6	22,158.21	77.67
Lao People's Democratic Republic	1	32	49	46	18	2	16,853.09	55.21
Malaysia	2	50	50	38	0	4	4,865.55	361.52
The Philippines	1	32	66	54	2	4	313,595.21	129.43
Singapore	2	55	45	31	0	4	323,907.23	2,462.39
Vietnam	3	47	50	45	2	6	223,779.87	122.84

GDP—Gross domestic product,
GGHE-D—Domestic general government health expenditure
CHE—Current health expenditure
PVT-D—Domestic private health expenditure
OOPS—Out-of-pocket health expenditure
EXT—External health expenditure
Current health expenditure per capita
Reference: World Bank national accounts data, and OECD National Accounts data files. World Health Organization Global Health Expenditure database

morbidities that necessitate expensive treatment. People are healthiest when measures are taken to avoid severe health problems to begin with. Of course, the primary and most obvious advantage of this is that people are healthier without NCDs compared to if they had minor conditions that were stopped before developing into serious ones. Not only does preventative care keep people generally more healthy, but in the context of providing healthcare to the poor, it also achieves the essential goal of ensuring that healthcare costs remain affordable. Hospital care costs necessary to treat diseases are extremely costly; once symptoms are discovered, and treatment is particularly difficult for the poor [7]. Compare this to preventative checkups with a primary care physician made possible by the video call module through PHC. Preventative care ensures not only healthier patients but is particularly important in making healthcare even more affordable for the poor.

Because PHC is designed as a healthcare strategy for the poor, its customizability can emerge as another major advantage [8]. Because of its modular design, PHC can be adapted to respond to common health-related problems in a given area. Diseases and illnesses that exist more prominently due to the prevalence of certain industries, for example, can be targeted more closely in a particular iteration of the PHC [9]. PHC treating unreached communities occupied in labor in coal mining, as an example, may focus on preventing the most common health hazards involved in the job, such as silicosis or other respiratory illnesses [10]. Not only can PHC be customized to aid populations suffering from diseases caused by a particular industry, but also those related to population trends within the demographic it attempts to treat. The study, "Applicability of Portable Health Clinic to Ageing Society" examines the effectiveness of PHC as a solution to the increasing pressure placed on public health system in a "super-aged society" [11].

References

[1] Office of Disease Prevention and Health Promotion. (2019, July 3). Access to Primary Care. Retrieved from https://healthypeople.gov/2020/topics-objectives/topic/social-determinants-health/interventions-resources/access-to-primar

[2] van Weel, C., Kassai, R., Qidwai, W. *et al.* (2016). Primary healthcare policy implementation in South Asia. BMJ Global Health, 1(2), e000057.

[3] Ahmed, A., Rebeiro-Hargrave, A., Nohara, Y. *et al.* (2015). Portable Health Clinic: A Telehealthcare System for UnReached Communities. Smart Sensors and Systems, 447–467.

[4] Weisgrau, S. (1995). Issues in rural health: access, hospitals, and reform. Health Care Financing Review, 17(1), 1–14.

[5] Dermish, A., Kneiding, C., Leishman, P., and Mas, I. (2011). Branchless and Mobile Banking

[6] Preventive Health Care Helps Everyone. (n.d.). Retrieved from http://wrf.org/preventive-healthcare/preventive-healthcare.php

[7] Amadeo, K. (2019, May 28). Preventive Care: How It Lowers Healthcare Costs in America. Retrieved from https://thebalance.com/preventive-care-how-it-lowers-aca-costs-3306074

[8] Solutions for the Poor: A Survey of the Literature. Innovations: Technology, Governance, Globalization, 6(4), 81–98.

[9] Shah, F.H., SehatMobile Primary Care Wellbeing Program: SE-BSP "Living Responsibility" by Reaching Out to Vulnerable Communities along Supply Chains, Concept Outline, Yunus Center AIT, 2 Apr 2014/v1-reviewed 1 Sep 2016.

[10] Donoghue, A. M. (2004). Occupational health hazards in mining: an overview. Occupational Medicine, 54(5), 283–289.

[11] Ahmed, A., Rebeiro-Hargrave, A., Maruf, R. I., Inoue, S., and Nakashima, N. (2014). Applicability of portable health clinic to ageing society. doi: 10.1007/978-3-319-07788-8_49

Chapter 7

Portable health clinic: concept, design, implementation and challenges

Ashir Ahmed[1], *Mehdi Hasan*[1], *Masuda Begum Sampa*[1], *Kazi Mozaher Hossein*[1], *Yasunobu Nohara*[2] *and Naoki Nakashima*[2]

Portable health clinic (PHC) is a remote healthcare system, jointly developed by Grameen Communications in Bangladesh and Kyushu University in Japan with the aim to providing affordable primary healthcare services to people who do not have regular access to healthcare facilities including the low-income population living in rural unreached communities.

This chapter introduces the basic concept and architecture of PHC; status of different pilot projects, findings, and observations; the technical and social challenges the projects faced during the implementation.

7.1 Basic concept and system architecture of PHC system

More than half of the world's population do not receive all the essential services they need. 100 million people are pushed into extreme poverty due to their health expenditures, forcing them to survive on just $1.90 or less a day [1]. Many of them live in areas where healthcare infrastructure (clinic, doctors, etc.) is not available. They are deprived of healthcare facilities for several reasons: (a) Poor healthcare facilities exist in rural areas—due to the scarcity of hospitals and clinics and absence qualified doctors, (b) Urban healthcare facilities are out of reach—because, of long distance takes long time and effort to go—need extra money to travel rather than treatment and female denies to show male doctors in person, and (c) Difficulties to access eHealth services—because village peoples' inability to measure basic health problems and do not have the measurement tools (Figure 7.1).

[1]Faculty of Information Science and Electrical Engineering, Kyushu University, Fukuoka, Japan
[2]Medical Information Center, Kyushu University Hospital, Fukuoka, Japan

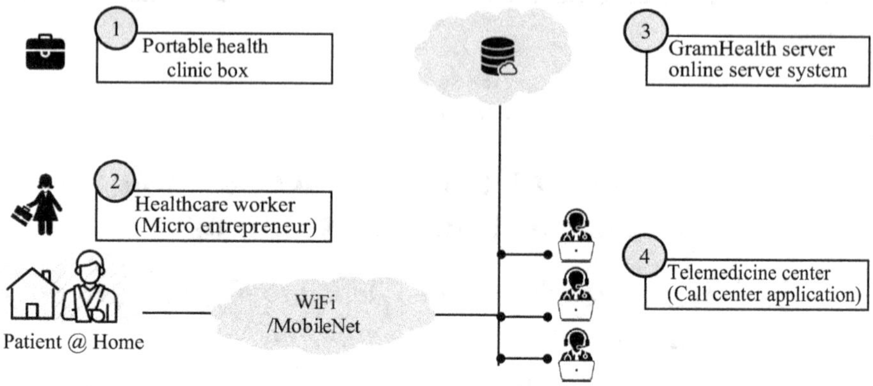

Figure 7.1 PHC service delivery model

We have prototyped "portable health clinic (PHC)", a compact telehealth system with diagnostic equipment and GramHealth software for archiving and searching patients' past health records. The back-end of the system consists of data servers and a medical call center. The front-end has the instances of portable briefcase consisting of medical sensors and measuring equipment operated by healthcare workers living in unreached communities. The front-end data transmission system and Skype telemedicine calls connect with the back-end using mobile network coverage and Internet. Doctors at the medical call center access GramHealth data cloud through the Internet or have a copy of the database in the call center server. Upon receiving a multimedia call from a patient, the doctor can find that patient's previous EHR record and then create and send an e-Prescription. The healthcare worker's PHC briefcase is designed to be low cost and portable. It is envisioned as costing less than US$300 (an amount an entrepreneur can borrow from micro-finance institutions such as Grameen Bank in Bangladesh) and light enough to be carried by a female health assistant. The PHC briefcase will be owned and operated by a village health assistant [2]. This will be a sustainable business model as the health assistant can build a professional relationship with her local clientele. We carried out experiments in different countries in different geographical and cultural settings.

PHC system comprising four modules: (a) a set of medical devices at the patient end, (b) a software system to collect and archive the medical records, (c) healthcare workers at the patient end to make the clinical measurements and explain the ePrescription, and (d) ICT-trained call center doctors (Table 7.1).

Services include basic health checkup and regular monitoring. Basic health checkup includes (a) a set of demographic questions, (b) fourteen clinical measurements, and (c) doctor consultancy with a prescription. The clinical measurements are: (1) blood pressure, (2) pulse rate, (3) body temperature, (4) oxygenation of blood (SpO_2), (5) arrhythmia, (6) BMI, (7) waist, hip, and W/H ratio, (8) blood

Table 7.1 Four major components for PHC system

Symbol	Name	Description
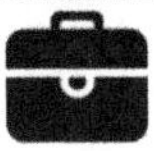	PHC Box	A set of sensors (thermometer, blood tester, urine tester, etc.) to measure health status and GramHealth Client software tool to collect health data and transmit to the server.
	Healthcare Worker	A licensed healthcare worker to operate the portable health clinic box, take health data, and explain the results and prescriptions from the doctor.
	GramHealth Server	A cloud-based software system to archive personal health records, produce statistics and provide healthcare tips to individuals.
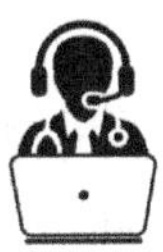	Telemedicine Center	A physical or virtual call center with connected licensed doctors.

glucose, (9) blood cholesterol, (10) blood hemoglobin, (11) blood uric acid, (12) blood grouping, (13) urinary sugar, and (14) urinary protein.

Every patient has a health account to access their past health history and health trends. The patients, as well as their authorized family members, can access the health account.

7.2 Evolution of technologies to adapt community needs

7.2.1 PHC for low-resource setting

PHC is designed to operate in rural areas [3]. The communication module of PHC can use mobile phone networks too. Fortunately, 98% of the geographical area has mobile phone network coverage in Bangladesh. However, the speed is not enough for smooth video conference. Power outage is a common phenomenon in rural areas. PHC added an offline mode so that it can operate when the network is poor. PHC also has a backup battery module so that it can run when there is no electricity.

PHC trains and employs local healthcare workers. There are pharmacies almost everywhere in the country. After receiving an ePrescription, a patient can purchase medicine if requires.

7.2.2 Toward improving the system efficiency

Remote healthcare systems, in general, carry medical errors. Most of them occur when a healthcare worker inserts healthcare data inside the system. In our PHC, we archived more than 45,000 records. We found 18% unusual data in five anthropometric items. All unusual data are not errors. It is a hard job to recheck, remeasure the data after we collect the data. We came up with a software-based approach to alert for unusual data during the measurement. An earlier detection saves time, cost, and assists for a better clinical decision. We analyze the past records to predict an acceptable value for each measurement for each individual patient. Unusual data are classified into impossible, suspicious and usual data based on age, gender, and personal health data profile. Impossible data are errors. Only suspicious data should be rechecked. This way, we can reduce errors, save recheck time and remote healthcare medical cost. The details are discussed in Section 7.4. The project has been partially funded by JSPS KAKENHI and the Future Earth Research Fund.

7.2.3 Trust of the consumers toward the PHC system

Traditionally a patient receives a face-to-face doctor consultancy. However, in remote healthcare systems, doctors appear on the screen. In this case, what would be the reaction of the patients? How can a patient trust whether the person on the screen is a real doctor? Can they trust the prescription that coming out from the cloud?

We carried out proactive monitoring of the patients to measure their trust. The idea was to check what do they do with the prescription provided by the PHC system. Six hundred patients were asked whether they are using PHC. 192 of them were PHC users. Ninety-five of them received a prescription. Seventy-one of them (75% of the prescribed patients) bought full medicine, 23% of them bought partially, and 2% did not buy medicine. It proves that people have trust in PHC prescription. However, this study has some limitations—it was carried out only in one location and only for one time. In order to draw an effective conclusion, we need to test the concept in different location and needs to be longitudinal to check whether the influential factors change over time. The details are described in Section 7.6. The project has been funded by Toyota Motor Corporation.

7.2.4 Geographical expansion of PHC concept

PHC concept has been introduced in several other countries including India, China, Pakistan, Cambodia, Liberia, and Thailand. PHC operation team has trained staffs in India, Pakistan, and Thailand. PHC has been piloting in India, Pakistan, and Cambodia. It is time we compared the results.

7.2.5 Modular expansion

Except for NCDs, PHC has been used in Bangladesh for other purposes, e.g., providing eyecare services, producing pathological reports, and taking care of maternal and child healthcare.

(i) Tele-Eyecare: This is a service for the patients of any age. We target rural areas where ophthalmologists are not available. A healthcare worker takes retinal images of the critical patients using a digital camera in a prescribed format and uploads the images to the PHC server together with physical observation report. A registered ophthalmologist from distance accesses the server to check the images, talks to the patient over a video call and finally writes a prescription for the patient. The report is also sent back to the patient for further consultancy with other doctors if needed in the future. We have served about 3,623 services for 2,997 patients in one vision center in Bogra district since 2017. The project has been funded by Grameen Healthcare Services Ltd.

(ii) Tele-Pathology: We have a crisis of pathologists in rural areas. PHC became a popular tool for pathological report generation. A trained PHC healthcare worker (Diploma in Laboratory Technologist) collects samples of blood, urine, stool, cough and/or skin, and prepares glass slides for microscopic analysis. Then he/she produces 6–10 difference microscopic images from different viewpoints and uploads to the PHC server. A PHC Pathologist in the urban area access to the images and produces a report. The report is preserved in the system and shared with the patients. So far, this system has produced 4,294 reports of 1,856 patients in four different healthcare centers in Barisal, Bogra, Manikgonj, and Thakurgaon district since 2016. Majority of the tests are of blood and urine. This project was jointly funded by Grameen Kalyan and Grameen Healthcare Services Ltd.

(iii) Maternal and child healthcare: The aim of this project is to help the rural pregnant women and newborn babies where access to a Obs and Gynae doctor is difficult. We are following the WHO guidelines to monitor a pregnant woman from the beginning of her pregnancy up to 6 weeks of the child age. A total of eight checkups are provided during this period with the help of PHC rural health workers followed by tele-consultancy by a gynecologist in the city. Besides, we are also monitoring all productive aged women between 15 and 49 years and provide basic health checkup by using PHC as preventive healthcare in the service area. The experiment started with a baseline survey in August 2018. We have started a pilot study from June 2019 for 439 subjects in one union of Shariatpur district. It will continue up to May 2020 at this phase. The project is funded by JSPS Bilateral Collaborations (Open Partnership) and Pfizer Health Research Foundation.

7.3 Target community for business: lessons learned

We have tried our PHC in different communities with different characteristics. The results are yet to be published.

7.3.1 Rural unreached community

People with low income. Access to hospitals is not easy. Almost 80% of them do not have a health checkup in their lifetime. NCDs are becoming common. Recently people became aware of diabetes. It is expensive for them to control diabetes. PHC is providing diabetes monitoring at one-third of the cost of other service providers. PHC is trying to provide a basic health checkup service to give them an early wakeup as a preventive measure. From our experience, we assume that a healthcare worker can serve 200 patients per month as a home delivery service. In the best setup, she can save 150 USD per month after the cost what is equivalent to a standard salary in rural Bangladesh. However, promotional activity is required before she starts a business. She needs about 2,000 USD to start a PHC community business which can be ideally funded by Grameen Nobin Uddyokta (new entre-preneurship development) program.

7.3.2 Urban aging community

Although the primary target of PHC was the low-income rural communities, we have found a good client segment in the urban aging community as well. The urban aging community has the same characteristics as developed countries. The rich urban patients are knowledgeable and most of them have their own blood pressure, diabetes test equipment, etc. However, sometimes it is not easy for them to take the checkup by themselves accurately and regularly as required for NCD patients. Besides, when they need to consult with a doctor, they need to visit a hospital through traffic-congested areas and stay in a long queue what is very laborious for an aged person. Now a PHC urban health worker visits registered patients at home at per preset schedule, conduct checkup professionally and if needed, connect to our call center doctor for a consultancy from patient's home. This low-cost service saves time, labor, and money of the aging clients. So far, we have approached to 34 urban apartments with 1,639 patients. We provide free health checkup first and then register to make them regular customers. The project was funded by Toyota Motor Corporation.

7.3.3 Urban corporate community

This community includes female employees mostly working at garments industries, and male workers working in the construction industries. Occupational health is rare at small medium enterprise. We carried out health checkup. Developing a business model for this sector has not been easy (Figure 7.2). The employers can understand the necessity of such service to enhance the productivity of their employees but are not interested in spending money for the preventive healthcare services. There is no health insurance for the employees. A third party agreed to pay from the buyer community for maintaining compliance as a requirement in the factories. This is not the case for all other industries.

7.3.4 Urban morning walkers community

Urban rich people gather and walk in parks in the morning hours. There were street small businesses to measure weight for few cents. However, looking at the demand of these morning workers, a different type of business has naturally grown in the park. They provide on-the-spot weight and diabetes measurements. They keep the

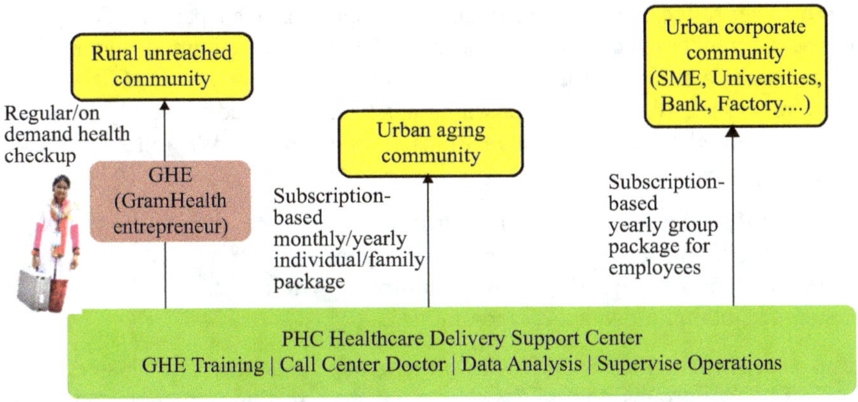

Figure 7.2 Business model to reach the target communities

records manually and are smart enough to remember everyone's history. PHC carried out a survey by providing healthcare services by collaborating with the existing business people. Morning walkers do not need doctors' services as they already have their own doctors at home. PHC needs to be customized to meet their demand.

7.4 Technical challenge: healthcare data errors

Remote healthcare systems carry errors. A wrong data leads to wrong clinical decision to be made by the remote doctor. It is also very complicated and expensive process to re-examine the error data for remote healthcare systems where the doctor checks the data after all the clinical measurements are measured and digitized [4]. Most of the errors occurred when a healthcare worker manually inputs the data in the system [5]. One way to reduce the error is to provide quality training to the healthcare workers or replace the manual data input mechanism to an automatic wireless data transmission mechanism. RFID-based wireless system can directly insert the measured data to the system. However, all the medical devices are not RFID-enabled and are not affordable at this point. Therefore, manual input mechanism will continue until the technology is ready and is affordable.

We propose a software solution to predict an acceptance range by analyzing the past records. It is relatively easy to predict a range for the patients who have plenty of past records. We call this range, personal acceptance range (PAR). If the patient does not have enough past record, we make a prediction for similar age and gender group. We call it group acceptance range (GAR). A hypothetical range is preset for all ages and gender. We call it a human acceptance range (HAR). All these acceptance range can be continuously updated based on experience.

In order to test our concept, we analyzed 40,391 health records, collected from different locations throughout Bangladesh. We identified the types of unusual/error data, the sources of the errors.

Human acceptance range: Human have biological growth pattern. The patterns would be different based on age and gender. HAR defines the minimum and maximum value of human anthropometric data (for example, *Height, Weight, BMI, Waist*, etc.).

We processed 40,391 raw data which has been collected randomly from 2010 to 2018, obtained from different locations in Bangladesh. We followed the following four steps:

- Step-1: Remove the records with partial data.
- Step-2: Classify the data according to the gender.
- Step-3: Remove unusual data from anthropometric items.
- Step-4: Obtain human acceptance range.

Group acceptance range: GAR shows the group tendency. The clusters can be identified by age groups. Figure 7.3 shows the steps to find out age-based GAR.

Our aim is to identify the cut-off points for different anthropometric items based on age. At first, we calculate the average of specific anthropometric items and analyze the growth pattern. And finally, we obtain the clear indication to identify the age groups by applying k-means cluster algorithm and Pearson correlation coefficient to formulate the GAR (Figure 7.4).

- Age level 20–49: An incremental pattern is observed at this age zone. Males gradually gain weight until the age of 50. This pattern is quite natural [6].
- Age level 50–79: A decremental pattern is observed. Males lose weight at this age level. This pattern is also quite natural.
- Age level 80–100: Exciting pattern is observed at this age level. According to the graph, the weight is increasing at this age level, which is not natural. It is assumed that the number of sample data is not representative at this age level. As described earlier, there are only 24 samples at age group 80–84, only nine samples at the 85–89 age group, eight samples at 90–94 age group and only two samples at 95–99 age group. Therefore, we need more samples to conclude.

Personalized acceptance range: PAR is applicable for any individual who has enough medical records in GramHealth server. We use machine learning algorithms to predict a range value for each anthropometric data. We will report the results elsewhere.

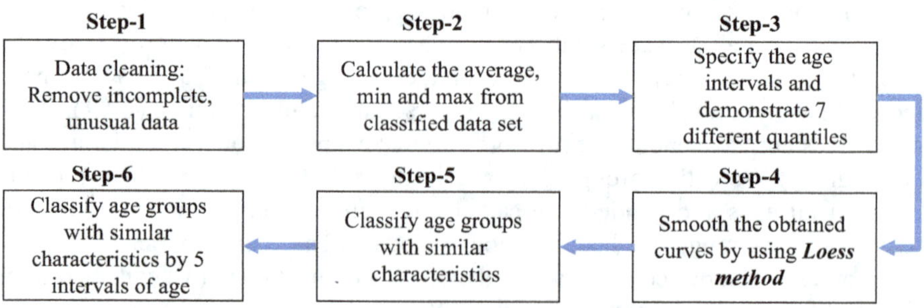

Figure 7.3 Steps to formulate GAR

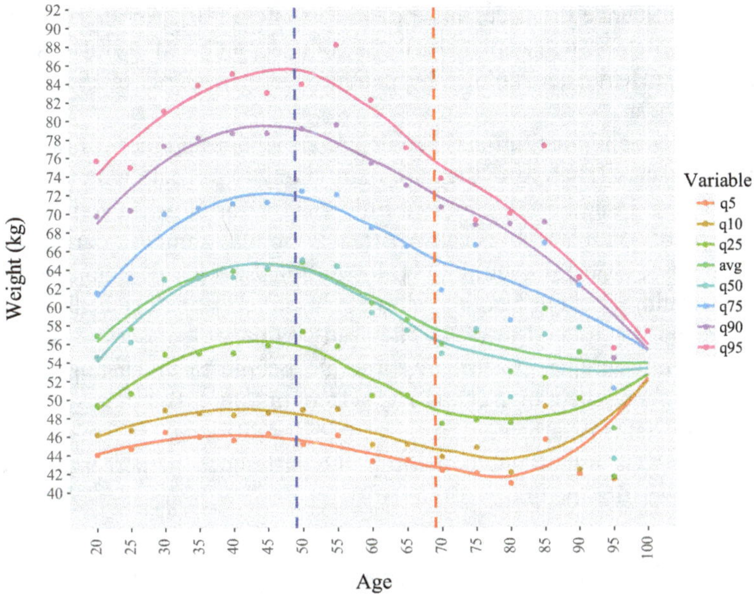

Figure 7.4 Group patterns of male weight from PHC data (N = 13,932) by 7 different percentiles (5 intervals age groups)

7.5 Social challenges: acceptance of remote healthcare service

The demand for remote healthcare systems is increasing day by day. Advanced technologies (IoT, BigData, Machine Learning, etc.) are being applied to improve the efficiency of the system. But, social adoption of these systems, especially in developing countries, has not been completely understood. It is necessary to increase the acceptability of remote healthcare systems.

There have been many previous studies targeted to explore the factors influencing the use behavior of a new technology. Technology acceptance model (TAM) is the major theory to understand how users come to accept and use a new technology/system. The first and second version of the TAM and Unified Theory of Acceptance and Use of Technology model act as the major informer to develop research hypotheses.

Based on TAM [7], TAM2 [8], UTAUT [9], and other existing user acceptance model previous studies developed PHC acceptance model that can investigate factors behind the actual use of PHC system in Bangladesh.

Most of the previous studies to enhance the acceptance of eHealth technology were conducted in developed countries. Though benefits of eHealth technology are very essential for developing countries where access to quality healthcare is hindered, very few studies were conducted in developing countries like Bangladesh.

A cross-sectional study in the rural area of Bangladesh identified social reference, advertisement, attitude toward the system, and perceived system effectiveness influence the acceptance of PHC system [10]. Another study identified influential factors such as perceived ease of use, perceived usefulness, and trust as adoption of eHealth technology by patients from hospitals of the capital city Dhaka, Bangladesh.

On the other hand, institutional people are very busy and most of the time they work sitting in seats. Therefore, they are more likely to develop noncommunicable diseases (NCDs). In addition, there is a little chance for physical activities among urban people of Bangladesh because of lack of playgrounds, parks, walkable footpath, and safe road for cycling [11]. Institutional people of Bangladesh do not have health insurance, high health awareness, routine mandatory health check-up, and they are not habituated to use ICT-based healthcare services. Therefore, we conducted a study among 264 urban corporate people to understand underlying factors that influence them to use the PHC system in future. But the psychology and socioeconomic status of urban and rural people are different.

Therefore, it is important to identify the difference in perception between urban people and rural people.

Methodology: We have been carrying out a survey inside Grameen Complex among 264 employees. The sample size was calculated based on "Sample size determination in Health Studies [12]. The data collection process is shown in Figure 7.5."

The survey collects following variables (data):

(a) Socio-demographic variables: age, sex, education, marital status, occupation, family size, individual monthly income, etc.
(b) Health-related variables: self-reported general health, family history of NCDs, Health needs, etc.
(c) Behavioral variables: tobacco use, dietary habit including fruits and vegetable consumptions, sugar, fat, and salt intake, physical activities, alcohol drinking, etc.

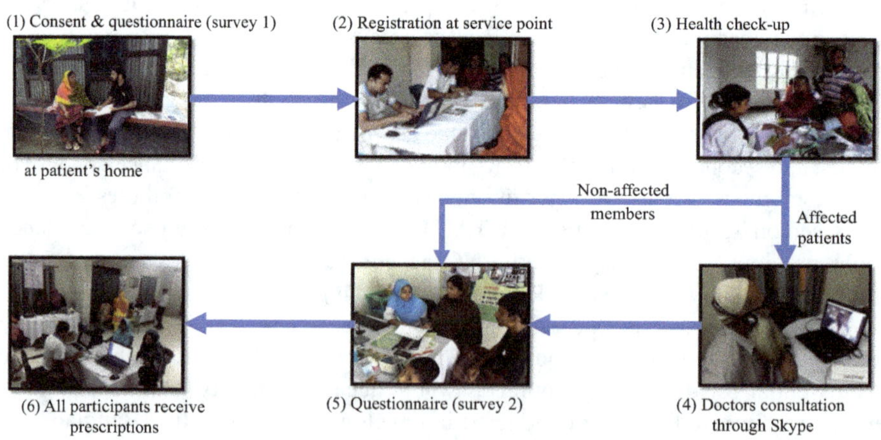

Figure 7.5 Data collection process

(d) Psychological variables: perception, attitudes, and intention to use PHC services, etc.
(e) Biological: clinical and anthropometric variables.

Results and discussion: Social influence was the significant factor for rural people to accept the PHC system but it did not appear as the significant factor for urban corporate people because corporate people are educated and they earn money that's why they take decision based on their own judgment. The acceptance of the PHC system by rural people depends on *social reference, advertisement, attitude toward the system, and perceived system effectiveness* [13]. The key to promoting the use of the eHealth technology among urban corporate people lies in the three factors: *perceived usefulness, intention to use, and health awareness* [13]. *Perceived usefulness* was the most important factor to urban corporate people to use the PHC system and understanding this factor can help developer or service providers in developing or improving the PHC system contents. Thus, increasing *perceived usefulness* in other words increasing perception of benefits of using the PHC system increase the use of the system. Moreover, we could increase use when we put efforts to increase health awareness among people, which positively and directly influences the *use*. The findings offer important practical guidelines to service providers, implementers, and policy makers in promoting the *use* of the eHealth system.

Perception to accept the PHC system is different between urban and rural people. Therefore, it is necessary to develop different model for rural and urban area because different factors may affect the acceptance of the same eHealth technology for different user groups.

7.6 Case study to increase the accessibility and reduce healthcare delivery cost

Currently, there are 3.2 billion adults at the BoP (Base of the Pyramid), comprising 68.7% of the world adult population [14]. The people at the BoP often pay higher prices for basic goods and services than wealthier consumers, either in financial or transaction costs, and often receive lower quality. The people at the bottom of the pyramid (BoP) often pay higher prices for basic goods and services than do wealthier consumers. This phenomenon is commonly known as BoP penalty. From a baseline survey in rural Bangladesh we have identified that BoP penalty is severe in the healthcare sector of developing countries. In this chapter we explain how ICT and mobility could reduce BoP penalty of a remote healthcare system.

Table 7.2 shows typical examples of BoP penalty and poverty premium in Bheramara, a rural area in Bangladesh.

Table 7.2 shows that receiving a healthcare service in a rural area has the biggest BoP penalty (2.00 times) in Bheramara. However, purchasing a typical medicine in Bheramara does not have a significant penalty. Both blood glucose test and paracetamol are in healthcare category. However, the supply chain network of drugstores is very strong even in rural areas in Bangladesh. Drug market became stable and formal with government regulation. However, there is an unavailability

Table 7.2 Examples of BoP penalty

Item	Price in Bheramara	Price in Dhaka	Poverty premium [times]	Category
Mineral water (500 ml)	20 taka	15 taka	1.33	Food and nutrition
Blood glucose test	**300 taka**	**150 taka**	**2.00**	Healthcare service (Blood Glucose Test)
Rice (per kg)	60 taka	50 taka	1.20	Food and nutrition
LP gas cylinder (12 kg)	1,000 taka	800 taka	1.25	Home appliance
Mosquito net (chemical coated)	950 taka	800 taka	1.19	Healthcare
T-shirt	400 taka	300 taka	1.33	Clothing
Renting a car	3,500	4,000	(0.87)	Mobility
Rickshaw fare	15 taka/km	20 taka/km	(0.75)	Mobility
Paracetamol (Medicine)	10 taka/10 tblts	10 taka/ 10 tblts	1.00	Healthcare/FMCG
Soap	20 taka	20 taka	1.00	FMCG

of advanced level of drugs in the rural areas. Due to strong regulation it is very difficult for the drug companies to charge premium price. In contrast, healthcare facilities such as hospitals and clinics lack in the rural areas. It needs to add additional transportation cost to receive healthcare services from urban and sub-urban hospitals. The architecture of the can be roughly sketched as consisting of a bottom sensor layer, a middle network layer, and a top application layer. As one of the primary information-acquiring means at the bottom layer of the tags have found increasingly widespread applications in various business areas, with the expectation that the use of RFID tags will eventually replace the existing bar codes in all business areas.

Field experiment: Toyota Motor Corporation and Kyushu University in Japan had been conducting this experiment since 2011 in Bangladesh. Grameen Communications in Bangladesh is supporting the experiment. A ten-seated Toyota Hiace vehicle is shared to carry ICT-based four major services such as: (1) Remote healthcare, (2) Female friendly transport using car sharing model, (3) E-learning, and (4) Last mile delivery service of online purchase. This research project is known as social services on wheels (SSW). Under SSW project there were two experimental sites in two districts in Bangladesh. One was in Kalihati Upazila under Tangail district (105 km away from the capital Dhaka city) and the other one was in Bheramara Upazila under Kushtia district (235 km away from the capital Dhaka city). In this research, we have used Bheramara Upazila as an experimental location. Bheramara is located in the western part of Bangladesh under Kushtia district and is close to the border of India. According to the census of Bangladesh Bureau of Statistics (BBS) 2011, the Bheramara sub-district has a population of 208,000 in six unions. We have found the existence of BoP penalty for healthcare

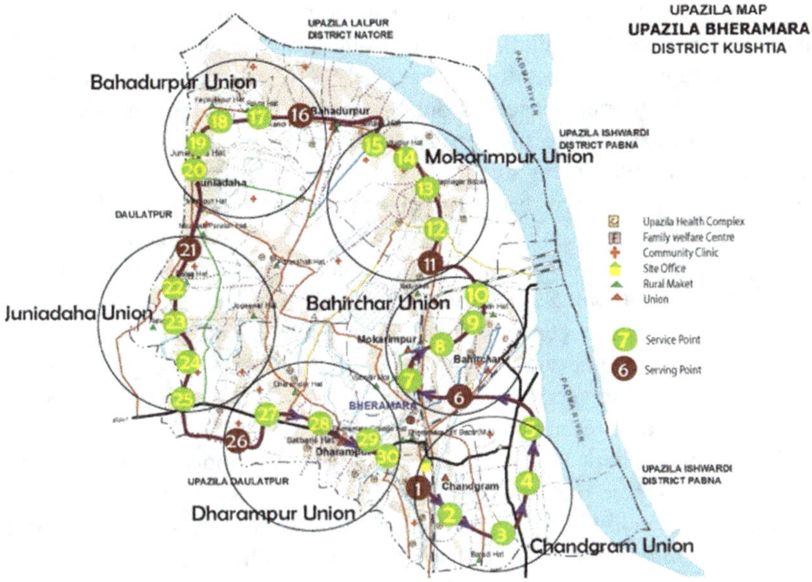

Figure 7.6 Mobility map of GramCar in Bheramara

Table 7.3 Demographic information of the experimental site

	Site: Bheramara
Population	0.2 million
Young adult population (Age 15–54)	0.12 million
Area (sq. km)	153.7
Population density (sq. km)	1,302
Distance from Dhaka city (km)	235
Number of mobile phones for young adult population*	0.09 million (75%)
Availability of Smart Phones among young adult*	0.072 million (60%)

*Estimated

service (Table 7.2) from a baseline survey conducted in a rural area (Bheramara Upazila) and an urban area (Dhaka city). However, we argue that, a shared delivery system of remote healthcare service.

In our model site, the GramCar visits different service points with multiple services in the community in a scheduled basis. Figure 7.6 shows a total of 30 service points in Bheramara sub-district dividing into six clusters of six unions. The service points are scheduled in such a way as one service point serves the rural people once a week (Table 7.3). Remote Healthcare Service is delivered once a week in a specific service point sharing the space of the GramCar. In this way, the operational cost at the last mile is shared among the multiple services.

A service point is a location where the SSW services are delivered. The location is usually an open space without any permanent settlement. We have used the space once a week or once in every 2 weeks with prior permission from the land owner or the local government authority. We did not pay any rent for using service point space. Rather, we have received logistics support from the local people such as chair, table to accommodate and display our service delivery components. Local community people who live within 2 km distance from the service point location get information about our SSW service day and time by receiving leaflets and listening to miking announcements through our promotional activities. Local people usually come to the service point on foot. On the service day we have been displaying banner at the service point which displays our services with price list. For healthcare service we bring the PHC package. For ICT connectivity we bring tablet PC, internet modem and a printer to print the prescription. We also displayed the profile of the remote doctor at our service point. For social goods delivery, we bring our product catalog in a printed version. We also display some physical items which are not available in the rural community such as chemically treated mosquito net, thermometer, blood pressure machine, umbrella, and so on.

Service point models: As mentioned in the previous section, GramCar visits a number of prespecified locations to deliver the services in a weekly or bi-weekly basis. Here, weekly and bi-weekly is the frequency of repeated service in the same service point. The GramCar with multiple services visited one place after every 2 weeks in a bi-weekly service delivery model. Similarly, the GramCar repeated one service point after 1 week in a weekly service delivery model. We could increase the number of new consumers when the number of service points was more. By increasing the number of service points we could cover more geographic areas. However, there were limitations as well of the bi-weekly service point model with the increased number of service points. As the same number of human resource visited increased number of service point the number of repeated consumers was less. On the other hand, when the number service point was less, the delivery frequency was more. In weekly service delivery model the GramCar repeated one service point after every week. Number of repeated consumers was more in weekly service delivery model compared to bi-weekly service delivery model. We wanted to find an optimum number of service points so that the overall performance would be higher. However, in weekly service delivery model there were less opportunity to serve new consumers. We have implemented three different service point models to deliver services at the last mile (Figure 7.7). According to the weekly service point model (model-1), the vehicle visited and delivered social services to five service points per month. One service point was repeated once a week. On the other hand, under the bi-weekly model (model-2) the vehicle visited ten service points in the community per month. One service point delivered social services once in every 2 weeks. Bi-weekly service point model served more new customers than weekly service point model while weekly service point model served more repetitive customers.

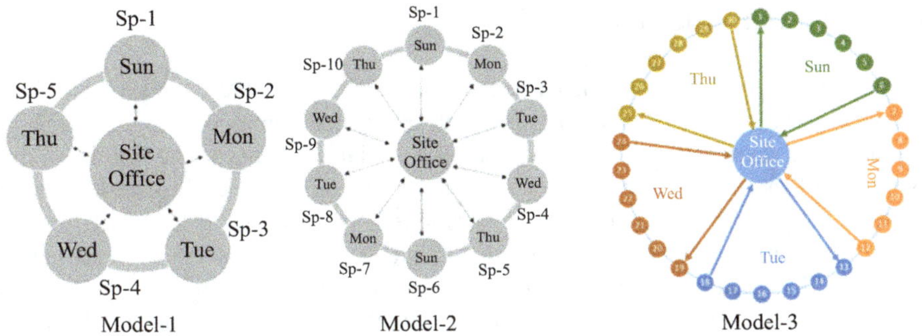

Figure 7.7 Remote healthcare service point models

Table 7.4 Remote healthcare delivery service point models

	Model 1	**Model 2**	**Model 3**
Visiting frequency (per month per service point)	4 times	2 times	4 times
Total service points in one site	5	10	30
Total customer (households) reach per month	1,000	2,000	6,000
Maximum product delivery time required	7 days	14 days	7 days
Human resource required	1 person	1 person	6 persons

In order to increase service frequency in the rural community, we have introduced a new service point model (Model-3). Under this model the vehicle touched six service points in 1 day. There were a total of 30 service points and every service point would be repeated after 1 week. Table 7.4 shows a comparison chart among different service point models.

Discussion: In this research, we have identified the practical examples of the existence of BoP penalty in healthcare in developing countries. We introduced the PHC, a remote healthcare system to provide healthcare service to the underserved communities. However, any service provided at the doorstep of the consumer ultimately increases the cost of service delivery. Therefore, the vehicle we have introduced to carry PHC service in the rural areas has increased the cost of service. We tested three different service point models with multiple social services to reduce the idle time of the vehicle to design a sustainable business model. Among three service point models, we have identified that model-3 is a combination of model-1 and model-2. It increased the number of service points and served more repeated consumers. We suggested the solution that a vehicle can be designed with multiple services and can be scheduled for different geographic locations to provide remote healthcare service in a sustainable way.

7.7 Chapter summary

In this chapter, we introduced the basic concept of PHC as a representative example of remote healthcare system that can operate in unreached community in a sustainable manner. We demonstrated the technical and social challenges and described the evolution of the technologies to meet the challenges one by one. Remote healthcare systems carry typical data errors. We introduced our mechanism to detect them at earlier stage and remove them before the data hits the server. The consumer behavior of remote healthcare services has not been studied for rural/urban inhabitants in developing countries. We initiated one project to continuously monitor their behavior and find out the influencing factors for practical use of such healthcare services.

It is interesting to observe that the poor people in remote areas pay more for the healthcare services. We initiated a joint project with Toyota Motor Corporation to see that how a vehicle service can extend social services in people doorstep to reduce the delivery cost.

References

[1] World Health Organization and International Bank for Reconstruction and Development. (2017). *Tracking Universal Health Coverage: 2017 Global Monitoring Report*. https://doi.org/ISBN 978-92-4-151355-5

[2] Ahmed, A., Inoue, S., Kai, E., Nakashima, N., and Nohara, Y. (2013). Portable health clinic: a pervasive way to serve the unreached community for preventive healthcare. In *International Conference on Distributed, Ambient, and Pervasive Interactions* (pp. 265–274).

[3] Kai, E., and Ahmed, A. (2012). Remote health consultancy service for unreached community: amazing facts and technical challenges. In *Proceedings of the First MJIIT-JUC Joint Symposium, MJIIT, UTM, Kulalumpur, Malaysia*.

[4] Hasan, M., Yokota, F., Islam, R., Hisazumi, K., Fukuda, A., and Ahmed, A. (2020). A predictive model for height tracking in an adult male population in Bangladesh to reduce input errors. *International Journal of Environmental Research and Public Health* 2020, 17, 1806. doi.org/10.3390/ijerph17051806

[5] Hasan, M., Fukuda, A., Islam R., Yokota, F., and Ahmed, A. (2017). Errors in remote healthcare system: Where, how and by whom? In *Proceedings of* TENCON 2017 – IEEE Region 10 Conference, Penang, 2017, pp. 170–175. doi: 10.1109/TENCON.2017.8227856

[6] Hasan, M., Nishikitani, M., Yokota, F., Fukuda, A., Islam, R., and Ahmed, A. (2019). Growth characteristics of age-based anthropometric data from human assisted remote healthcare systems. *International Journal of Advanced Computer Science and Applications(ijacsa)*, 10(3), pp. 615–619.

[7] Fred, D., Richard, P., and Paul, R. (1989). User acceptance of computer technology: a comparison of two theoretical models. *Management Science*, 35(8), 982–1003.

[8] Venkatesh, V., and Davis, F. D. (2000). A theoretical extension of the technology acceptance model: four longitudinal studies. *Management Science*, 46(2), 186–205.

[9] Venkatesh, V., Morris, M. G., Davis, G. B., and Davis, F. D. (2003). User acceptance of information technology: toward a unified view. *MIS Quarterly*, 27(3), 425–478.

[10] Hossain, N., Yokota, F., Sultana, N., and Ahmed, A. (2018). Factors influencing rural end-users' acceptance of e-health in developing countries: a study on portable health clinic in Bangladesh. *Telemedicine and E-Health*, 25(3), 221–229.

[11] Zaman, M. M., Rahman, M. M., Rahman, M. R. *et al.* (2016). Prevalence of risk factors for non-communicable diseases in Bangladesh: results from STEPS survey 2010. *Indian Journal of Public Health*, 60(1), 17–25.

[12] Lwanga, S. K., and Lemeshow, S. (1991). Sample size determination in health studies: a practical manual. *World Health Organization*. https://apps.who.int/iris/handle/10665/40062.

[13] Sampa, M. B., Hossain, M. N., Hoque, M. R., Islam, R., Yokota, F., Nishikitani, M., Fukuda, A., and Ahmed, A. (2020). Influence of factors on the adoption and use of ICT-based eHealth technology by urban corporate people. *Journal of Service Science and Management*, 13(1), 1–19.

[14] London, T., Anupindi, R., and Sheth, S. (2010). Lessons learned from ventures serving base of the pyramid producers. *Journal of Business Research*, 63, 582–594.

Chapter 8

Modular expansion of PHC in Bangladesh

Rafiqul Islam Maruf[1,2], Kimiyo Kikuchi[3], Yoko Sato[4], Rieko Izukura[1] and Mariko Nishikitani[3]

Portable health clinic (PHC) has been designed for providing primary healthcare service to the rural communities by telemedicine with the support of remote doctor [1,2]. However, when the health workers visit rural areas with PHC for primary care, they face many patients who needs secondary or tertiary level of treatment for various diseases. That leads for the modular expansion with various specialized features of the basic PHC system. Besides, adding new healthcare features for specific diseases, PHC also aims to add new service approaches for better treatment in PHC. Thus, the concept of self-reported health outcomes is to be added in PHC and this chapter gives a light on it. Also, the living environment as well as the working habit highly influences the health status. Thus, the occupational and environmental health becomes so important these days, and this will be covered in the last part of this chapter.

8.1 Requirement of modular expansion of PHC

The prevalence of noncommunicable diseases like diabetes mellitus and hypertension has increased to a cautious extent in Bangladesh. However, these diseases and the consecutive complications can be effectively prevented by taking cautions beforehand. Preventing such diseases to occur or diagnosing it at early stage can help people to save a lot on medical bills. For this, regular screening of health status is important, which can be facilitated by PHC. Thus, PHC system has been developed with a special focus on noncommunicable diseases in preventive way [3,4].

Besides NCDs, we find patients coming with a wide range of complaints that includes eye care problem, maternal and child healthcare problem, dental problem, skin program, and communicable diseases. Many cases our call center doctors refer them to nearest sub-district hospitals but still too far for them. So they try to insist

[1]Medical Information Center, Kyushu University Hospital, Kyushu University, Fukuoka, Japan
[2]Global Communication Center, Grameen Communications, Dhaka, Bangladesh
[3]Institute of Decision Science for Sustainable Society, Kyushu University, Fukuoka, Japan
[4]Department of Health Sciences, Faculty of Medical Sciences, Kyushu University, Fukuoka, Japan

the call center doctors for consultancy and sometimes they need to respond having no other alternative. Otherwise, the patient may remain with this problem without visiting distant doctor. Here comes a requirement from the call center doctor's side. They need more investigation and pathological reports of the patients for better diagnosis. So the first module we have added to PHC is the Tele-Pathology module. Later, we have added the Tele-EyeCare module and the Maternal and Child Health (MCH) module in PHC for advanced support in these areas as a priority due to the highest level of demand in the rural communities.

8.2 Tele-Pathology system in PHC

8.2.1 Introduction

Like other developing countries, Bangladesh has a huge shortage of pathologist and it is just 0.024 for every 10,000 patients. In other words, there is 1 pathologist for every 416,000 patients. However, there are many pathological laboratories operated by unskilled laboratory technologists (2 to 3 years' diploma graduate in pathology) in the remote villages. They play a significant role in the rural community with their services in absence of professional pathologist but many times their wrong diagnosis causes huge trouble to patients. Therefore, it is very much needed to empower them and thus, PHC has added this Tele-Pathology module.

8.2.2 Tele-Pathology system structure

The tele-pathology module of the PHC system enables the rural diagnostic centers operated by laboratory technologists for producing quality pathological report with the support of the qualified remote pathologist (Figure 8.1). At present, this system is capable of blood hematological (CBC) test, routine examination of urine, routine examination of stool, and skin scarping test [5,6].

In this system, the rural laboratory technologist (1) collects the sample, prepare the physical report, produce test slide, (2) take a number of microscopic image of

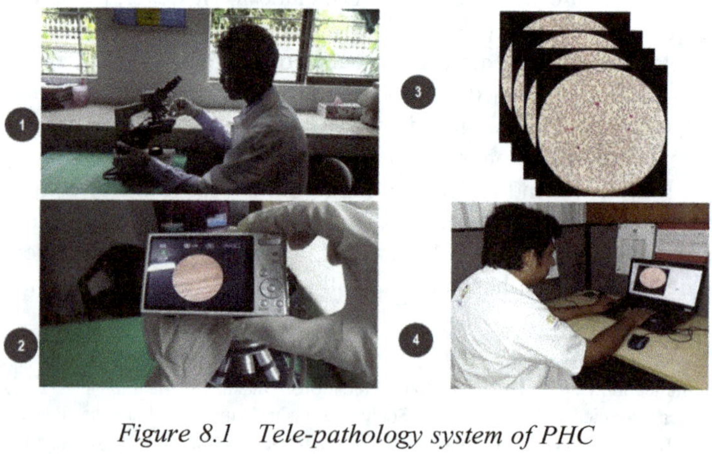

Figure 8.1 Tele-pathology system of PHC

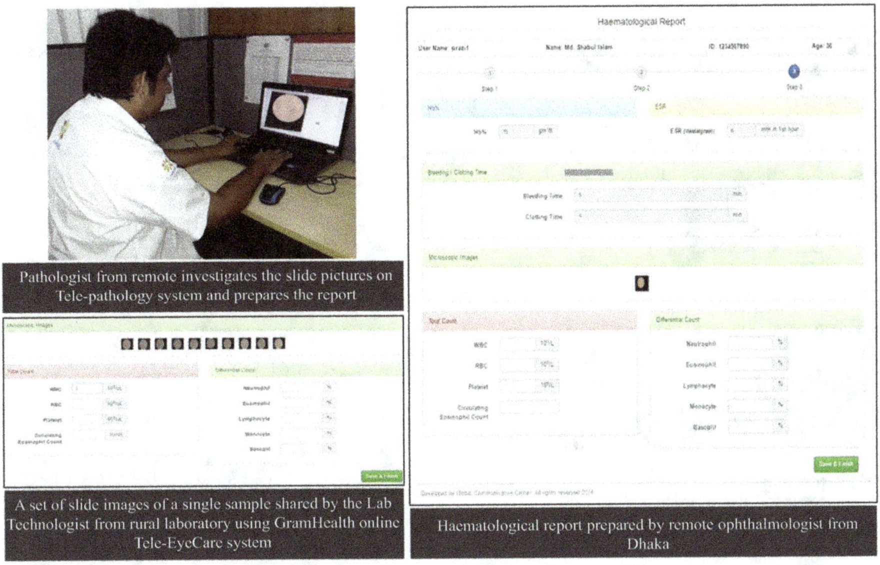

Figure 8.2 Pathology report preparation by a remote pathologist

the slides with varying position, and then (3) upload the images together with the physical report to the online server. The remote pathologist then (4) diagnoses the sample based on the cell counts of the microscopic slide images with the reference of physical report, finalize the pathology report, and upload to the online server (Figure 8.2).

In line with the PHC protocol, the Tele-Pathology system uses simple, low cost, and available devices for its operation. The microscope used in this system is Optima G-302 that is often used in local pathology laboratory.

Optima G-302
Eyepiece: WF10×
Objective: 4×, 10×, 100×
Light source: 6 V, 20 W halogen
Power Supply: 220 V

For taking microscopic images, SONY Cyber-shot DSC-W320 (14.1 mega-pixel camera with 4× optical zoom lens; starting at a wide 26 mm equiv., and a 2.7″ screen) camera has been used. However, other commonly available devices were also tried and found significantly workable.

8.2.3 PHC service delivery process with Tele-Pathology system

In case a pathological report is required by a call center doctor (physician) for tele-consultancy in PHC service, the doctor advises the local health worker to send the patient to the nearest pathological laboratory under PHC service, give the sample

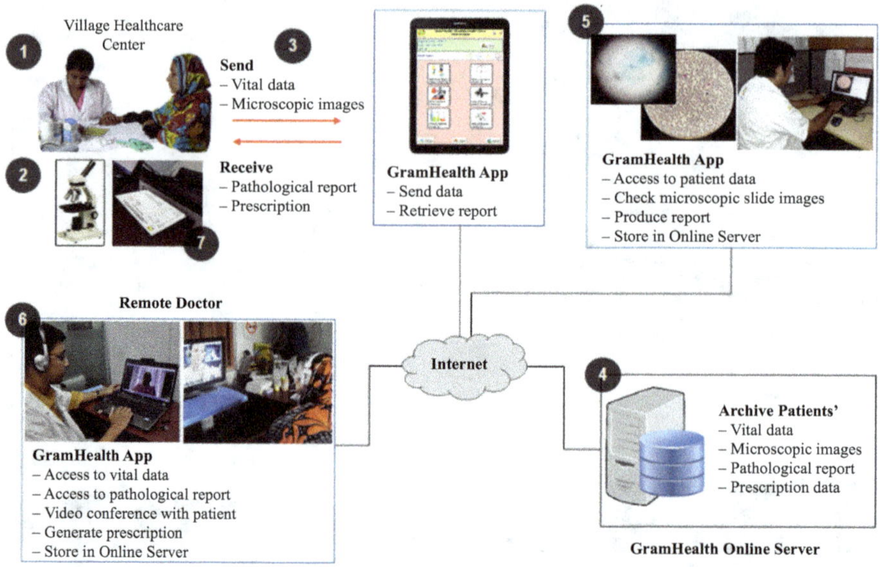

Figure 8.3 PHC service delivery process with tele-pathology system

and come for the telemedicine next day. By that time, the laboratory technologist completes the report with the support of remote pathologist. Next day when the patient comes, the doctor can get access to the report from the online server, interview the patients once again and prepare the prescription (Figure 8.3).

In case of emergency, the PHC pathology laboratory can produce urgent report with urgent support from the remote pathologist. If needed, the laboratory technologist can also download this report from the server to deliver to the patient directly.

8.3 Tele-EyeCare system in PHC

8.3.1 Introduction

Like many other developing countries, ophthalmic disease is at a very high risk especially in the rural areas of Bangladesh. Bangladesh sources states that 20% of the rural population are affected by ophthalmic diseases where glaucoma is a leading cause. The main causes of these diseases are unhygienic environment, dust in the air, uncleaned water, and risky jobs besides the usual aging problem. There are only 1,000 ophthalmologists for a population of 160 million resulting only 0.063 doctors per 10,000 people. Thus, it becomes impossible for the existing facilities to cover all patients with quality services.

When we provide primary healthcare services in rural Bangladesh by PHC system, many patients irrespective of their age and gender come with ophthalmic diseases. Considering this huge demand in rural Bangladesh, a module called

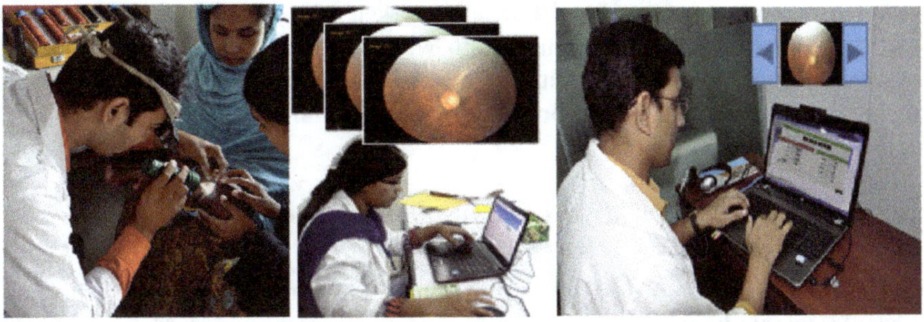

Figure 8.4 Tele-EyeCare service system of PHC

"Tele-EyeCare" system has been added to PHC for ensuring better eye care services (Figure 8.4). The aim of this system is to conduct primary checkup of the patients at the rural area and classify the patients as per severity of the problem using a triage system. Low risk patients with simple problems are supported by the trained local health workers. However, in case of doubtful cases, the patients' vital information, initial primary checkup report, and ophthalmic images are shared with a remote ophthalmologist using the cloud-based data-server, and then establish a direct video conference between the patient and the ophthalmologist. The ophthalmologist directly talks to the patients, reconfirm his/her status, and finally, provide online prescription. However, as all the doubtful cases are now referred to ophthalmologist, the ophthalmologist is burdened to respond to all those patients. Thus, it causes misuse of a significant amount of his/her valued resources for comparatively simple cases. So it is very much needed not to refer all doubtful cases but diagnosis them further and only the critical ones to be referred to the ophthalmologist so that the people really in need get priority attention.

8.3.2 Tele-EyeCare system structure

The Tele-EyeCare module of the PHC system ensures primary eye care services for the rural communities [6]. This module has added a Digital Fundus Camera to the PHC box for capturing retinal images (both mydriatic and non-mydriatic) of the patients. This enables the health workers to have a better view of the retina and the peripheral for identifying the problem with certainty. Thus, the trained local health workers check and classify the patients as per severity of the problem. Low risk patients with simple complications are served by the health workers. However, in case of doubtful cases, the patients' vital information, initial primary checkup reports, and ophthalmic images are stored in the online server and share with a remote ophthalmologist.

The ophthalmologist then checks the initial checkup reports produced and shared by the local health worker, investigates the ophthalmic images, directly talks to the patients over video conference system, reconfirms their status, and finally, provide online prescriptions. If needed, the ophthalmologist can ask for further investigation of the patient by the health worker and can also provide glasses prescription with the support of the health workers. Thus, this system enables to provide basic eye care to the ordinary patients by the health workers and special care for the critical patients by professional ophthalmologist who really deserve special attention.

8.3.3 Automated Tele-EyeCare system using AI technologies

The Tele-EyeCare system is a step up for providing eye care service to the rural patients by telemedicine support of the distanced ophthalmologist. However, since the number of ophthalmologist is too limited and the resource is too valued, there is a need to make possible best use of it. Thus, there is an urgent need to use advance technologies to support the ophthalmologist (Figure 8.5).

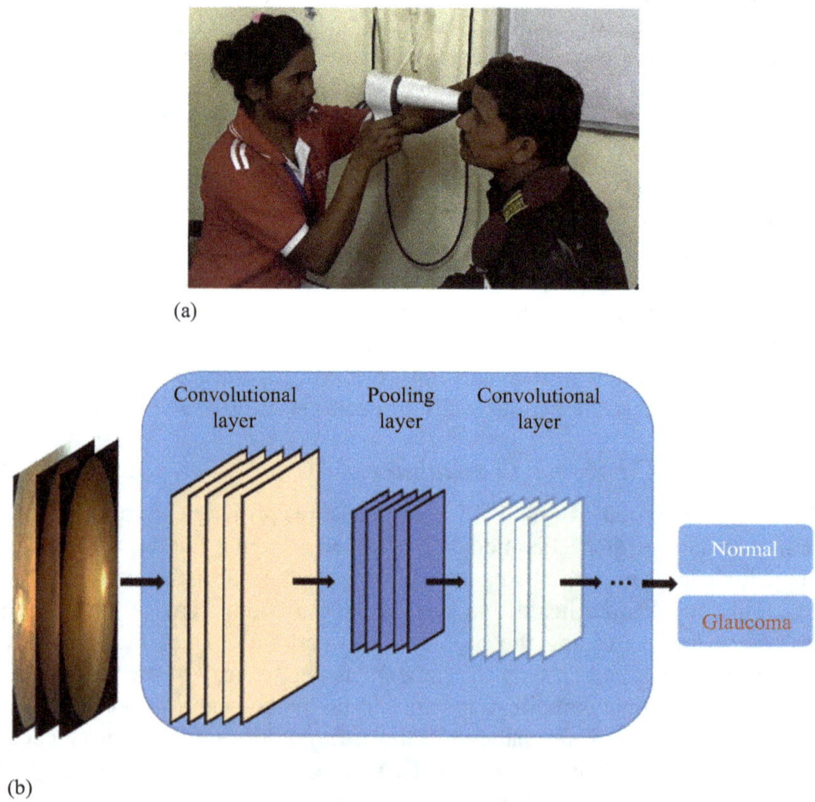

Figure 8.5 (a) Digital fundus camera and overview of a common glaucoma detection framework using deep learning and (b) digital fundus camera and overview of a common glaucoma detection framework using deep learning

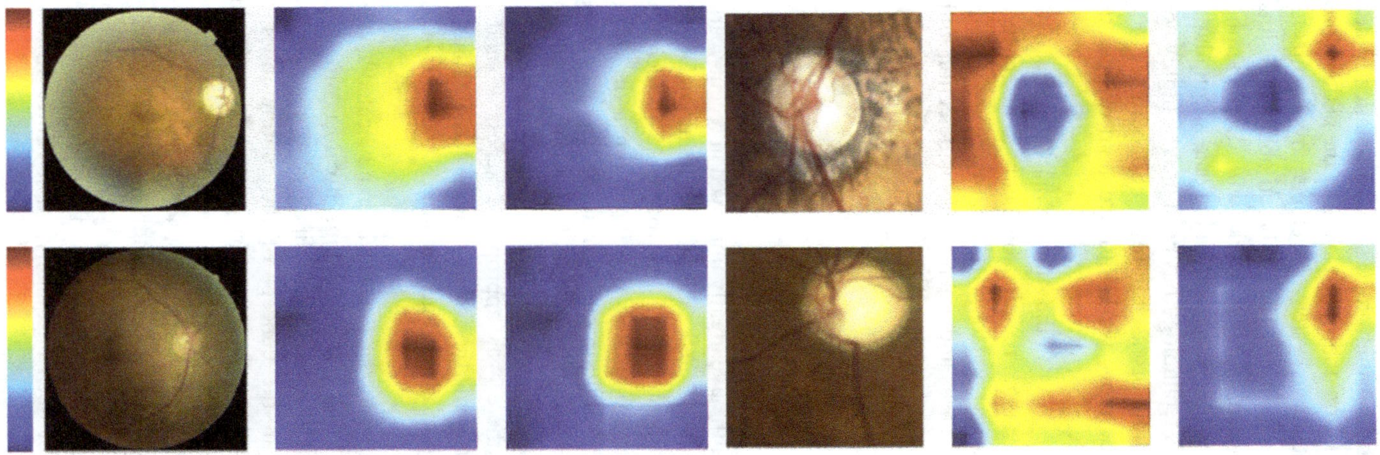

(a) (b)

Figure 8.6 (a) Class activation map for glaucoma detection on the full images and (b) class activation map for glaucoma detection on the optic disc images

PHC Tele-EyeCare system aims to use a smart technology involving artificial intelligence (AI) with Deep Learning process for automatically detecting diseases by ophthalmic image recognition and rightly classify the patients based on severity. The ophthalmic image detection system developed by Japan Ophthalmological Society will be used for this purpose. The AI-based ophthalmic image recognition system uses deep convolutional neural networks with deep learning technology to identify ophthalmic disorders comparing with a big data accumulating from various medical facilities. So far this technology has been proved highly accurate to detect glaucoma and other ophthalmic diseases in research laboratory (Figure 8.6). PHC aims to incorporate this laboratory work into real field of operation and see the effect on Tele-EyeCare system performance.

There is a significant progress on the study of diabetic retinopathy using retinal fundus photographs but there is no mentionable study to detect heart diseases and atherosclerosis using retinal image data. PHC Tele-EyeCare system may initiate a new study trend for heart diseases and atherosclerosis detection with retinal image recognition technology.

8.4 MCH care system in PHC

8.4.1 Introduction

Both maternal and child health have greatly improved in recent years, primarily due to the implementation of the United Nation's Millennium Development Goals. Though great progress has been made, the worldwide incidence of preventable deaths still remains high; approximately 303,000 women die of maternal causes annually [7]. Meanwhile, 5.6 million children under 5 years of age die [8], with 40% of these deaths occurring within the first 28 days of life or during the neonatal period [9]. Most of these deaths occur in low- and middle-income countries, and should be preventable if there was appropriate access to and availability of healthcare [10,11]. Because of this, the United Nations has called to end preventable deaths among mothers and children by 2030 in its Sustainable Development Goals [12].

The concept of the continuum of care has been advocated as a way to globally improve the status of MCH [7]. The continuum of care is an integrated series of care steps, composed of both time and space dimensions, that women and children access continuously [13]. In the concept of the continuum of care, the time dimension of the continuum is composed of service delivery during multiple stages throughout life; adolescence/pre-pregnancy, pregnancy, delivery, postpartum, childhood, and motherhood. Meanwhile, the space dimension of the continuum is composed by three care stages; clinical care, outreach–outpatient care, and family–community care [14]. Because of its ability to reach patients across multiple touchpoints, use of the continuum of care is an effective strategy to improve MCH. However, to date, it has not been adequately implemented in low- and middle-income countries [12].

8.4.2 Maternal and child health system structure

8.4.2.1 New Aspects in the PHC for MCH

In order to address this problem, a new module on MCH has been developed. Basically, the concept of the system itself has not changed; the clinic is composed of an eHealth system that comprises a set of sensor devices in an attaché case, a data transmission system linked to a mobile network, and a data management application. The health status of patients checked at the clinic is automatically categorized into four stages once the examination data is entered in the identification system: healthy, caution, affected, and emergent. The new aspects in the PHC for MCH as compared to the original clinics is the inclusion of particular objectives; to improve the continuum of care of mothers and children and, by doing so, to improve their health status. To attain these objectives, the system structure has also been modified: health checkup devices specific for mothers and children have been added, and the criteria of the categorization of health status were modified to suit that needed for MCH (Figure 8.7).

8.4.2.2 Implementation procedures

An implementation team is used in the clinic, consisting of one local pharmacist and one traditional birth attendant. The team provides regular health checkups for mothers during their preterm and postpartum period, as well as for their children during the 6 weeks from their birth (Figure 8.8). The components of the PHC for MCH are presented in the Table 8.1. The timings of care are: at the fourth month, sixth month, eighth month, and ninth month of pregnancy, immediately after birth, and 2 days, 6 days, and 6 weeks after delivery/birth. At these times, the implementation team examines the check points presented in Table 8.2 at mother's

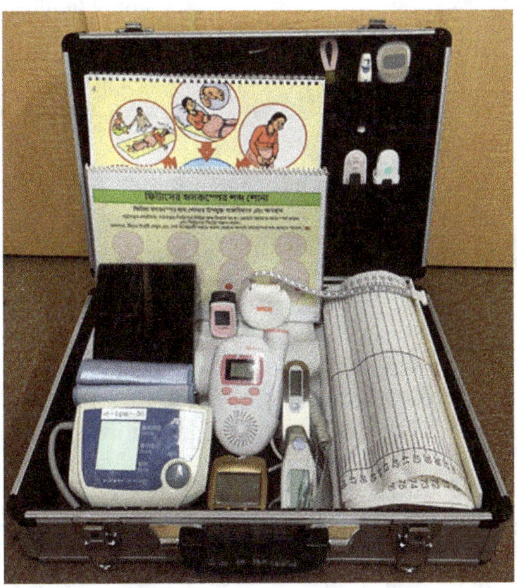

Figure 8.7 Portable health clinic for maternal and child health

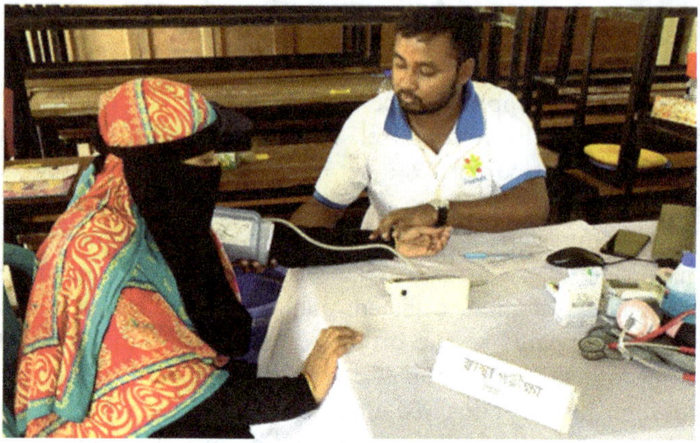

Figure 8.8 Health checkup of a local woman

Table 8.1 Components of PHC for maternal and child health

No.	Target	Name of devices and strips
1	Mother	Weigh scale for adult
2	Mother	Digital sphygmomanometer
3	Mother	Manual sphygmomanometer
4	Mother	Blood glucose test sensor
5	Mother	Pulse oximeter
6	Mother	Height measurement tape
7	Mother	Hemoglobin test sensor
8	Mother	Digital thermometer for woman
9	Mother	Portable ultrasounds
10	Mother	Fetus heartbeat sound meter
11	Mother	Urine test strip
12	Mother	Adult stethoscope
13	Mother	Flip chart for health education
14	Child	Newborn stethoscope
15	Child	Handy digital weight measure
16	Child	Newborn weight-scaling hammock
17	Child	Height measurement for newborn
18	Child	Digital thermometer for child

home. Once data from the examinations of the mother or child shows that they have an abnormal health status, the mother is connected to a medical doctor by Skype in order to receive consultations or necessary prescriptions (Figure 8.9).

8.4.2.3 MCH record book

At the same time as receiving health checkups, mothers also receive a so-called "Maternal and Child Health Record Book," where their health status alongside their child's is chronologically recorded. This record book is usually kept by the mother and is referred to by health workers to determine the mother/child's health status history.

Table 8.2 Health check points of mothers and children during various stages

Pregnancy period of mother	Blood pressure, pulse, temperature, hemoglobin, urine protein, urine sugar, blood glucose, body-mass-index, fetus beat per minute, height of uterus, edema, position of baby, interview of health check points
Postpartum period of mother	Blood pressure, pulse, temperature, hemoglobin, urine protein, urine sugar, blood glucose, body-mass-index, interview of health check points
Postnatal period of child	Weight, height, temperature, cyanosis, interview of health check points

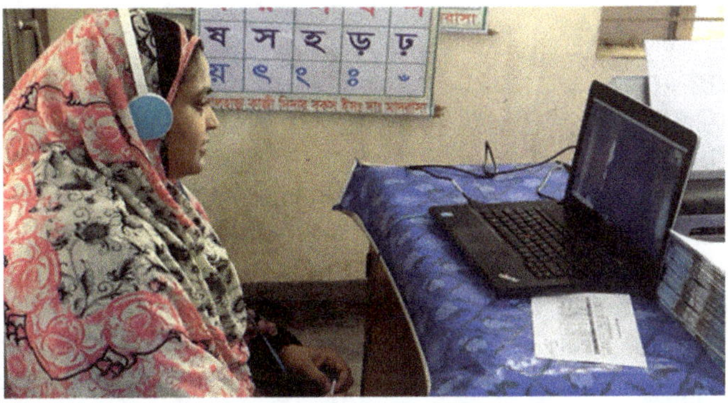

Figure 8.9 A local woman is consulting a doctor in Dhaka

8.4.3 Expected outcomes of the maternal and child health system

Using the PHC for MCH, multiple positive outcomes are expected. First, there would be an increase in number of mothers who receive MCH continuously from pregnancy to the postpartum/postnatal period, in particular in rural areas where access to health services is limited. Second, by receiving care continuously, pregnancy-induced diseases and perinatal infections in both mothers and children may be detected earlier or even prevented. Because of this, the PHC for MCH should be explored further to improve the health status of both mothers and children in resource-limited areas of any country.

8.5 Self-reported health outcomes in PHC

8.5.1 Introduction

The measurement of self-reported health outcomes, i.e., patient/resident-perceived health status and quality of life (QOL), is crucial for successful intervention. Conventionally, therapeutic efficacy tends to emphasize the survival and life expectancy rates. However, at present, it is generally acknowledged that evaluation of health care should be examined by QOL, as well as its quantity. With the change in disease structures, socioeconomic environment, and lifestyles, immediate response to a variety of health care needs is vital. Typical health outcomes, such as blood pressure and serum glucose values, neither cover a wide range of primary care services, nor adequately explain their quality improvement. In contrast, QOL can be useful in evaluation or improvising efforts for better health care services [15]. Further, the evidence-based primary care services will be requested to prevent and manage diverse chronic conditions. Nowadays, many scientific validated measurements of self-reported health outcomes have been published and used worldwide.

This instance thus reports the current tendency of QOL measures as one of the self-reported health outcomes. It also indicates the future issues applicable to portal health clinic (PHC).

8.5.2 Bangladeshi population trends in QOL or health-related QOL (HR-QOL): a study focused on the Bangladeshi population (brief summary)

The QOL measuring instruments are briefly divided into disease-specific and generic scales, and the latter are preferred when measuring health-related QOL (HR-QOL) in people with or without chronic conditions [15]. Table 8.3 displayed the literature in terms of measurements of QOL, focusing on the Bangladeshi people in the last 5 years. Further, a brief online search was performed using PubMed. In all, 24 literature searches, which matched the description of "*Bangladesh**," "*quality of life*," "*health-related quality of life*" seen in abstract, were found. Out of the 24 literatures found, 17 adopted HR-QOL scales such as SF-36 and WHO quality of life brief scale (WHOQOL-BREF), etc. As these HRQOL scales have been translated into many languages, it is possible to examine HR-QOL between countries.

8.5.3 Expected outcome and future issues

PHC is a primary health care system including telemedicine. It is expected that the self-reported health outcomes contribute as a complementary resource to primary health services using PHC. In particular, assessing HRQOL, which covers a concept of health (components of health such as physical, mental and social domains, etc.), could be clarified the interventional approach to specific health issues.

Regarding the use of self-reported health outcomes, the following could be considered: (1) It could be used properly after understanding the conceptual basis and psychometric properties in the scales of self-reported health outcomes [15]. (2) Assessing generic QOL, which will be applicable across a range of conditions, is desirable in primary care settings such as screening. (3) Additionally, the translated scales should be examined for reliability and validity. (4) Finally, researchers should be thoroughly trained for measuring self-reported health outcomes; researcher-led assessment may create misinterpreted facts, resulting in

Table 8.3 Summary of QOL or HR-QOL studies for Bangladeshi population

Authors	Study design	Instruments	Sample (No., participant's features)
Ahammed *et al.* [16]	cross-sectional	ADDQOL	$n = 164$, type 2 diabetes
Saleh *et al.* [17]	cross-sectional	EQ-5D	$n = 500$, type 2 diabetes
Safita *et al.* [18]	cross-sectional	EQ-5D, EQ-VAS	$n = 591$, type 2 diabetes vs non-type 2 diabetes
Mahumud *et al.* [19]	cross-sectional	EQ-5D-5L, EQ, VAS	$n = 465$, pregnancy (age 18–42 years)
Bashar *et al.* [20]	cross-sectional	MENQOL	$n = 435$, with or without menopause (age ≥ 17 years)
Hassan *et al.* [21]	cross-sectional	PAQOL	$n = 162$ with asthma (7–17 years old)
Rahman M *et al.* [22]	cross-sectional	PedsQL	$n = 50$, children with nephrotic syndrome (age 2–12 years old)
Jahan *et al.* [23]	cross-sectional	PedsQL	$n = 149$, children with institutionalized autism spectrum disorder
Mitry *et al.* [24]	cross-sectional	PedsQL	$n = 180$ (57 children with visual acuity impairment and 95 with some patient reported perceptual visual dysfunction)
Rahman *et al.* [25]	longitudinal	QLQ-C30, QLQ-BR23	$n = 250$, primary breast cancer
Rahman *et al.* [26]	longitudinal	QLQ-C30, QLQ-BR23	$n = 251$, surgery of breast cancer
Hossain *et al.* [27]	cross-sectional	QLQ-C30, QLQ-CX24	$n = 109$, cervical cancer
Hossain *et al.* [28]	mixed retrospective-prospective	SF-12	$n = 350$, spinal injuries
Hossain *et al.* [29]	cross-sectional	SF-12	$n = 260$, spinal cord injuries
Walker *et al.* [30]	observational retrospective	SF-36	$n = 17$ (14 women with irreparable obstetric fistulas and 3 with bladder exstrophy)
Quadir *et al.* [31]	cross-sectional	SF-36	$n = 338$, Rana Plaza survivors
Imoto *et al.* [32]	cross-sectional	SF-36	$n = 78$ women with surgery of obstetric fistula out of $n = 113$
Hossain *et al.* [33]	cross-sectional	WHOQOL-BREF	$n = 1326$, Chikungunya infection
Uddin *et al.* [34]	cross-sectional	WHOQOL-BREF	$n = 280$, older adults (age 60–75 years)
Uddin MN *et al.* [35]	cross-sectional	WHOQOL-BREF	$n = 1500$ adults (age 18–59 years) and 1200 older adults (age 60–90 years)
Tsutsumi *et al.* [36]	cross-sectional	WHOQOL-BREF	$n = 189$, leprosy vs. without leprosy

(Continues)

Table 8.3 (Continued)

Authors	Study design	Instruments	Sample (No., participant's features)
Laskar *et al.* [37]	cross-sectional	WHOQOL-BREF	$n = 104$ with arsenicosis vs without arsenicosis
Gomez-Olive *et al.* [38]	cross-sectional	WHOQOL-BREF	$n = 4{,}004$ Bangladeshi out of $n = 43{,}935$ at 8 countries
Imam *et al.* [39]	cross-sectional	WHOQOL-HIV BREF	$n = 82$, HIV infection

MENQOL: menopausal-specific QOL, PAQOL: pediatric asthma Quality of Life,
PedsQL: pediatric quality of life Inventory, ADDQOL: Audit of diabetes-dependent quality of life
QLQ-C30: European Organization for Research and Treatment of Cancer Quality of Life Questionnaire
QLQ-BR23: European Organization for Research and Treatment of Breast Cancer Quality of Life Questionnaire
QLQ-CX24: European Organization for Research and Treatment of Cervical Cancer Quality of Life Questionnaire
WHOQOL-BREF: WHO quality of life brief scale, WHOQOL-HIV BREF: WHO HIV quality of life brief scale

inappropriate responses to people needs. It seems that the future PHC will capture both the subjective and objective health outcomes for the improvement of the quality of primary healthcare.

8.6 Occupational and environmental health module

8.6.1 Introduction

As the main target of PHC activities is noncommunicable diseases, a health check-list is often designed for preventive medicine. In developed countries, preventive concepts and activities are well accepted. Medical services have developed from treat and cure approaches to injuries and diseases to try to resolve the causes of such health problems. Currently, these countries are addressing not only the management of injury and disease, but also the promotion of health in the population.

The health check-list system is a practical way to improve social health. A preventive action can identify the health problem at a very early, subclinical stage, and the health check system enables us to provide behavioral guidance to avoid health problems developing to the clinical level. Once injuries and diseases have occur, the remediation costs often exceed the interventions costs to avoid the adverse condition and, more importantly, people's QOL will be negatively affected. If people maintain their individual best possible health status in a community, they may keep and increase the productivity and capability of that community. Such a benefit has often been found indicated in the studies of a company or industry [40].

Among developed countries, Japan is known for the longevity of its population and the fast-paced economic growth of the last half-century. At the same time, this country has been known for its unique and active occupational health services [41]. The system of occupational health legislated by the Industrial Safety and Health Act includes a scheduled health check for individual workers, the provision of this check which is duty required of employers. Also, the occupational health regulations specify the level of atmospheric concentration of hazardous materials at the working place, not the level of exposure for human. Due to this country experience of environmental damage caused by industrial activities during the era of high-speed economic growth, these unique restrictions have been developed over a considerable period.

As another unique point of Japanese occupational health, many people, including employees and their families, can receive free health checkup services in Japan. Additionally, other types of health checkup systems also cover other people, who do not belong to employees' programs, with low cost coverage based on National Health Insurance. Historically, Japan has introduced medical insurance that includes all of the citizens, and this system also provides the regular health checkup system. These whole health check systems have been developed and introduced to contribute to equitable economic development and the stability of society. As a result, this public health policy of Japan may be seen as contributing to enhancing people's healthy life and longevity.

One characteristic of the Japanese universal health coverage system is implemented by main both the Employees' Health Insurance and the National Health

Insurance. When considering the promotion of universal preventive action, we should know the difference between these two systems as a good example. While the Employees' Health Insurance is funded by premiums from both employees and employers, the National Health Insurance is funded only by subscribers' premium in principle. However, in most situations, the latter insurance system needs government subsidies and tax refunds because some subscribers cannot afford to pay full premium due to their low income or unemployment. In case of shortage of fund resources, it is difficult to expend the insurance money for nonurgent health problem, like health checkups. Preventive action often comes after necessary medical treatments. People and the government are not willing to pay for such health preventive services unless they are aware of impending health problems, especially in developing countries where resources are insecure and economy is limited. Instead, PHC activities can offer in the field of occupational health. It has a lot of possibilities to benefit many people and develop sustainability.

8.6.2 Measurements of workers' health and environmental condition

When the health checkup is provided to workers at the work place, the items of PHC do not need to be changed from the usual style which targets noncommunicable diseases. However, it would be more desirable if it contained the measurement for work-related health problems. For example, if the task is visually demanding, an eye test may be highly recommended. Similarly, if the work place involves the use of lead, an anemia test, or the assessment of the nervous system should be required.

At the same time, the environmental assessment is necessary in case hazardous materials are often released into the air, and others are often discarded in waste fluid or soil around the workplace. The accurate and highly reliable way to evaluate possible contaminants at the workplace is by laboratory test after sampling. However, given the features of PHC system, which include portability and easy of approach, the assessment of the environment should be equally mobile and accessible. Here, we can use a water pack-test (Figure 8.10) [42] or a hand-held electrochemical detector (Figure 8.11) [43] to measure materials in water solutions. This hand-held electrochemical detector called the DEPSOR utilizes a voltammetric technology to determine Pb, Cu, Cd, Zn, As, Hg, and other metals in ppb level at the site in real time [44]. The use of these devices to assess environmental materials especially with a health checkup is beneficial in the context of promotion of disease preventive actions.

In any case, the items of health check should be decided by industrial hygienists and health care professionals with the opinions of employees and employers with consideration of industrial types and working conditions. Environmental assessment is also a useful tool to support the enhancement of worker's health.

8.6.3 Expected outcome and future issues

If the PHC and environmental assessment systems are included in the occupational health service, business owners could more readily manage their health effectively

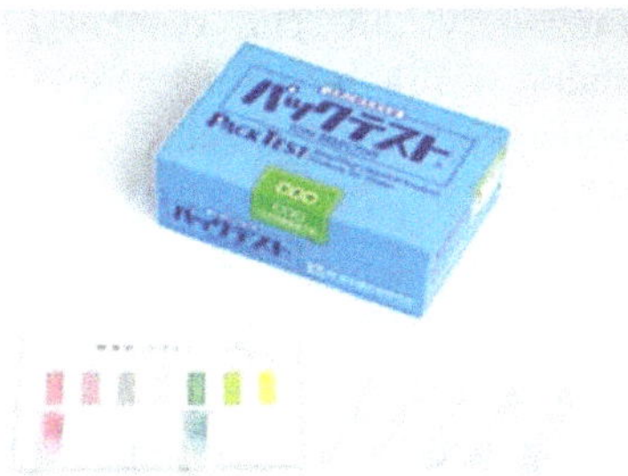

Figure 8.10 PackTest by KYORITSU CHEMICAL-CHECK Lab., Corp. [42]

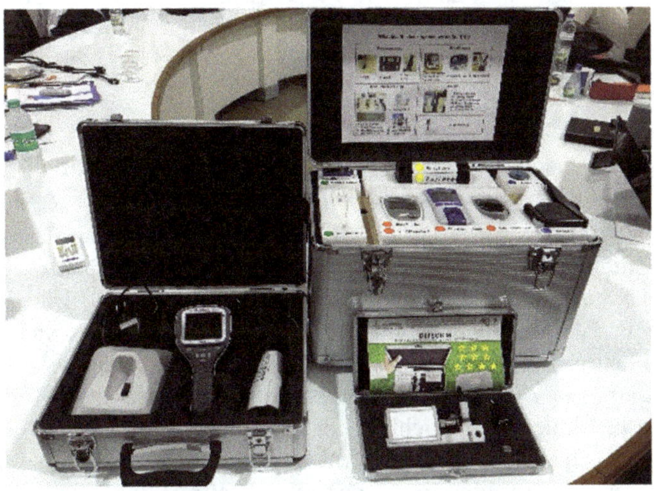

Figure 8.11 PHC with eye camera and DEPSOR [43]

together with workers, and preserve ecological safety. Preservation of the environment can enable workers and their families to keep developing the region by providing better living conditions and thus nourishing the next generation. As a result, much productive labor power can be available sustainably.

Moreover, the medical insurance system can be established in developing countries if preventive actions such as health checkups are introduced in the occupational health field. Because some countries have implemented a medical insurance system on the bases of workers, and this mutual assistance system is acceptable for regions whose economic status is chronically insecure and shortage. This system can achieve the idea of Universal Health Coverage [45]. Based on the example of Japan which makes the universal insurance and world's best longevity, the approach of PHC and environmental assessment on occupational health can effective to promote people's health in the countries having immature health care system and medical insurance system. This type of PHC activities should contribute to keeping sustainable health for many people, and it may be a key that employers collaborate with workers and their families, and the surrounding environment.

8.7 Conclusion

Being a modular system, new medical service features will be gradually added to PHC system. There is a huge demand of new specialized services from the local communities as they face a wide range of diseases in their daily life. In the next step, we hope to add skin care and dental care module as a priority. Gradually, it will also add some communicable diseases support system. This will increase patient's satisfaction as well as trust to PHC because they will be able to receive even secondary level services for a wide range of common diseases. Finally, this advancement will contribute to the sustainability of the PHC business model in remote communities.

References

[1] Ahmed A, Hargrave AR, Nohara Y, *et al.* "Portable health clinic: a Telemedicine system for unreached communities" in *Smart Sensors and Systems, Springer International Publishing*, 447–467, 2015.

[2] Ghose P, Islam R, Nakashima N, Nohara Y, Ahmed A, and Shimizu S, Effectiveness of preventive healthcare through Telemedicine in Bangladesh, *Proceedings of 18th ISfTeH International Conference*, 2013.

[3] Yokota F, Ahmed A, Kikuchi K, Nishikitani M, Islam R, and Nakashima N, Diabetes, obesity, and hypertension in Bheramara Kushtia District, Bangladesh – results from portable health clinic data, 2013–2016, *Proceeding of Social Business Academia Conference*, 2016.

[4] Nohara Y, Kai E, Ghosh P, *et al.* Health checkup and telemedical intervention program for preventive medicine in developing countries: verification study. *J Med Internet Res*, 2015; 17(1).

[5] Islam R, Ahmed A, Nakashima N, and Shimizu S, GramHealth: an integrated Tele-Healthcare system for unreached communities, *Proc. of 11st Asian Telemedicine Symposium*, 2017.

[6] Islam R, Nohara Y, Rahman MJ, Sultana N, Ahmed A, and Nakashima N, Portable health clinic: an advanced Tele-Healthcare system for unreached communities, Ebook: MEDINFO 2019: Health & Wellbeing e-Network for All, Volume 264, 416–419.

[7] Kerber KJ, de Graft-Johnson JE, Bhutta ZA, Okong P, Starrs A, and Lawn JE. Continuum of care for maternal, newborn, and child health: from slogan to service delivery. Lancet. 2007; 370(9595): 1358–1369.

[8] WHO. Global health observatory data 2015 [cited 2017 June 1]. Available from: http://who.int/gho/en/

[9] The Partnership for Maternal N, and Child Health. Newborn death and illness 2011 [cited 2017 June 1]. Available from: http://who.int/pmnch/media/press_materials/fs/fs_newborndeath_illness/en/

[10] Bhutta ZA, Das JK, Bahl R, *et al.* Can available interventions end preventable deaths in mothers, newborn babies, and stillbirths, and at what cost? Lancet. 2014; 384(9940): 347–370.

[11] Froen JF, Friberg IK, Lawn JE, *et al.* Stillbirths: progress and unfinished business. Lancet. 2016; 387(10018): 574–586.

[12] UN. Sustainable Development Goals [cited 2017 June 1]. Available from: http://un.org/sustainabledevelopment/

[13] The Partnership for Maternal N, and Child Health. PMNCH knowledge summary #02 enable the continuum of care. Geneva, Switzerland: The Partnership for Maternal, Newborn, and Child Health; 2010.

[14] WHO. Pregnancy, childbirth, postpartum and newborn care: a guide for essential practice. Geneva, Switzerland: WHO; 2003.

[15] Hand C. Measuring health-related quality of life in adults with chronic conditions in primary care settings. Can Fam Physician 2016; 62(7): e375–e383.

[16] Ahammed A, Pathan F, Afsana F, *et al.* The burden of severe hypoglycemia on quality of life among diabetes mellitus patients in a tertiary level hospital of Bangladesh. Indian J Endocrinol Metab 2018; 22(4): 499–504.

[17] Saleh F, Ara F, Mumu SJ, and Hafez MA. Assessment of health-related quality of life of Bangladeshi patients with type 2 diabetes using the EQ-5D: a cross-sectional study. BMC Res Notes 2015; 8: 497.

[18] Safita N, Islam SM, Chow CK, *et al.* The impact of type 2 diabetes on health related quality of life in Bangladesh: results from a matched study comparing treated cases with non-diabetic controls. Health Qual Life Outcomes 2016; 14(1): 129.

[19] Mahumud RA, Ali N, Sheikh N, *et al.* Measuring perinatal and postpartum quality of life of women and associated factors in semi-urban Bangladesh. Qual Life Res. 2019.

[20] Bashar M, Ahmed K, Uddin MS, *et al.* Depression and quality of life among postmenopausal women in Bangladesh: a cross-sectional study. J Menopausal Med 2017; 23(3): 172–181.

[21] Hassan MR, Kabir S, Basher AE, *et al.* Quality of life in children with asthma in Bangladesh. Mymensingh Med J 2017; 26(3): 471–476.

[22] Rahman M, Afroz S, Ali R, and Hanif M. Health related quality of life in children with nephrotic syndrome in Bangladesh. Mymensingh Med J 2016; 25(4): 703–709.

[23] Jahan MU, Karim MR, Rahman A, and Akhter S. Cognitive functions and health related quality of life of institutional autism spectrum disorder children in Dhaka city. Bangladesh Med Res Counc Bull 2015; 41(3): 151–159.

[24] Mitry D, Williams C, Northstone K, *et al.* Perceptual visual dysfunction, physical impairment and quality of life in Bangladeshi children with cerebral palsy. Br J Ophthalmol 2016; 100(9): 1245–1250.

[25] Rahman MM, Hossain AFMA, Ahsan A, *et al.* Moving beyond cancer: immediate impact on-the health-related quality of life of breast cancer patients after mastectomy. Bangladesh Med Res Counc Bull 2015; 41(2): 52–58.

[26] Rahman MM, Ahsan MA, Monalisa NN, and Rahman K. Influence of socioeconomic status and BMI on the quality of life after mastectomy in Bangladeshi breast cancer patients in a public hospital. Jpn J Clin Oncol 2014; 44(12): 1150–1157.

[27] Hossain N, Akter QM, Banu F, and Mahmud S. Quality of life of cervical cancer patients after completion of treatment–a study among Bangladeshi women. Bangladesh Med Res Counc Bull 2015; 41(3): 131–137.

[28] Hossain MS, Rahman MA, Bowden JL, *et al.* Psychological and socio-economic status, complications and quality of life in people with spinal cord injuries after discharge from hospital in Bangladesh: a cohort study. Spinal Cord 2016; 54(6): 483–489.

[29] Hossain MS, Islam MS, Rahman MA, *et al.* Health status, quality of life and socioeconomic situation of people with spinal cord injuries six years after discharge from a hospital in Bangladesh. Spinal Cord. 2019.

[30] Walker SH, Ambauen-Berger B, Saha SL, and Akhter S. Quality of life among women in Bangladesh following ileal conduit urinary diversion operations for irreparable vesicovaginal fistula and bladder exstrophy: observational study. BJOG 2018; 125(5): 616–622.

[31] Quadir MM, Lee YJ, Hoque R, Karim MM, and Alamgir H. How are the surviving workers of the Rana Plaza factory collapse in Bangladesh doing: quality of life, participation restriction, income and occupation. Disabil Rehabil 2019; 18: 1–7.

[32] Imoto A, Matsuyama A, Ambauen-Berger B, and Honda S. Health-related quality of life among women in rural Bangladesh after surgical repair of obstetric fistula. Int J Gynaecol Obstet 2015; 130(1): 79–83.

[33] Hossain MS, Hasan MM, Islam MS, *et al.* Chikungunya outbreak (2017) in Bangladesh: clinical profile, economic impact and quality of life during the acute phase of the disease. PLoS Negl Trop Dis 2018; 12(6): 1–16.

[34] Uddin MA, Soivong P, Lasuka D, and Juntasopeepun P. Factors related to quality of life among older adults in Bangladesh: a cross sectional survey. Nurs Health Sci 2017; 19(4): 518–524.

[35] Uddin MN, Bhar S, Al Mahmud A, and Islam FMA. Psychological distress and quality of life: rationale and protocol of a prospective cohort study in a rural district in Bangaladesh. BMJ Open 2017; 7(9): 1–10.

[36] Tsutsumi A, Izutsu T, Islam AM, *et al.* The quality of life, mental health, and perceived stigma of leprosy patients in Bangladesh. Soc Sci Med 2007; 64 (12): 2443–2453.

[37] Laskar MS, Rahaman MM, Akhter A, *et al.* Quality of life of arsenicosis patients in an arsenic-affected rural area in Bangladesh. Arch Environ Occup Health 2010; 65(2): 70–76.

[38] Gomez-Olive FX, Schröders J, Aboderin I, *et al.* Variations in disability and quality of life with age and sex between eight lower income and middle-income countries: data from the INDEPTH WHO-SAGE collaboration. BMJ Glob Health 2017; 2(4): 1–11.

[39] Imam MH, Karim MR, Ferdous C, and Akhter S. Health related quality of life among the people living with HIV. Bangladesh Med Res Counc Bull 2011; 37(1): 1–6.

[40] Forastieri V. Improving health in the workplace: ILO's framework for action. Fact Sheet. International Labour Organization. !6 October 2014. https://ilo.org/safework/info/publications/WCMS_329350/lang–en/index.htm (accessed on Aug 15, 2019)

[41] Horie S. Sangyo Hoken no Seisaku to Gakujutu no Kokusai Doko (Global trend of occupational health policy and academia). Kousei no Shihyo (Journal of health and welfare statistics) 2015. 62(13): 1–8. (Japanese)

[42] KYORITSU CHEMICAL-CHECK Lab., Corp. Simplified Water Analysis Products. https://kyoritsu-lab.co.jp/english/index.html (accessed on Aug 15, 2019)

[43] Bio Solutions. DEPSOR-M. Available from: http://biyanibiosolutions.com/ (accessed on Aug 15, 2019)

[44] Biyani M, Biyani R, Tsuchihashi T, *et al.* DEP-on-go for simultaneous sensing of multiple heavy metals pollutants in environmental samples. Sensors (Basel). 2017; 17(1): 45.

[45] World Health Organization. Universal health coverage. Available from: https://who.int/westernpacific/our-work/universal-health-coverage

Chapter 9

PHC and case studies of remote healthcare services in Asian countries

Fumihiko Yokota[1], Manish Biyani[2], Yuandong Hu[3], Kimiyo Kikuchi[1], Faiz Shah[4], Junko Yasuoka[5], Keiko Nanishi[6], Rowena Alcoba[4] and Amina Noureen[4]

This chapter introduces the case studies of remote healthcare services in Cambodia, China, India, and Pakistan, aimed at preventing noncommunicable diseases (NCDs). In Cambodia, India, and Pakistan, the portable health clinic (PHC) has been customized or modified to fit specific needs of the various targeted populations; whereas in China, it relies on government-initiated systems. Case studies from each country describe processes at different stages of designing, planning, implementing, monitoring, and evaluating remote healthcare services, and outline challenges and future courses.

9.1 Processes of co-design and co-implementation in a portable health clinic research project in Jaipur District, India (March 2016–August 2019)

In India, the PHC research project started in March 2016 as a community-based health check-up service project under a collaboration among Kyushu University (KU) in Japan, Grameen Communications (GC) in Bangladesh, and Biyani Group of College (BGC) in India as part of the Future Earth Research Project (Figure 9.1). The initial collaboration on India PHC project began in 2012, when a research director of the BGC expressed his strong interest in the PHCs, which were presented by professors from the KU at the sixth Asia Telemedicine Symposium in

[1] Institute of Decision Science for a Sustainable Society, Kyushu University, Fukuoka, Japan
[2] Biyani Group of Colleges, Rajasthan, India
[3] Institute of Chronic Disease, Guizhou Provincial Center for Disease Control, Guizhou, China
[4] Yunus Center, Asian Institute of Technology, Bangkok, Thailand
[5] Research and Education Center for Prevention of Global Infectious Diseases of Animals, Tokyo University of Agriculture and Technology, Tokyo, Japan
[6] Office of International Academic Affairs, Graduate School of Medicine, The University of Tokyo, Tokyo, Japan

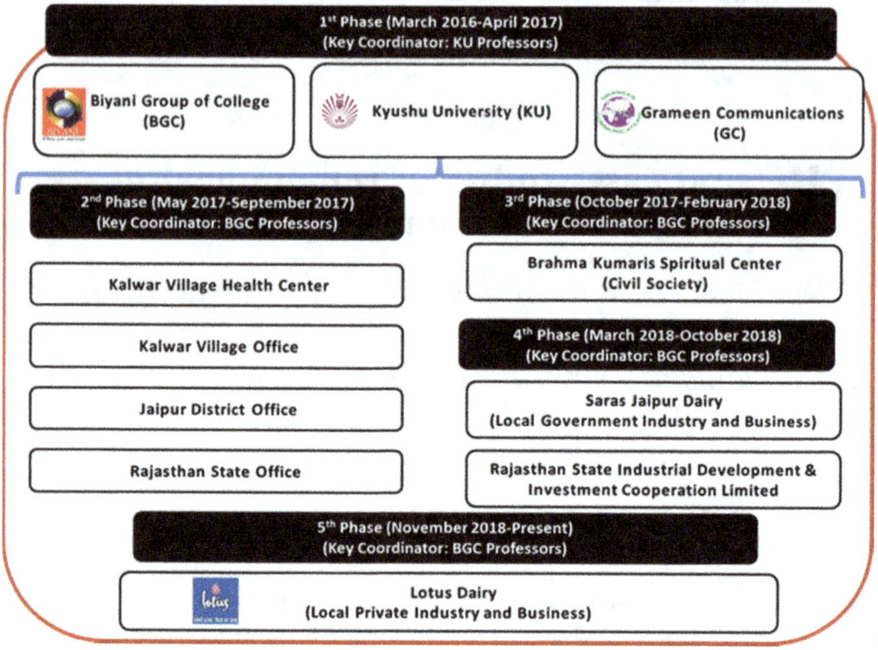

Figure 9.1 Stakeholders and key coordinators for the PHC project in India

Japan. India PHC project aimed to provide sustainable mobile health check-up services in collaboration with local government agencies, industries, and communities in Rajasthan, India.

9.1.1 First phase (March 2016–April 2017)

During the first phase, these objectives related to the sustainable development goals (SDGs) such as "Good health and wellbeing (goal #3)" and "Partnerships for the goals (goal #17)" were shared and agreed among the KU, the GC, and the BGC. In the first phase as a pilot phase, development of research plan, training workshops, implementation of research, data analysis, and result feedback workshop were conducted in collaboration with the KU, the GC, and the BGC. The key person who locally coordinated these pilot activities was BGC research director (Figure 9.1).

9.1.2 Second phase (May 2017–September 2017)

In the second phase, the KU and the BGC research teams visited the following agencies in Rajasthan state in May 2017: the Government of Rajasthan's & Jaipur's Department of Medical, Health, and Family Welfare; the Kalwar Village Office; and the Kalwar Health Center (Figure 9.1). This process was smoothly facilitated by the BGC having pre-established relationships with the mayor of Kalwar Village and a director of Rajasthan's Department of Medical, Health, and Family Welfare. We have visited these agencies at least two times in 2017 to discuss and understand about their needs, priorities, and local regulations related to health issues, which can be supported by our PHC projects. As a result, we could receive the official agreement and approval letter from these agencies, which facilitate us to implement our PHC activities in Rajasthan, India.

9.1.3 Third phase (October 2017–February 2018)

The third phase began in October 2017, when the KU and the BGC signed an official academic collaborative agreement. Based on the revised research plan and protocol which was based on the needs and priorities from Rajasthan, Jaipur, and Kalwar village offices (second phase), we decided to investigate the health needs, priorities, and effects of the PHC services among different populations in Jaipur District. To achieve these objectives, it was necessary to provide check-up services to the same individuals over a period of time in order to monitor long-term changes in their health status, behaviors, needs, and priorities. We recognized that it was easier to follow up with members of civil society organizations than with general community residents over the years. Consequently, the BGC conducted first PHC service at the Brahma Kumaris World Spiritual University (BKWSU) for more than 200 members of the BKWSU (Figure 9.1).

9.1.4 Fourth phase (March 2018–October 2018)

The fourth phase started in March 2018. However, unlike members of civil society organization in the third phase, the target population was government industry employees, because we found insufficient needs for health check-up services among the BKWSU and they were not able to sustain our PHC project neither as health insurance scheme nor as a business due to their financial issues. Therefore, in the fourths phase, we aim to develop our partnership with local business industries. First, the BGC staff searched local industries to schedule a meeting explaining our PHC project. After several industries were contacted, one of the largest milk product enterprises in Rajasthan State, Saras Jaipur Dairy (SJD), expressed strong interest in providing health check-ups for their employees, and agreed to let us use their facility rooms (Figure 9.1). In March 2018, PHC services were conducted for a total of 205 employees who participated in both the check-up and survey interview. The process of PHC services provided at the SJD during the fourth phase was the same as previous phases (Figure 9.2). However, our PHC services could neither continue as a business model nor as a health insurance scheme in a sustainable manner.

From the previous phases, we learned that there were needs for eye check-up and traditional Indian doctors (Ayurveda) among factory employees in Jaipur district, India. In addition, factory employees needed more detailed blood tests including HbA1c for diabetes and HDL/LDL cholesterol. Therefore, the Indian PHC services were customized according to specific population's needs.

We also learned difficulties to implement long-term sustainable health check-up services for government factory employees due to following reasons: (1) low

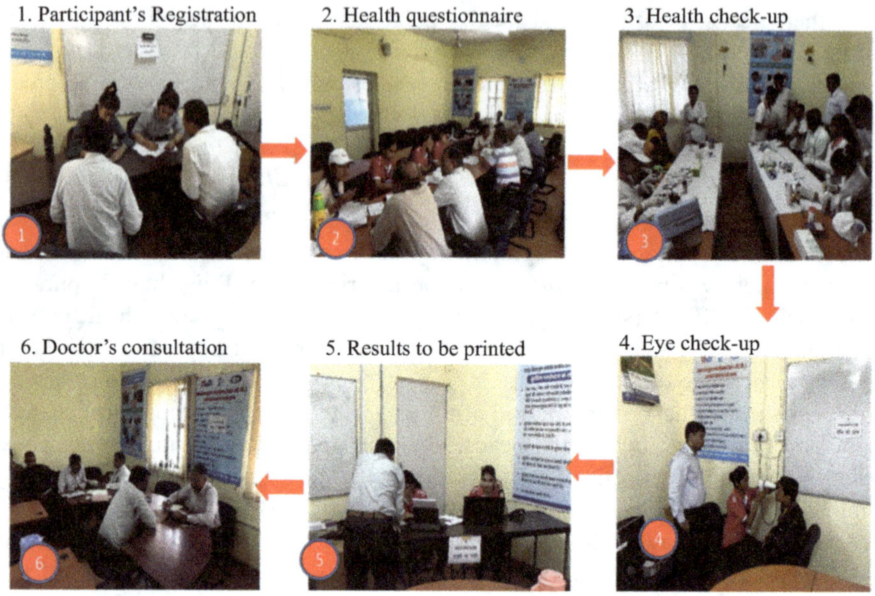

Figure 9.2 Processes of PHC health check-ups for government industry employees in India

awareness for health, (2) low perceived needs for PHC, (3) very slow government approval process and required paper works, and (4) low accountability to initiate new sustainable health check-up system. In the fifth phase, therefore, we changed our collaborative partners from government company to private companies.

9.1.5 Fifth phase (November 2018–Present)

From September to October 2018, we have searched any potential private companies who are interested in implementing PHC for their employees in a long term as a health insurance scheme or as a social business. From the BGC's principle's network, we found that Lotus Dairy (LD) Milk Company is interested in the PHC health check-up services for their employees and they were willing to provide their own factory's facility room as a PHC and willing to pay for a cost for medicines. The KU, the GC, the BGC, and the LD had several meetings to discuss "how can we continue to implement PHC health check-up services for LD's employees even after research funds finish?" Based on the discussions, all four (the KU, the GC, the BGC, and the LD) could have official agreement on implementing sustainable PHC health check-up services for LD's factory employees in Jaipur district, India (Figure 9.3). The sustainable health check-up scheme is a cost-sharing scheme as below:

- The LD is to provide a cost for their factory clinic, electricity, water, and other clinic maintenance cost as well as cost for medical drugs.

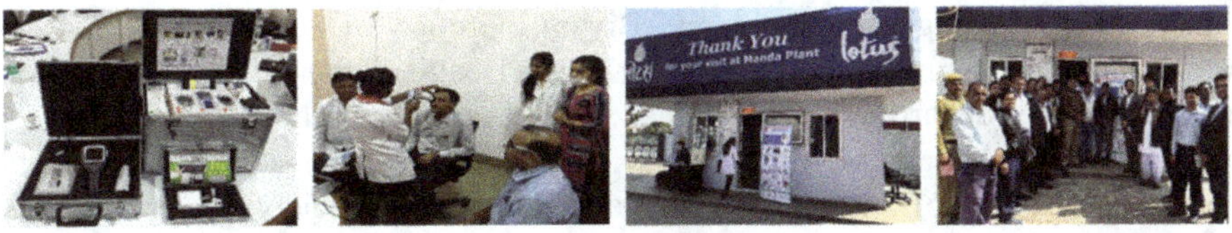

Figure 9.3 Newly customized PHC provided for factory employees by the KU, the GC, and the BGC, at Lotus Dairy and Lotus Manda factory clinic in phase 5 (November 2018–Present)

- The BGC is to provide a cost for human resources (coordinator, Ayurveda doctor, health workers, and IT technicians).
- The GC is to provide technical assistances on data management and software for PHC system.
- The KU is to provide scientific knowledge and evidence on effects and impacts of health check-up and tele-consultation services (data collection, data analysis, publish academic papers, etc.), and provide consumables for health check-up for first 1 or 2 years.

9.1.6 Summary of co-design and co-production processes in all five phases

In all phases that we described in this section, we utilized the seven processes for co-design and co-implementation with stakeholders: (1) jointly develop and revise a research plan and protocol which includes research objectives, methods, timelines, activity schedules, and budgets; (2) reach collaborative agreement and consensus on the research plan and protocol with both academic and nonacademic stakeholders through meetings, consultations, and workshops; (3) conduct local research staff training workshops based on the protocol in order to improve the quality of services and quality of data jointly with stakeholders; (4) implement the pilot PHC health check-up research involving all stakeholders; (5) analyze, disseminate, and provide feedback on the results with all stakeholders through presentations, seminars, workshops, and conferences; (6) revise the research plan and protocol based on feedback such as local needs, priorities, and requests from stakeholders, and (7) develop and implement sustainable PHC social business model (business partners, staff, customers, business services and products, service delivery process and activities, business resources, cost structures, time frame, target locations, and marketing plan).

Acknowledgments

This research was funded by the Future Earth Research Fund, grant number 18-161009264; and the Kyushu University QR Program, grant number 30105. Special thanks to following stakeholders: Biyani Group of Colleges, Grameen Communications, Kalwar village office, Kalwar Health Center, Jaipur District and Rajasthan state department of medical, health, and family welfare, Brahma Kumaris Spiritual Centers, Saras Dairy, and Lotus Dairy, India, and Kyushu University, Institute of Decision Science and Sustainable Society.

9.2 All-in-one health machine project in rural area of China

9.2.1 Introduction

40.4% of Chinese population, about 564 million people, live in the rural area [1]. The Chinese central government has implemented several national projects to improve the primary healthcare of rural area, such as the essential public health service (EPHS) and the new rural cooperative medical system (NRCMS) [2]. With huge investment in the last two decades, 632,057 village clinics were built to provide primary healthcare to every village of China (Figure 9.4(a)) [3].

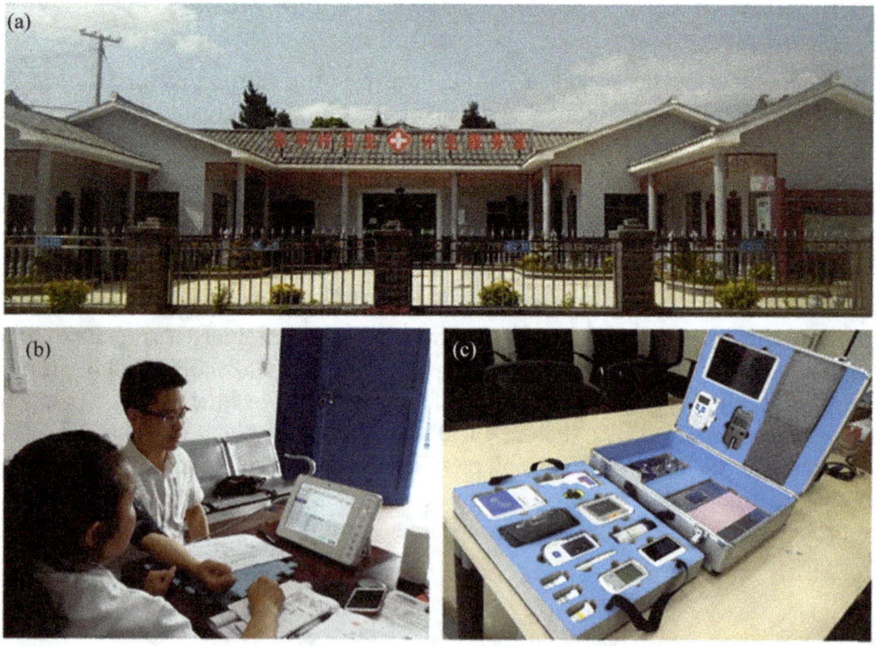

Figure 9.4 (a) A newly built village clinic; (b) the village doctor is using AIO Health Machine to measure a resident's blood pressure; (c) the new generation of AIO Health Machine

Medical information technology has been considered as one of the 12 key fields of China's National Informatization Strategy from 2016 to 2020, according to the State Council of China [4]. To empower the healthcare service of village clinics, the central government of China and most of its provincial governments have implemented the all-in-one (AIO) Health Machine project since 2014 [5].

9.2.2 Implementation of AIO health machine project

9.2.2.1 Functions of AIO Health Machine

According to the provincial procurement notices, AIO Health Machine has at least seven essential functions: (1) 12-leads electrocardiogram; (2) heart rate; (3) blood glucose; (4) blood pressure; (5) blood oxygen; (6) urine test; and (7) body temperature. The second category was requirements for data management, for AIO Health Machine is considered as an important part in the national strategy of building electronic personal health record of every Chinese resident [6]. Besides browsing and saving the health check-up results, AIO Health Machine is required to support data exchanging with the personal health record system of EPHS through the Internet. It was also required to read the personal information from the ID cards of Chinese residents, which have a unique 18-digit number for every resident [7,8]. Some manufactures have added optional modules, such as blood urine acid and blood lipid test into their product to make it more competitive [9].

9.2.2.2 Procurement of AIO Health Machine

The provincial government plays the key role in the procurement of AIO Health Machine. The government needs to release a notice of invitation for bids on certain government procurement website to declare its demands, including the purchase amount, expected bidding price, etc.

9.2.2.3 Allocation and supervision of AIO Health Machine

After the procurement, the AIO Health Machine will be allocated to each village clinic. Training of how to use of AIO Health Machine was conducted by the engineer of manufacturer. The engineer will display how to do health check with AIO Health Machine, and how to maintain and calibrate the machine.

9.2.3 Challenges and problems in the application of AIO Health Machine

As of this writing, the central and provincial governments of China have purchased and allocated about 60,000 AIO Health Machine. The price of one single machine has dropped from 20,000 Chinese Yuan to 8,000 Chinese Yuan in last 5 years [5,7,8].

Although there is no official statistics data of the actual application situation, the AIO Health Machines have not lived up to the government's expectation according to sporadic reports. In one investigation conducted by the local government of Zhuzhou, Hunan Province, in 2017, the average monthly use frequency was 34.53 times for each AIO Health Machine. In some investigated village clinics, their machines were still in sealed condition at several months after allocation. In the unsealed ones, some never upload any data either [10].

There are several reasons for this problem. The first one is the inadequate medical training of village doctors, most of which only received a 3-year or even 6-month medical training before working in the village clinic. Because the rural resident doctor's salary is not as attractive as other jobs for young people, only elders are willing to be village doctor in most village. Since their age and education level, many village doctors have very little knowledge of electronic device and the Internet.

Besides the shortage of qualified primary healthcare staff, the defects of the AIO Health Machine themselves exacerbate the problem. To use the machine properly, there are dozens of parameters to be set, and several types of docking port to connect. Though the manufacturer has conducted a brief training when allocating the machine as referred, many village doctors still got lost in the maze of setting network parameters, import, and export of data.

9.2.4 Possible solutions for better usage of AIO Health Machine

Many provinces of China have started to improve the education, working condition, and payment of village doctor in recent years. According to "the 3-year Medical Service Promoting Project, 2016–2018" of Guizhou Province, if a staff of primary medical agency has passed the entrance examination of medical college for further education and promised working in the same agency for certain years after graduation, the local government will pay for his tuition fee [11]. In another ambitious plan of Guizhou Province, 3,500 of directional training medical students, 3,000 general practitioners, and assistant general practitioners will be introduced to primary healthcare agency within 3 years. The Guizhou Province's target is to allocate at least one qualified doctor in 30% of villages clinics by 2022 [12].

In 2019, the local government of Anqing, Anhui Province, has implemented an experimental "Smart Medical Assistant" project. One aim of this project is to realize the real-time remote consultation between primary medical agency and superior hospital. Consultant of superior hospital can review the health-check data of AIO Health Machines and give his advice online. Smart medical assistant can also give computer aide diagnosis (CAD) suggestion by using a AI decision-making module. The government hopes that this technology will compensate the inadequacy of village doctor's education and experience [13].

As a large-scale reform of information technology in primary medical care, the advanced nature and technique potential of AIO Health Machines are admitted by all the stakeholders, including medical staffs, researchers, and government officials. Other than the developing and purchasing, the major challenge is to find a sustainable mode of application. In the ideal mode, qualified medical staff can receive reasonable payment by offering cheap and convenient heath-check service to the residents of rural areas with AIO Health Machines.

9.3 Remote monitoring to improve the continuum of care in mothers and newborns in Cambodia

9.3.1 Introduction

Following the millennium development goals from 2001 to 2015, SDGs have called for reducing the maternal and child mortality and morbidity rates [14]. These rates have shown measurable reduction. However, the incidence of preventable deaths remains high in low- and middle-income countries in Southeast Asia [15]. One of the main reasons could be the inadequate uptake of care for mothers and newborns during the antenatal, delivery, and postnatal periods. In this context, the concept of "the continuum of care" has been promoted in the field of global health to improve the maternal and newborn's health status [16]. The concept calls for increasing the uptake of care for mothers and newborns successively from the antenatal to postnatal periods. However, in most remote areas, realizing the successive uptake of care faces such challenges as long distance and lack of transportation from the home to the health facilities. To address this problem, the Integrated Continuum of Care Project has been conducted in Ratanakiri, Cambodia, in collaboration between National Center for Parasitology, Entomology and Malaria Control, Cambodia (CNM), Ratanakiri Provincial Health Department, Kyushu University, Tokyo University of Agriculture and Technology, and the University of Tokyo. The project aimed to realize the continuum of care in remote areas by designating village malaria workers the role of providing the health services to mothers and newborns using ICT. This ICT component was elaborated by Kyushu University and CNM. This study aimed to introduce the mechanism of this system and the challenges to promoting it as a standard monitoring system in Cambodia.

9.3.2 Intervention

The project conducted the intervention in the catchment area of seven selected health centers in Ratanakiri Province (Figure 9.5). The study population was approximately 380 women and their newborn who lived in the study area. Women who were between 16 weeks pregnant and 6 weeks in the postnatal period were included in the study. In the framework of the project's intervention, the village malaria workers visited the homes of women and newborns and provided health examination for them using a portable health kit, which was composed of a mobile internet communication device (tablet type personal computer) and medical equipment: sphygmomanometer, thermometer, weighing scale for the mother and newborn, height meter for the newborn, malaria rapid diagnostic test kit, and urine sugar and protein test slips (Figures 9.6–9.7). By registering the collected examination data in the triage software, the risk of complication in women and newborns could be detected. Those who were identified as at risk for complication received health workers' consultation through the internet video system and were referred to the nearest health facility.

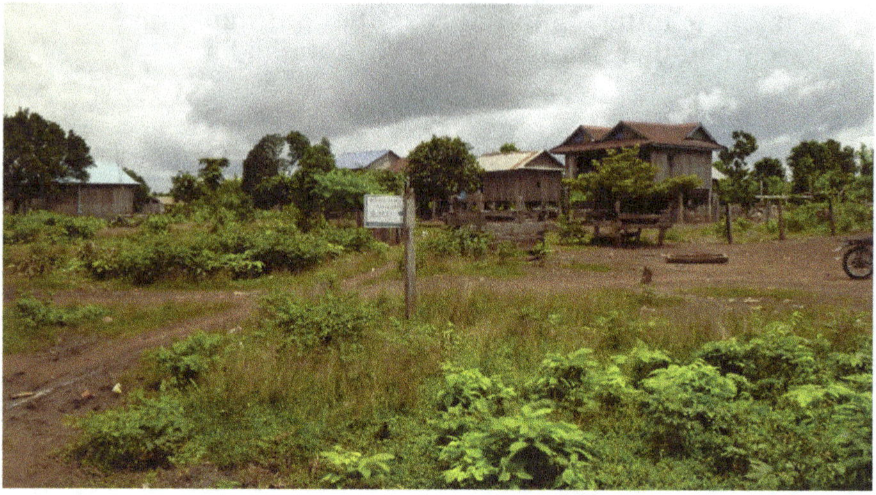

Figure 9.5 Local houses in Ratanakiri region

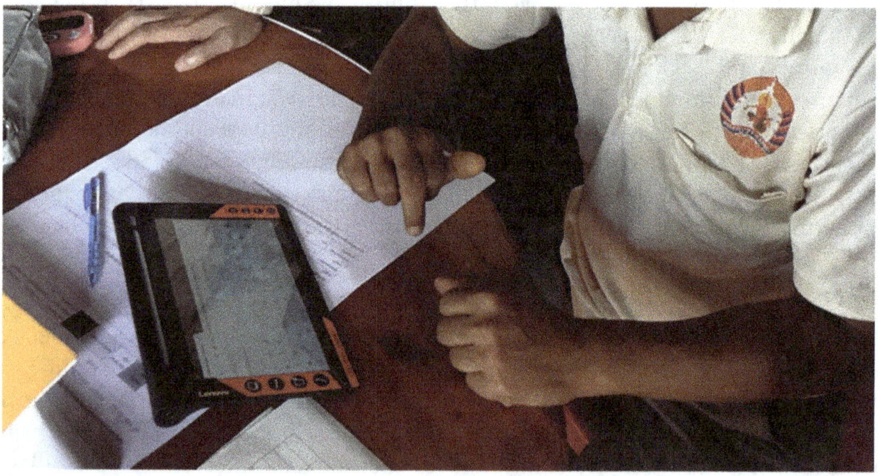

Figure 9.6 Computer devise training for village malaria workers

9.3.3 Identified challenges

During the intervention, the following challenges were observed. Village malaria workers needed basic internet and equipment knowledge, which requires advanced training. They need also technical follow-up supervision for their usage of the Internet and equipment. Moreover, countermeasures are needed to address their difficulty in visiting women's homes during the rainy season, when roads become impassable (Figures 9.8–9.9).

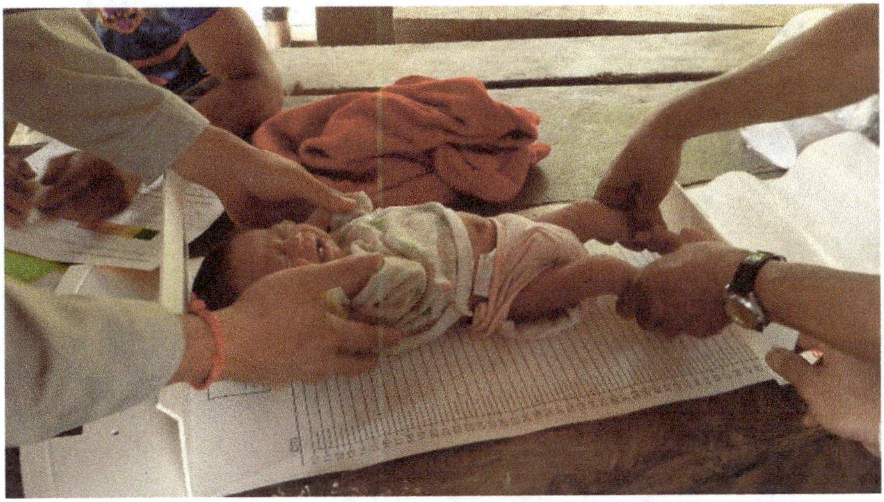

Figure 9.7 Height measurement of baby by village malaria workers

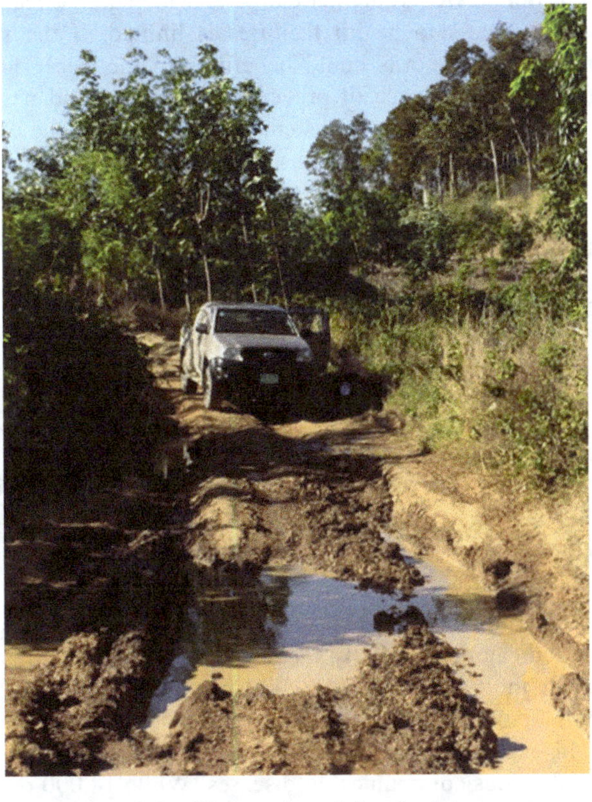

Figure 9.8 The road sunk by the heavy rain

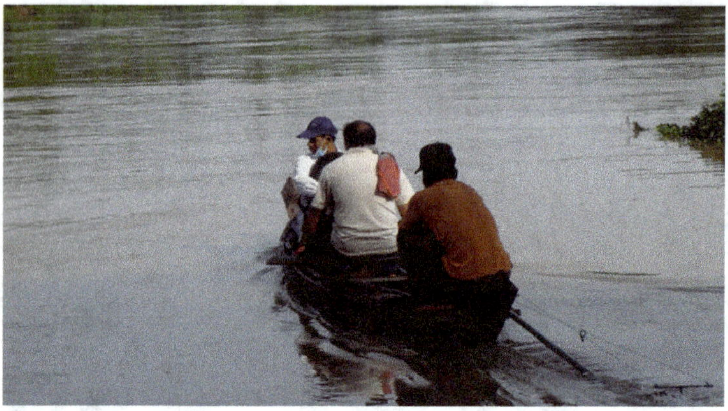

Figure 9.9 People often need to use a boat to get to the home of mothers

9.3.4 Conclusion

This ICT-based health service system could be considered an effective system for remote areas where access to health facilities is limited. If the system is well organized, women and newborns could benefit from the stable health services, which could reduce the incidence of preventable maternal and newborn complications. However, to disseminate the system to many areas, some challenges need to be addressed. Efforts are required to ensure the stability and accessibility of the health services system to enhance the continuum of care among women and newborns.

Acknowledgments

This study was funded by JSPS KAKENHI Grant Number JP15H05284.

9.4 Mobile health care for migrant workers along corporate supply chains in Kasur District, Pakistan

9.4.1 Introduction

Rural areas in Pakistan, home to almost 60% of its 204.596 million citizens, continue to carry a higher burden of disease, and as a result, a depressed quality of life. Pakistan's health indicators, especially for women and children, are comparatively low, with maternal mortality at 178/100,000 live births and infant mortality at 52/10,000, placing it 154th among 195 countries on the Healthcare Access Quality Index. With healthcare spending at 2.75% of GDP, almost 40% of the burden of disease is from infectious/communicable diseases. While 14,000 doctors graduate every year, 70% of them being women, there is only one doctor for every 1,475 persons. 70% healthcare delivery personnel and infrastructure are concentrated in big cities, and emphasize curative care, while 60% of the rural population across the country is served by under-qualified health practitioners.

Health conditions most commonly associated with poor rural communities, such as malnutrition and developmental deficiencies, diarrheal disease, respiratory infections, viral hepatitis, malaria, and tuberculosis, also significantly affect women and children. The high maternal mortality rate stems from unsafe childbirth practices carried out by untrained midwives. Likewise, morbidity rates among children reflect poor health-awareness among mothers and caregivers. More importantly, these are all conditions that can be addressed by preventive strategies.

The conventional response to insufficient healthcare facilities and lack of medical professionals in rural areas has been to make heavy investments in static infrastructure and a mobile health workforce. While there is evidence of initial success, these investments typically wither over time due to lack of budgetary support and staff attrition. As a result, many gains in grassroots healthcare delivery turn out to be financially, or programmatically unsustainable. On the other hand, even in the remotest rural communities in Pakistan, the nongovernmental sector bridges the gap in public-sector services. Private clinics, medical laboratories, pharmacies, domiciliary care facilities, physiotherapy centers, ambulance services, and allied healthcare providers are present in Pakistan's farthest communities. Such services are frequently provided by welfare or donor-funded initiatives; but as a rule, rural communities rely on fee-for-service providers for their immediate healthcare needs. Sadly, not all entrepreneurial service providers, particularly traditional healers or under-qualified practitioners, actually relieve the burden of disease because of mal-practice. Quality of care, therefore, remains a challenge.

Ensuring healthcare access to vulnerable and remote communities, particularly seasonal migrants, presents a multi-faceted challenge because of the sheer diversity of cultural, behavioral, and financial contexts that often escape macro-level planning. Exacerbated by nonavailability of trained healthcare professionals, and "distance decay effect," which is described in terms of the distance between patient households and healthcare service providers. This means that traditional responses, which typically comprise curative services delivered from static healthcare service hubs, sidestep communities that are most in need, and must be augmented by innovative preventive responses that are cost-effective and scalable.

In recent years, a number of healthcare delivery innovations have emerged in Pakistan, whose success indicates the ready uptake for enterprise-driven mobile health solutions. These illustrate the transforming landscape of access by introducing affordable and user-friendly options to hitherto un-reached patient segments, overcoming driven by disruptive technologies that sidestep technological gaps, social-cultural nuances, societal trust and skepticism, and data security integration. Of particular interest is the integration and inclusion of women into the healthcare delivery mainstream, whether doctors pulled away from clinical careers, or women patients restrained in mobility.

One such initiative, doctHERs capitalizes on home-based women doctors to offer telemedicine consultations, and charges 20% service fee. The program serves

250,000 slum residents in Karachi, partnering with government, as well as expanding into overseas markets, particularly in the Middle East. Another mobile health initiative, Sehat Kahani, specifically targets disadvantaged communities, offering to "democratize" healthcare through its 14 e-health clinics spread across urban and rural locations all over Pakistan, and having reached 600,000 people. Interestingly, Sehat Kahani and doctHERS are collaborating to capitalize on the potential of 15,000 home-based women doctors to provide consultation, health awareness, and health caregiver training. Start-up, Marham, has a mobile phone application allowing users to search for doctors, book appointments, and provide feedback on an open forum. More particularly, it offers a repository of retrievable patient records for attending physicians. With 12,000 doctors and 300,000+ subscribers, Marham processes 50,000 appointments and 20,000 reviews, every month, serving 5 million patients from within and outside Pakistan.

9.4.2 PHC as delivery system integrator

Within this fast-moving yet selective healthcare delivery context, the GramHealth Portable Health Clinic (PHC) was chosen as the core component of a corporate pilot project. Named SehatMobile, the project sought to mitigate health risks for seasonal migrant workers engaged in the collection and sorting of agricultural and nonagricultural waste that form the raw material for the company's primary product. Migrant agri-waste workers are a marginalized community that follows the sowing-cropping cycle along a well-defined geographical axis, yet typically subsists outside community-based social nets. Often ignored by the national welfare system, they are exposed to health hazards associated with "tuberculosis, asthma, cough, skin diseases, allergies and other contagious diseases." The PHC was seen to fit the need for an out-of-the-box solution for the following rationale:

- Focus on preventive rather than curative care, so that financial and opportunity cost of curative care is reduce.
- Affordable access to qualified practitioners, so that workers are less exposed to mal-practice and quackery.
- Entrepreneurial model of service, so that the budgetary burden on corporate resources is minimized.
- Technology-driven triage that is independent of practitioner discretion, so that quality of care is higher.
- Integration of patient data across service delivery tiers, so that healthcare outreach strategies can be optimized.
- Real-time, remote, and data-rich decision support for practitioners, so that the quality of care professional remains high.
- Portability and scalability, so that mobile fieldworkers to take preventive healthcare services to the very doorstep via ubiquitous mobile networks.

For SehatMobile, PHC became a delivery system integrator, for an integrated service platform offering preventive care, clinical services, screening, referral and follow-up, with added elements for social empowerment through education on health and nutrition, reproductive rights, and citizenship. Design criteria included service innovation, need-responsiveness, demonstrability, and value-for-money. As the core technology platform for the SehatMobile outreach model, the PHC ties together a custom-built vehicle platform equipped with specialized modular service consoles to deliver:

A. *Primary Care Ambulatory, Tertiary Referral, & Follow up*: Full-time SehatMobile staff conducting outpatient clinic supported by the PHC's 16-parameter tele-medicine protocol, and triaging patients by color-coded results. Data of specialist physicians designated by their host institute available online during agreed time-slots to backstop the outpatient clinic. Medical records centralized online to help referrals and followed up.

B. *Health Education, Preventive Care, & Occupational Safety*: Specialists from collaborating partners conducting awareness and education in preventive medicine, nutrition, hygiene and sanitation practices, and occupational health. Awareness and behavior change communication materials and staff provided by program partners to run sessions and demonstrate personal protective equipment (PPEs) and emergency response drills.

C. *Rights & Citizenship Awareness & Community Organization*: Collaborating community or citizens organizations using SehatMobile as platform for existing programs on citizenship awareness and community action for human rights, access to justice and community empowerment as part of the SehatMobile schedule.

D. *Social Business Skilling & Entrepreneurship Training*: Invited specialists offering training and pre-incubation, and community champions promoting independent and entrepreneurial thinking among migrant communities, motivating workers' families and friends to organize into social businesses, such as recycling cooperatives, so that members claim social security benefits or workers' compensation under existing law.

9.4.3 SehatMobile design and implementation

The pilot was designed for implementation at two distinct but integrated levels. The first phase included the design and fabrication of one SehatMobile vehicle installed with PHC and ancillary service delivery systems, training of project staff, induction of delivery partners and the establishment of a field-based clinicians' referral network, and handing over the tested SehatMobile to the corporate partner in Kasur, Pakistan. The second phase included technical backstopping, over a 12-month pilot phase, and the implementation of a hand-over strategy toward a successor arrangement. The advantage of such a phased approach was that it the pilot was able to seamlessly integrate into future programs in response to emerging demand. The SehatMobile unit was delivered in mid-2017, and since the culmination of the backstopping phase, is now fully rolled out.

The unit, as designed, carries one primary care house physician, one nurse or medical auxiliary, one ICT data technician, and one driver-assistant. There is room for up to two visiting specialists, contributed by program partners according to an

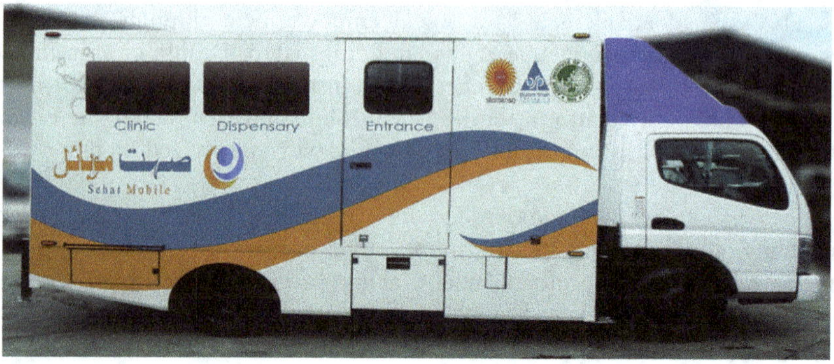

Figure 9.10 The SehatMobile vehicle platform ready for deployment

agreed schedule, to provide consultations in medical specialties, screening and diagnostics, ambulatory procedures, as well as health education, reproductive health services or citizenship and mobilization (Figure 9.10).

9.4.4 Opportunities and challenges

The original design illustrates the PHC's value beyond simply a mobile health technology platform. The Pakistan experience indicates its utility as a hub for a variety of wellbeing initiatives. The piloted model demonstrates a ready interface with target populations, zero-cost mobilization, and high-impact penetration of ideas, services, and products through partnerships leveraging mutual benefit. Delivery partners chosen for the pilot were a select few, but the potential for involving wider stakeholder participation makes SehatMobile a reliable coordinating hub for healthcare and wellbeing services at the doorstep to under-served communities.

The challenge specific to the SehatMobile vehicle platform is the high-cost of fabrication and maintenance. However, the pilot confirmed that the PHC technology core lends itself to numerous adaptive uses, which can be tailored to fit a variety of terrain, and tighter budgets. The follow-up being planned for Pakistan's Balochistan Province aims to apply learnings from the Kasur pilot into designing a need-responsive fee-for-service model that requires less start-up investment.

9.4.5 Conclusion

Within Pakistan's context, SehatMobile serves to address two challenges. First, it enables remote and underprivileged populations with poor access to healthcare and wellbeing services to be included in the national mainstream using expanding and ubiquitous technology. Second, online availability of healthcare providers, augmented with face-to-face engagement with key service providers, skill-teachers, and opinion leaders, empowers marginalized communities to expand horizons, integrate with the mainstream, and acquire new insights and experiences that enhance novel livelihood opportunities for more and more people.

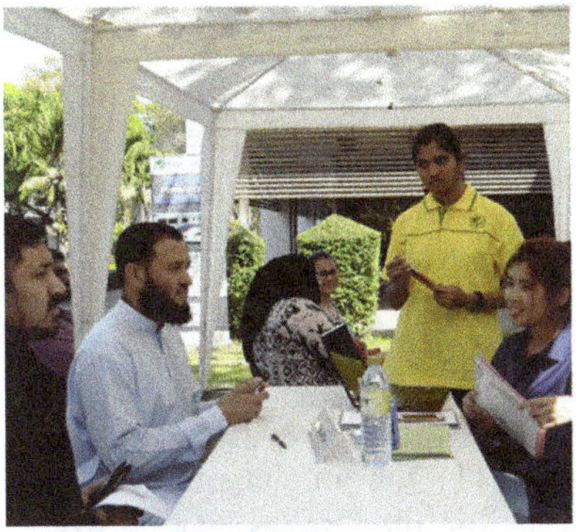

(a) Registration interview

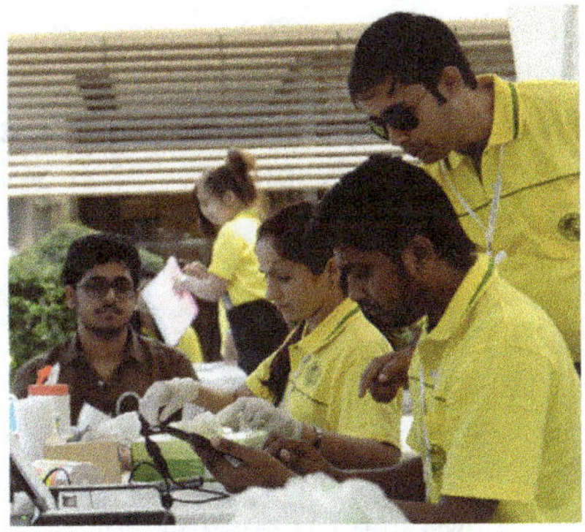

(b) Data entry & cross-check

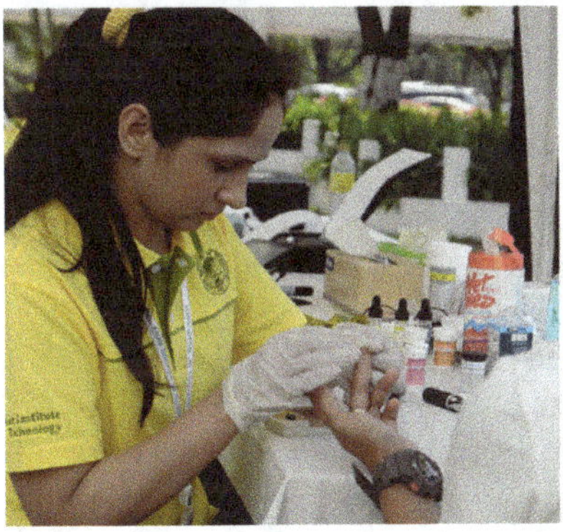

(c) Lab test on site

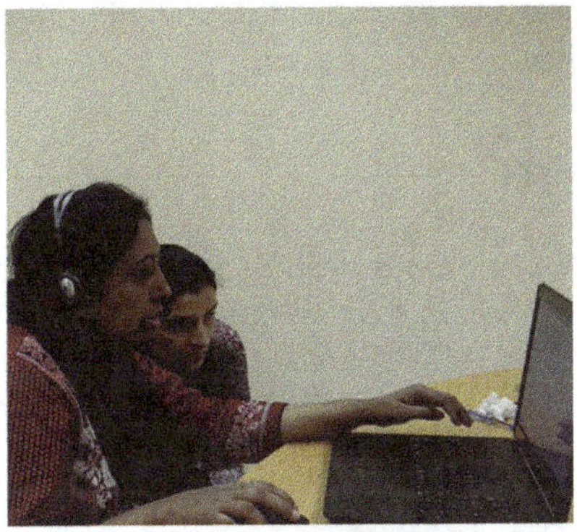

(d) Doctors in call center

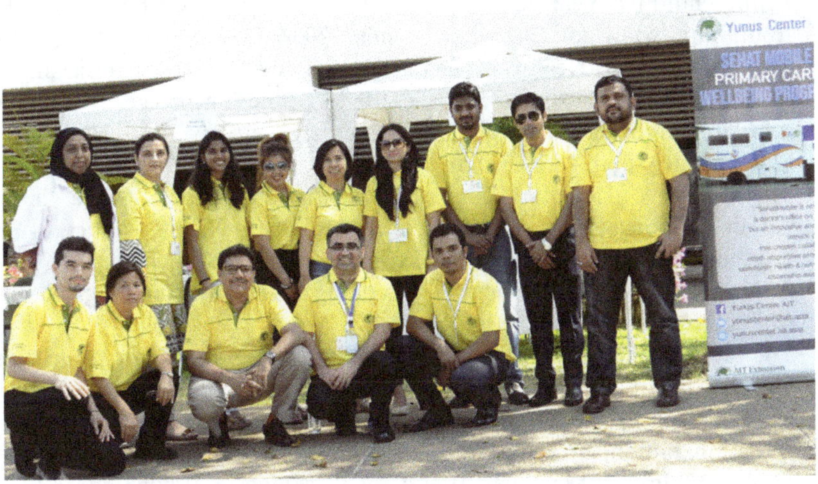

(e) Yunus Center AIT and Stora Enso-Bul;leh Shah teams at the SehatMobile pilot

Figure 9.11 SehatMobile pilot under way

Acknowledgements

This pilot was supported by Stora Enso and Bulleh Shah Packaging, Pakistan through project agreement with Yunus Center, Asian Institute of Technology, Thailand.

9.5 Summary

This chapter described the case studies of remote healthcare services in India, China, Cambodia, and Pakistan, focusing on (1) the implementation process, (2) challenges, and (3) possible solutions. Based on the lessons learned from each country's case study, remote healthcare services including PHC will be further improved to be more user friendly, culturally and socially appropriate, and more sustainable in the future.

References

[1] National Bureau of Statistics of China. Nation Data of China, 2018. Chinese. Available from: http://data.stats.gov.cn/.

[2] Yu, H., Universal health insurance coverage for 1.3 billion people: What accounts for China's success? Health Policy, 2015. 119(9): p. 1145–52.

[3] The Ministry of Health of China, 2018 China Health Statistical Yearbook. 2019. Chinese.

[4] The State Council of China, National Informatization Strategy during the "Thirteenth Five-Year Plan" period. 2016 December 15. Chinese. Available from: http://www.gov.cn/zhengce/content/2016-12/27/content_5153411.htm

[5] The Ministry of Health of China, Notice of Properly Purchasing and Allocation of Medical Device of Village Clinics in Year 2014. Chinese. Available from: http://www.nhfpc.gov.cn/zwgkzt/xxjy/201611/1f3864190355473d82ae42dbd24d36ca.shtml

[6] The Ministry of Health of China, the Ministry of Finance of China, the State Administration of Traditional Chinese Medicine of China, Notice of properly conducting the work of EPHS in year 2018. 2018 June 13. Chinese. Available from: http://cps.nhfpc.gov.cn/zjjgzx/zzzl/201806/30fe8a4bd8fb45c3a2190fe6b1aa3c14.shtml

[7] The Sichuan Provincial Ministry of Health, Notice of Invitation for Bids of Health All-In-One Machine. 2016. November 19. Chinese. Available from: http://www.ccgp.gov.cn/cggg/dfgg/gkzb/201611/t20161109_7555438.htm

[8] The Jilin Provincial Ministry of Health, Notice of Invitation for Bids of Health All-In-One Machine. 2019 April 17. Chinese. Available from: http://www.ggzyzx.jl.gov.cn/jyxx/005002/005002001/20190417/20e6efef-a363-49be-b608-bb94308fb67c.html

[9] Qingdan, Z., Digital Health All-In-One Machine Becomes Village Doctor's "Treasure", in Chinese Science Daily. 2019 September 10. Chinese. Available from: http://news.sciencenet.cn/sbhtmlnews/2014/9/291749.shtm

[10] The Zhuzhou Municipal Ministry of Health, Report of AIO Health Machines Application Status. 2018 January 22. Chinese. Available from: http://www.zzx.gov.cn/c9714/20180122/i619272.html

[11] The Guizhou Provincial Ministry of Health, Provincial Education Promotion Program of Primary Healthcare Staffs in Year 2018. 2018 September 4. Chinese. Available from: http://www.gzhfpc.gov.cn/xwzx/tzgg/201809/t20180904_3543453.html

[12] The Guizhou Provincial Ministry of Health, Work plan of "Eight Major Projects" for Improving Healthcare Service, 2019–2022. 2019 February 1. Chinese. Available from: http://www.guizhou.gov.cn/zwgk/zcfg/szfwj_8191/qfbh_8197/201902/t20190201_2234698.html

[13] The Anhui Provincial Ministry of Health, Experimental Application of "Smart Medical Assistant" to Make up the Weak Points of Rural Healthcare Service. 2019 May 5. Chinese. Available from: http://wjw.ah.gov.cn/news_details_50415.html

[14] United Nations. Sustainable Development Goals [online]. New York, USA; United Nations; 2019. Available from https://www.un.org/sustainabledevelopment/sustainable-development-goals/ [Accessed Sep 2019]

[15] World Health Organization. Global Health Observatory data [online]. Geneva, Switzerland; World Health Organization; 2019. Available from https://www.who.int/gho/en/ [Accessed Sep 2019]

[16] Kerber K. J., de Graft-Johnson J. E., Bhutta Z. A., Okong P., Starrs A., and Lawn J. E. Continuum of care for maternal, newborn, and child health: from slogan to service delivery. Lancet, 2007. 370(9595): p. 1358–69.

Chapter 10

Personal health record in Japan, China, and Bangladesh

Naoki Nakashima[1], Yuandong Hu[2], Rafiqul Islam Maruf[1,3] and Ashir Ahmed[4]

The personal health record (PHR) is known not only as a self-healthcare/disease management tool by the citizens/patients but also as a communication tool between patients and the medical staff. Moreover, recently the PHR has been considered as an indispensable tool for patient engagement in the area of noncommunicable diseases (NCD) and has gained importance. In this chapter, we aim to introduce Asian PHR especially focusing on those in Japan, China, and Bangladesh, in three different situations.

10.1 PHR, a powerful tool for healthcare and patient engagement

10.1.1 What is PHR?

Today, there are several applications in smartphones that help manage personal clinical data about NCDs generated in clinics and drugs dispensed by pharmacies. We generally call them "Personal Health Record (PHR)." We expect that a PHR can manage information regarding an individual's vital signs, exercise pattern, behavior, and location at home or at the office using built-in sensors in the smartphone or using sensor networks based on internet of things (IoT) technology.

The PHR is considered an indispensable tool for patient engagement and is rapidly spreading worldwide. Patient engagement enables NCD patients to access their personal health/medical data using the PHR, monitor the disease, and decide the treatment policy. This not only increases the rate of concordance regarding the

[1]Medical Information Center, Kyushu University Hospital, Fukuoka, Kyushu University, Fukuoka, Japan
[2]Institute of Chronic Disease Prevention and Treatment, Guizhou Center for Disease Control and Prevention, Guiyang, China
[3]Global Communication Center, Grameen Communications, Dhaka, Bangladesh
[4]Faculty of Information Science and Electrical Engineering, Kyushu University, Fukuoka, Japan

treatment policy between the physician and the patient but also provides the physician a trigger to change the policy and intervene [1].

Generally, it is important that the patient and/or family ask questions and share their subjective concerns with the medical staff. Patient-reported outcome (PRO) is another area for which there are applications on smartphones. The PHR can function in coordination with the PRO for greater generation of data and accuracy [2].

In the PRO, the patients input data on items, such as healthcare/medical service satisfaction, subjective feeling of symptom and function, health-related quality of life (HR-QOL), and treatment adherence. Scientifically appropriate indicators that can guarantee reliability and relevance, considering the characteristics of the subjective indicator [3], should evaluate these.

For elderly patients, the PHR providers (including insurers, care providers, medical institutes, etc.) should improve the environment of the patients and their families, educate them about NCD treatment, train them on how to input information into the PHR, and empower them, instead of giving up to involve them in patient engagement. However, to avoid imposing too much burden on the healthcare/medical staff because of a rapid increase in communication with patients and families, application and service system should be considered before they are developed and provided.

The WHO promotes the installation of patient engagement, especially for the developing countries, and highlights the importance of using the PHR [4].

10.1.2 Recommended configuration for PHR

It is expected that a large-size database related to NCD, such as that for diabetes mellitus and hypertension, will be generated in daily clinical services. However, database generation without standardized data item sets would be limited in their usefulness. To address this, six Japanese academic associations have cooperatively developed core item sets and self-management item sets for diabetes mellitus, hypertension, dyslipidemia, and chronic kidney disease, as well as recommended configuration for the PHR, detailing the specifications for implementing the four self-management item sets in PHR applications to facilitate risk stratification, the generation of alerts using information and communications technology systems, the avoidance of data input errors, and the generation of reminders to input the self-management item set data [5]. The approach developed by the committee may be useful for combining databases for various purposes (such as for clinical studies, patient education, and development/maintenance of electronic medical record systems) and for facilitating collaboration among PHR administrators.

10.2 Japanese PHR

10.2.1 Japanese situation of healthcare and medical informatics

The Japanese public medical insurance system was launched in 1961. This system covered all citizens and allowed free access to any medical institution. There are many commercial insurers in Japan (3,418 in March 2015), and these can be classified into the following three categories: those providing insurance for self-employed individuals (1,880 insurers, matching the number of local governments, i.e., cities, towns, and villages), those providing employee insurance (1,491 insurers), and those providing insurance for those aged $\geq$ 75 years (47 insurers, matching the number of prefectural governments).

Medical services are provided by 8,442 hospitals (defined as medical institutions with $\geq$ 20 beds); 101,529 clinics (medical institutions with < 20 beds); and 68,940 dental clinics as of October 2016. Additionally, there were 58,678 functional dispensing pharmacies on March 2015.

These institutions employed 318,480 medical doctors; 104,533 dentists; 1,210,665 nurses; 62,118 public health nurses; 39,613 certified midwives; and 301,323 pharmacists as of December 2016.

Japanese medical costs have been increasing with the aging of its population. The costs reached JPY 42.2 trillion in 2017, and this amount may continue to increase. Thus, improving the cost-effectiveness of medical services is an urgent national task.

Insurance claims data began to be digitized at the beginning of the twenty-first century, and currently (2019), 99% of the data has been digitized. All the medical procedures covered by insurance have been recorded in the claims data, allowing the insurers to evaluate what procedures were performed for which insured person by the medical institutions they visited.

In 2008, the nationwide standardized health checkup system (NSHC) was implemented as a duty of the insurer to detect and prevent NCDs, such as diabetes mellitus, hyperlipidemia, dyslipidemia, and chronic kidney diseases. The target age group for NSHC is 40–74-year-olds (52 million people). The number of NSHC examinees has increased from 38% during the implementation to 52% (27 million) in 2017. The results of the NSHC are shared with both the examinee (the insured) and the insurer.

In the analysis of medical Real World Data (RWD), electronic health record (EHR) data that includes clinical outcome data, such as results of lab tests and diagnosis data, are more useful than the insurance claim data that only show the clinical procedures that were performed. However, the EHR has been not yet globally integrated in Japan; they remain distributed in medical institutions as electronic medical records (EMR). The EMR is limited to data from only those who had visited clinics and hospitals but not from healthy subjects. The NSHC database includes the data on healthy subjects; however, these data are maintained separately by the 3,418 insurers and are not integrated, except in the form of an anonymous national database, only available for secondary use.

In sum, by October 2017, only 34.4% of the medical records from clinics and hospitals in Japan were digitized; however, the number has been gradually increasing.

10.2.1.1 PHR in Japan

The concept of the PHR is expected to gain more popularity in the near future, and the PHR is expected to become the main data source for the EHR together with the EMR in medical institutes, with higher use of smartphones.

Japan has a long history of the PHR. Although, it is a paper system, maternal-baby notebook, including records of maternal and baby statuses during pre- and post-delivery periods, neonatal health checkup, and vaccination records, was launched in 1942 and is used until today. Drug notebook, another spread paper PHR, used by every generation, has been available since 2000 when insurance companies started to cover it and has contributed to reduce duplicated prescription among clinics. Several millions of disease-specified notebooks, such as those for diabetes mellitus and hypertension, have been published annually even with the paper system for self-management and/or data sharing among medical institutions.

However, paper PHR has certain limitations in functions and purpose of secondary use. Therefore, several research projects have attempted to develop electronic PHR, by digitalization and integration of paper PHR, to be installed and managed in individual smartphones in Japan, as smartphones gain greater distribution.

Simultaneously, the IoT concept has gained popularity and is expected to contribute to the collection of vital and behavior data using sensor devices around patients and the accumulation in the PHR.

In the near future, the PHR will accumulate data for the entire day, including caregiving data for elderly patients. Thus, we expect the PHR to provide complete health and medical data of an individual from the time of birth till the time of death.

Additionally, we expect that the secondary use of PHR data can be a main and powerful solution to overcome many health issues that are generated due to the aging of the population.

However, ideas around digitalized PHR are still in the research stage, and the PHR service model has not yet been established and used in Japan.

Herein, we have introduced our experiment using the PHR with business models paid by insurers (Figure 10.2) [6]. In this PHR project, the recommended configuration for the PHR was installed (Figure 10.1). Personal clinical data were collected from hospitals, clinics (or regional clinical laboratory centers), and pharmacies.

Insurers outsource data input of NSHC, disease management of NCD, including "data health plan," which means that the insurer intervenes the insured person based on the matching results of personal insurance claim data and NSHC data.

In this project, we assumed that the government establishes a backup data center for the PHR. Users can keep a backup of their personal data using the backup system in case the smartphone is broken or lost, and clinics/hospitals can retrieve the data from the backup system. Users can change the PHR provider to another if the latter complies with the recommended configuration for the PHR via the backup database.

Accumulated data can be used by researchers and industries after anonymization, with patient consent.

Insurers may pay for this PHR business model in Japan because they have the motivation to improve the health of the insured persons and thus reduce their

ID of SMIS	Item	Unit, expression	SMIS for Diabetes Mellitus			SMIS for Hypertension			SMIS for Dyslipidemia			SMIS for CKD		
			from Medical	from health checkup	from home	from Medical	from health check-up	from home	from Medical	from health check-up	from home	from Medical	from health check-up	from home
1	Height	cm	○	○		○	○		○	○		○	○	
2	Weight	kg	○	○		○	○		○	○		○	○	
3	Systolic Blood Pressure	mmHg	○	○		○	○		○	○		○	○	
4	Diastolic Blood Pressure	mmHg	○	○		○	○		○	○		○	○	
5	LDL Cholesterol	mg/dL	○	○		○	○		○	○		○	○	
6	HDL Cholesterol	mg/dL	○	○		○	○		○	○		○	○	
7	Smoking	Yes, No, Yes in the past	○	○		○	○		○	○		○	○	
8	Serum Creatinine	mg/dL	○			○			○			○		
9	Urine Protein	−, ±, +, 2+, 3+or over	○	○		○	○		○	○		○	○	
10	Blood Glucose	mg/dL	○	○		○	○		○	○				
11	Age diagnosed as Diabetes Mellitus	under 10y.o, 10's, 20's, , , 70's, 80y.o. or over, Not yet, Unknown	○											
12	HbA1c	%	○	○								○	○	
13	ALT	IU/L	○	○					○	○				
14	Diabetic Retinopathy	Yes, No, Unknown	○											
15	Age diagnosed as Hypertension	under 10y.o, 10's, 20's, , , 70's, 80y.o. or over, No, Unknown				○								
16	Serum Potassium	mEq/L				○						○		
17	Abnormality on ECG	Yes, No, Unknown				○								
18	Triglyceride	mg/dL	○	○		○	○		○	○		○	○	
19	Age diagnosed as Dyslipidemia	under 10y.o, 10's, 20's, , , 70's, 80y.o. or over, No, Unknown							○					
20	Past History of Coronary Diseases	Yes (by contrast study), Yes (by another study), No, Unknown							○					
21	Age diagnosed as CKD	under 10y.o, 10's, 20's, , , 70's, 80y.o. or over, No, Unknown										○		
22	Serum Albumin	g/dL										○	○	
23	Hematuria	−, ±, +, 2+, 3+or over (Micro hematuria), Macro hematuria										○	○	
24	Total Cholesterol	mg/dL	○			○			○			○		
25	Urine Albumin/Creatinine	mg/gCre	○											
26	AST	IU/L	○	○										
27	Waist	cm		○			○			○				
28	Urine Glucose	−, ±, +, 2+or over	○	○										
29	γ GTP	IU/L	○	○										
30	Diabetic neuropathy	Yes, No, Unknown	○											
31	Regular visit at Dental Clinic (*1)	Yes, No, Unknown	○											
32	Uric Acid	mg/dL				○						○	○	
33	Systolic Blood Pressure at home	mmHg						○						
34	Diastolic Blood Pressure at home	mmHg						○						
35	Family History of Renal Failure(*2)	Yes, No, Unknown										○		
36	Urine Protein /Creatinine	g/gCre										○	○	
37	Urine Protein / Day	g/day										○	○	
38	Serum Total Protein	g/dL										○	○	
39	BUN	mg/dL										○		
40	Hemoglobin	g/dL										○	○	
41	Cystatin C	mg/L										○		

CIS for Diabetes Mellitus · CIS for Hypertension · CIS for Dyslipidemia · CIS for CKD

Figure 10.1 Six Japanese clinical societies developed a set of self-management items for use in the recommended configuration for the PHR

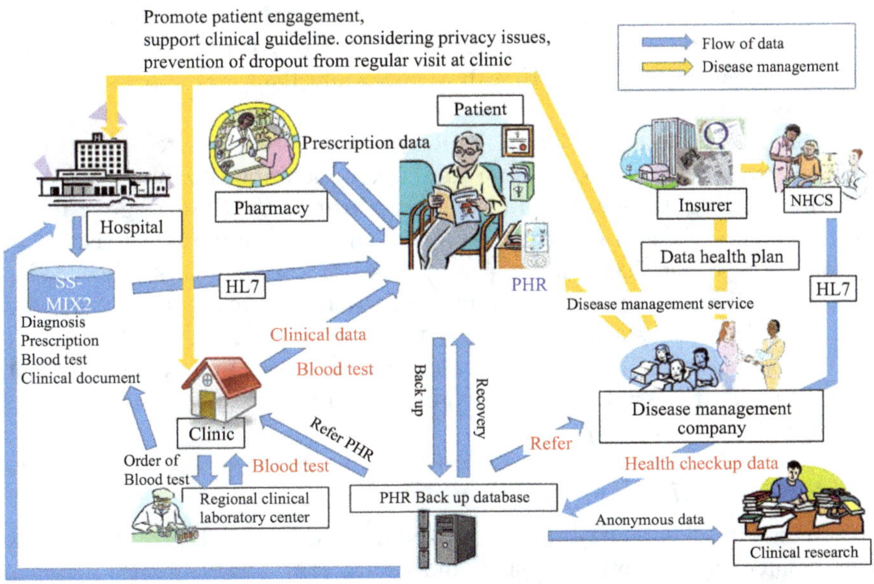

Figure 10.2 The Japanese cabinet and six clinical societies have been promoting the PHR social experiment with chronic disease management since 2014 [5]

medical expenses. Another incentive would be to avoid the economic penalty based on insufficient outcomes of the NSHC and data health plan. The penalty system was launched in 2018 by the Ministry of Health, Labor, and Welfare.

As shown earlier, the Japanese PHR is still in the startup stage, although the importance has been recognized widely. There are insufficient PHR providers, and standardization of the PHR protocol is still not achieved, although the recommended configuration for the PHR has been recently published as described earlier.

Compared to other countries, the Japanese PHRs (even in the trial phase) were poor in terms of gaming sensation/entertainment and had a less attractive graphic user interface. In contrast, DialBetics by Waki *et al.*, which captures all pictures of daily dishes by smartphone, followed by nutritionist's advices, have been evaluated using scientific methods [7]. Evidence-based development of PHR is a requirement in Japan.

10.3 Chinese PHR

10.3.1 History of PHR in China

Before 2009, there is national PHR system in China. In 2009, the central government of China implemented an ambitious national project called "Essential Public Health Service (EPHS)," aiming to provide primary health service to all Chinese residents [8]. The content of EPHS increased from 9 items to 14 items in last 10 years [9,10]. Among all the items, the PHR is always considered as the fundamental and most important one, because almost all the other service items are related to health record. The target of this part of EPHS is to build PHR of every permanent resident who have lived for more than 6 months in the same community.

Though no basis of a national PHR system before, this project was completed in several years. Considering the huge population of China, this speed was quite amazing. Besides the financial support from the Chinese government, this preliminary success should be contributed to two important reasons: the first one was China has built a primary health care network since 1950s, including millions of township hospitals and village clinics. The second reason was China already has a national ID system, which called "Shenfenzheng" in Chinese. Begun at 1984, this system allocated an 18-bit unique code to every adult and make it possible for the government to management the huge population in many aspects [11].

10.3.2 Mechanism of the Chinese PHR

The administrative structure of China can be divided into six levels: central, province, municipality, county, township, and village [12]. For the EPHS, the levels from central government to the county are mainly in charge of designing annual working plan, direction, and examination. Township hospitals and village clinics are the main force to provide the EPHS to all residents [13].

Specific to the PHR, the village doctor is required to do the home visit to all the families in his/her village, to communicate the residents about their recent health situation and fill the PHR forms, then the village doctor needs to handle these forms to the staffs of township hospital. In the period which used paper as recording medium of the PHR, every township hospital had an archive to store the PHR documents of all residents of this town. All the health records of one individual were put into a book; then, the PHRs of all members of the family were put into the same document box; then, the names of all family members and code of this family were marked on the spine of the box. Document boxes from the same village were put in the same cabinet [14].

The ownership of the PHR data is a controversial topic. So far, there is no law or regulation to define the ownership of health data in China. Some jurists suggest: (1) even if the PHR system is invested by the government, permission from the individual for using his/her data is essential in any occasion; (2) if the government needs to use the data for public benefits, the part of private information in the PHR should be removed or anonymized; and (3) government employee's access to the PHR should be carefully authorized and supervised.

10.3.3 Content and format of the Chinese PHR

The National EPHS Regulation, which is compiled and published by the Chinese Ministry of Health, is the most authoritative document for the EPHS. This regulation lists all the required content and standard operation procedure of the PHR. The basic content, including the socioeconomic information and a physical examination form, is same for every resident. Besides the basic content, residents are divided into different groups according to their age and gender: children, maternal, elder, and patients of hypertension or diabetes. Every group has its specific content: appraisal forms of growth and development for the children, maternal health records for the pregnant women, free annual health check record for the elders, seasonal follow-up records for the chronic disease patients [15].

At the beginning, the recording medium of the PHR in most areas was paper forms. The disadvantages of paper record are obvious: it needs enormous space to store the paper records. It is almost impossible to duplicate, do statistical calculation, and analyze the data on paper effectively. To change this situation, the Chinese government aimed to build electronic PHR for more than 75% resident in its 12th five-year plan [16]. In 2019, all the province has achieved this goal, and in some of them, the ratio could be more than 90% [17].

10.3.4 Improvement of the Chinese PHR

As most areas have changed their PHR systems to electronic ones, the further improvement of the PHR was put on the agenda. The main purposes of improvement are to make it available to exchange data between the PHR and other database, and to make it more convenient to use the PHR data.

In Zunyi, Guizhou Province, the local government has connected the hospital information system (HIS) with the PHR system. Once a doctor diagnosed a new hypertensive or diabetic patient, a notice will be pushed to the healthcare provider who is in charge of the patient's community to remind him/her to do the follow-up after the patient is back from hospital. Correspondingly, a doctor can review a prediagnosed hypertensive or diabetic patient's PHR in the interface of the HIS to give medical advice and prescription more precisely.

In Qingzhen, another county of Guizhou Province, all the medical information system within this area have been integrated together. If a patient received a blood routine test or a chest X-ray in any hospital, the results of the laboratory information system (LIS) or the picture archiving and communication systems (PACS) can be reviewed on the PHR system at real time. Because Guizhou is an undeveloped inland province, many young people go to work in the rich coast province for higher salary. The local government also developed a smartphone app, which allowed the residents to check their family members' PHR on the cellphone. This app is welcome by the mobile workers because it helps them to know the health situation of their family members, no matter where they are.

10.3.5 Challenges for the Chinese PHR

Though the first step for building electronic PHR has been completed, many big challenges remain. First, there is no uniformed national platform yet, each province needs to build its own PHR system, the PHR system were developed by different IT companies, data exchange is not available even between counties in one province, which hinders the advanced analysis of health data and the decision-making of health policy. As a solution, the Chinese government has made a national standard for health data in 2009 [18]. This standard defined the format of all health data involved in the PHR. The first stage is to create a provincial health data network, and then a nation network in the end.

The second problem is the shortage of qualified data scientist, most medical staffs are trained as traditional healthcare provider, only a few of them has experience of taking advantage of massive data. The National CDC of China and some provincial CDCs have regular training programs to teach investigation and analysis skills, but this is enough, compared to the huge demand.

The major barrier for the improvement of the PHR is never technical issues; the real challenge for the government is to find out what is people really need and coordinate all its resources to solve the problem. Fortunately, with better understanding of the PHR, the policy-makers of China are going to designing more creative and flexible policies.

10.4 Bangladeshi PHR

10.4.1 Bangladeshi situation of medical informatics

Healthcare sector is one of the most prior sector in any country. Bangladesh is not an exception. However, the healthcare infrastructure and qualified human resources in the sector are still inadequate. There is a huge shortage of hospitals all over the country. Other than few private hospitals of the capital city, none of them keeps any records of the patients' health status for more than few months; so, maintaining the EHR is far behind. Whenever a patient needs healthcare service, the patient visits a hospital, clinic, or a general practitioner, gets consultancy, and purchases medicine; once cured, the patients don't care to preserve the records. So, when they need to go to hospital next time, they start everything from the beginning. This is a huge loss of the limited invaluable resources.

Fortunately, against many other odds, Bangladesh has started her journey to Digital Bangladesh. Under this initiative, the government is trying to use Information and Communication Technologies (ICT) in every sector including healthcare for faster development of the country. Now, the Ministry of Health is working for policy-making involving healthcare service, telemedicine, data management, and data sharing. However, it will take more time to see all public health facilities with the EHRs keeping system as well as PHR services.

In Bangladesh, there are some private hospitals with global standard facilities, which are only accessible to the rich people of the society and they have their own EHR system. However, the PHR is not yet there. In this context, when the portable health clinic (PHC) system was designed in 2009, the EHR was there from the beginning where patients' information was preserved in electronic format to the online server (Figure 10.3). Later, the PHR service was added as a personal service to the patients. Now, the PHC call center doctor can access to the patients' data for providing consultancy. The patients can also access to their password-protected personal health records anytime, anyplace using online application and share with the doctors in need. As per our study, a limited number of the urban-conscious PHC patients show their interest and personally access to their personal data to monitor the progress of their health status. The graphical analysis of the PHR data in the PHC system is very easy for the patients to understand the progress and they become anxious if there is any irregularity in the data. This is very helpful as patients will be more careful of their health before it goes worst.

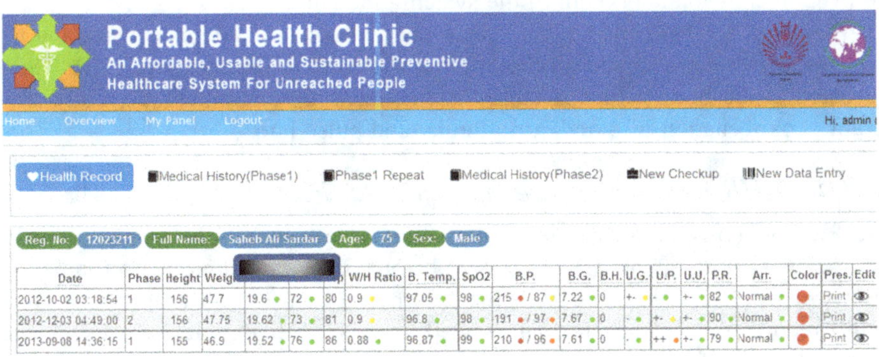

Figure 10.3 The EHR system of the PHC

10.4.2 Content of PHR in PHC system

PHC was originally designed for basic primary healthcare. However, the current trend of common diseases in Bangladesh shows that 67% goes under NCDs, especially hypertension and diabetes. Therefore, the test items were designed keeping hypertension and diabetes in mind so that these problems are screened out. The basic test items are:

1. Body temperature
2. Blood pressure
3. Pulse rate
4. Arrhythmia
5. Height, weight, and BMI
6. Waist, hip, and W/H ratio
7. Oxygenation of blood
8. Blood glucose (random)
9. Blood grouping
10. Urinary sugar
11. Urinary protein
12. Hemoglobin
13. Cholesterol
14. Uric acid

10.4.3 Comparison of PHC-PHR with Japanese PHR

Although there is no recognized global standard for the PHR, Japan has proposed one for this purpose. This can be considered as a base document for now. Compare to the total self-management item sets (SMIS) of this Japanese standard, the PHR for primary health checkup of the PHC system has covered most of it, as shown in Figure 10.4. As the PHC system has a special focus of NCDs like diabetes mellitus and hypertension, it covers most of the items of SMIS for diabetes mellitus and SMIS for hypertension of the Japanese PHR proposal. For missing items, being a functionally modular system where new modules are added in needs time to time, the PHC intends to adopt them in the system gradually.

However, the PHR of the PHC has some additional test items considering the local needs in rural Bangladesh that are not included in the Japanese PHR. These are listed at the bottom of this table that includes hip circumference, body temperature, oxygenation of blood, arrhythmia, and pulse rate.

10.4.4 PHR monitoring user interface in PHC

The PHC system has a very important feature to monitor the personal health record. Every user can access to his/her personal data using unique username and password from anywhere through the Internet. The user can monitor previous health record both in data format as well as in simple graphical representation (Figure 10.5). This graphical presentation is very easy to understand if any particular vital status is improving or deteriorating. This makes the patients

ID of SMIS	Item	Primary Health Checkup			SMIS for Diabetes Mellitus			SMIS for Hypertension		
		from Medical	from Health Check-up	from Home	from Medical	from Health Check-up	from Home	from Medical	from Health Check-up	from Home
1	Height		•		•	•		•	•	
2	Weight		•		•	•		•	•	
3	Systolic Blood Pressure		•		•	•		•	•	
4	Diastolic Blood Pressure		•		•	•		•	•	
5	LDL Cholesterol				○	○		○	○	
6	HDL Cholesterol				○	○		○	○	
7	Smoking		•		•	•		•	•	
8	Serum Creatinine				○			○		
9	Urine Protein		•		•	•		•	•	
10	Blood Glucose		•		•	•		•	•	
11	Age diagnosed as Diabetes Mellitus		△		△					
12	HbA1c				○	○				
13	ALT				○	○				
14	Diabetic Retinopathy				○					
15	Age diagnosed as Hypertension		△					△		
16	Serum Potassium							○		
17	Abnormality on ECG							○		
18	Triglyceride				○	○		○	○	
19	Age diagnosed as Dyslipidemia		△							
20	Past History of Coronary Diseases		△							
21	Age diagnosed as CKD		△							
22	Serum Albumin									
23	Hematuria									
24	Total Cholesterol		•		•			•		
25	Urine Albumin/Creatinine				○					
26	AST				○	○				
27	Waist		•			•			•	
28	Urine Glucose		•		•	•				
29	γ GTP				○	○				
30	Diabetic neuropathy		△		△					
31	Regular visit at Dental Clinic (*1)		△		△					
32	Uric Acid		•					•		
33	Systolic Blood Pressure at home		△							△
34	Diastolic Blood Pressure at home		△							△
35	Family History of Renal Failure(*2)									
36	Urine Protein /Creatinine									
37	Urine Protein / Day									
38	Serum Total Protein									
39	BUN									
40	Hemoglobin		•							
41	Cystatin C									
	Hip		•							
	Body Temperature		•							
	Oxygenation of Blood		•							
	Arrhythmia		•							
	Pulse Rate (bit/min)		•							

Figure 10.4 Comparison of the PHR of the PHC with Japanese standard

interested to check the progress status often and they become more conscious to maintain once it goes wrong.

This is very important for the patients from the point of preventive healthcare approach. Once they see any negative development, they become conscious and try to follow the medication or advice from the doctors or health workers. And,

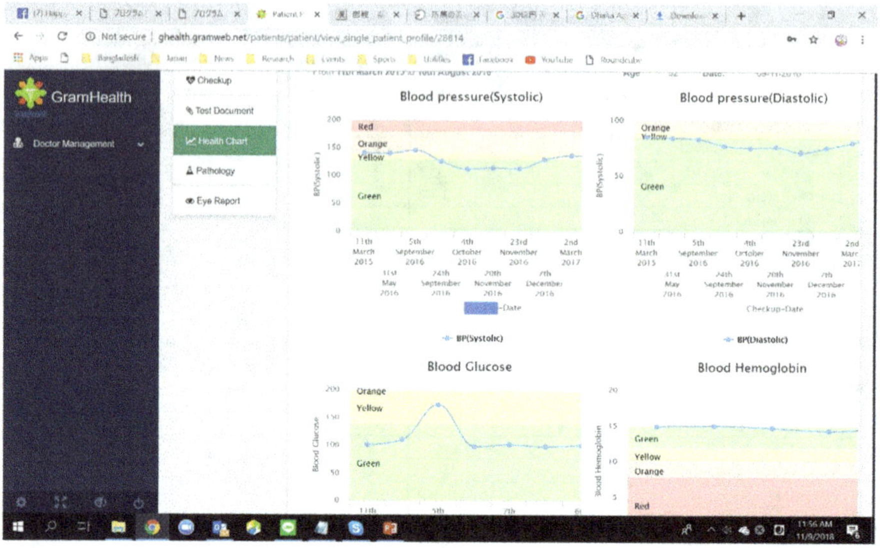

Figure 10.5 Graphical representation of PHR data

they also try to see the progress hereafter to ensure that the situation has been improved.

References

[1] Bombard Y, Baker GR, Orlando E, *et al.* Engaging patients to improve quality of care: a systematic review. Implement Sci. 2018;13(1):98. Published 2018 Jul 26. doi: 10.1186/s13012-018-0784-zTechnology and Tools for Patient Engagement

[2] Bae WK, Kwon J, Lee HW, *et al.* Feasibility and accessibility of electronic patient-reported outcome measures using a smartphone during routine chemotherapy: a pilot study. Support Care Cancer. 2018;26(11):3721–3728. doi: 10.1007/s00520-018-4232-z. Epub 2018 May 7.

[3] Innominato PF, Komarzynski S, Palesh OG, *et al.* Circadian rest-activity rhythm as an objective biomarker of patient-reported outcomes in patients with advanced cancer. Cancer Med. 2018;7(9):4396–4405. doi: 10.1002/cam4.1711. Epub 2018 Aug 7.

[4] WHO Regional Office for Europe. Health literacy: The solid facts. http://www.euro.who.int/__data/assets/pdf_file/0008/190655/e96854.pdf

[5] Nakashima N, Noda M, Ueki K, *et al.* Recommended configuration for personal health records by standardized data item sets for diabetes mellitus and associated chronic diseases: a report from collaborative initiative by six Japanese associations. Diabetol Int. 2019;10:85–92 https://doi.org/10.1007/s13340-019-00389-7

[6] Nakashima N, Yoshida M, and Yamamoto R. Personal health record system based on standardized item sets generates personal advice in accordance with clinical guidelines. Diab Tech Therap. 2018;20(S1):349–349.

[7] Yamaguchi S, Waki K, Tomizawa N, *et al.* Previous dropout from diabetic care as a predictor of patients' willingness to use mobile applications for self-management: a cross-sectional study. J Diabetes Investig. 2017;8 (4):542–549. doi: 10.1111/jdi.12613. Epub 2017 Feb 22.

[8] The State Council of China. Key implementation plan of medical and health system reform in the near future (2009–2011).2009 March 18. Chinese. Available from: http://www.gov.cn/zwgk/2009-04/07/content_1279256.htm

[9] The Ministry of Health of China, the Ministry of Finance of China, the National Population and Family Planning Commission of China. Opinions concerning stepwise promoting equalization of EPHS. 2009 July 7. Chinese. Available from: http://www.gov.cn/ztzl/ygzt/content_1661065.htm

[10] The Ministry of Health of China, the Ministry of Finance of China, the State Administration of Traditional Chinese Medicine of China, 2018 June 13. Chinese. Notice of properly conducting the work of EPHS in year 2018. 2018 June 13. Chinese. Available from: http://www.nhc.gov.cn/jws/s3577/201806/acf4058c09d046b09addad8abd395e20.shtml

[11] Wikipedia. Shenfenzheng[Internet]. Available from: https://en.wikipedia.org/wiki/Shenfenzheng

[12] Wikipedia. Administrative divisions of China[Internet]. Available from: https://en.wikipedia.org/wiki/Administrative_divisions_of_China

[13] Liu YF, Zhang XF, Xiang YX, *et al.* Analysis on the present responsibility division of township and village in national essential public health service project. Chinese Health Economics. 2013,(9):72–75. Chinese. Available from: http://med.wanfangdata.com.cn/Paper/Detail?id=PeriodicalPaper_zgwsjj201309022

[14] The Ministry of Health of China. Residents Health Records Management Service Standard. Chinese. Available from: http://www.nbphsp.org.cn/jbgw/jkda/

[15] The Ministry of Health of China. National EPHS Regulation (3rd Edition). Chinese. Available from: http://www.furong.gov.cn/service/bmfw/health/prevention/mbzhfzyjsws/201811/P020181123646040312634.pdf

[16] The State Council of China. The plan and implementation plan for deepening the reform of the medical and health care system. 2009 March 14. Chinese. Available from: http://www.gov.cn/zwgk/2012-03/21/content_2096671.htm

[17] The State Council of China. The 13th Five-Year Plan For National Informatization. 2016 December 15. Chinese. Available from: http://www.gov.cn/zhengce/content/2016-12/27/content_5153411.htm

[18] The Ministry of Health of China. Basic framework and data standards for health records. 2009 May 15. Chinese. Available from: http://www.gov.cn/gzdt/2009-05/19/content_1319085.htm

Chapter 11

Telemedical education in Asia

Shuji Shimizu[1], Kuriko Kudo[1], Tomohiko Moriyama[1], Shunta Tomimatsu[1], Shintaro Ueda[1] and Naoki Nakashima[1,2]

11.1 Telemedicine

11.1.1 Definition and advantages

Telemedicine refers to medicine-related activities performed remotely using communication technology such as the Internet. Demand for telemedicine has been growing in various fields of medicine because it reduces time and cost. In addition, telemedicine is efficient and scalable, as it can be easily repeated and allows participants from multiple locations.

11.1.2 Classification

Telemedicine can be classified into two major categories, namely telemedicine that includes doctors and patients and telemedicine that includes only doctors. The former includes remote consultation with patients, which is becoming increasingly popular worldwide. It also includes remote surgery, where the patient is operated on by a remote surgeon [1]. The latter includes remote consultation by a doctor with a specialist in fields such as radiology and pathology. It also includes remote medical education, where medical students remotely attend classes, and joint case discussions between doctors at multiple locations.

This chapter focuses on remote medical education.

11.2 Remote medical education

11.2.1 History

Remote education was first tried in the 1990s, in the early years of the Internet. However, doctors were unsatisfied with these attempts because the transmitted image quality was insufficient for medical purposes. Anatomy was difficult to show

[1]Telemedicine Department Center of Asia (TEMDEC), International Medical Department, Kyushu University Hospital, Fukuoka, Japan
[2]Medical Information Center, Kyushu University Hospital, Fukuoka, Japan

properly and video was often choppy due to limited bandwidth. Satellite networks could send higher-quality images, but the cost was prohibitive for regular use.

Compression algorithms are applied to images to reduce the required transmission bandwidth. However, compression inevitably deteriorates image quality. With the high available bandwidth added between Japan and Korea when they co-hosted the FIFA World Cup in 2002, it is now possible to transmit uncompressed images between the two countries. A technology for transmitting video, called the digital video transport system (DVTS), which is free video conferencing software, made it possible to send video without costly videoconferencing equipment; all that was needed was commercially available personal computers and digital cameras [2].

Broadband internet cables have been installed throughout Asia. With the development of technologies that improve image quality and reduce cost, telemedicine has expanded rapidly into Asia, which includes many developing countries with unmet medical needs. China joined our programmes in 2004, followed by Thailand and Singapore in 2005, Vietnam and Indonesia in 2006, and the Philippines in 2007 [3].

11.2.2 Programmes in Asian countries

Figure 11.1 depicts the cumulative numbers of remote education programmes by year in selected countries in Asia. All countries show a steady increase in the number of programmes. Of note is the very rapid increase in Indonesia, the reasons for which are described in Section 11.5.3.

Some attractive programmes have been introduced. One is a regular endoscopic case teleconference organised by a Malaysian doctor, which connects around 20 hospitals and medical colleges throughout Asia [4]. Because the programme is very educational, it was endorsed by the Asian-Pacific Society for

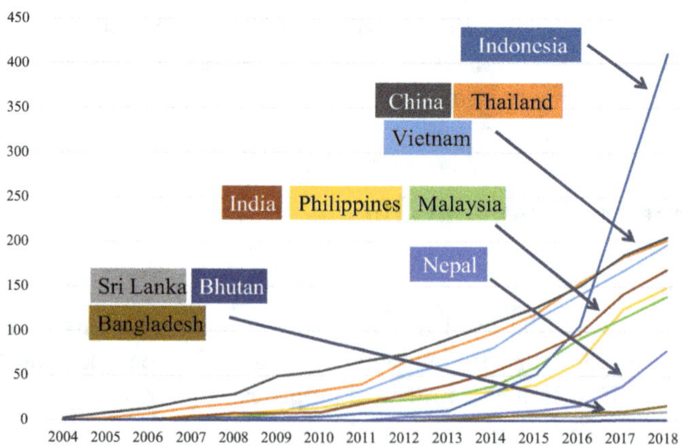

Figure 11.1 Cumulative numbers of remote medical programmes in Asian countries

Digestive Endoscopy in 2018. Another is a surgical teleconference where recorded operations are shared in an active discussion among multiple sites (Figure 11.2).

Live demonstrations are another type of remote education. Live urology surgery was transmitted from Korea to a large congress in Japan, and a live class between Japan and Korea was well accepted by medical students [5,6]. A live demonstration of minimally invasive surgery has been reported in China [7]. The usefulness of live endoscopy was documented based on the experiences in a Japanese congress [8].

11.2.3 Beyond Asia

One-fourth of our programmes are operated outside Asia (Figure 11.3). Latin America is the next most active continent, even though it is the farthest from Asia [9]. In Russia, a programme that started with four sites near Moscow in 2017 expanded to ten sites in just 8 months, covering the whole country. In Africa, although activity is not yet at full scale, we started some programmes with 13 institutions in seven countries.

The expansion of our remote medical education programmes beyond Asia has coincided with FIFA World Cup events. In 2010, when the FIFA World Cup was organised in South Africa, we broadcasted the first live surgery from Japan to the University of Cape Town [10]. After several years of trials, we organised the first successful teleconference with Latin American countries in 2013, around the time the FIFA World Cup was held in Brazil. In 2017, we started our remote education programmes in Russia with satisfactory quality, 1 year before Russia hosted the FIFA World Cup. The Internet links installed in the host countries facilitated these telemedicine programmes.

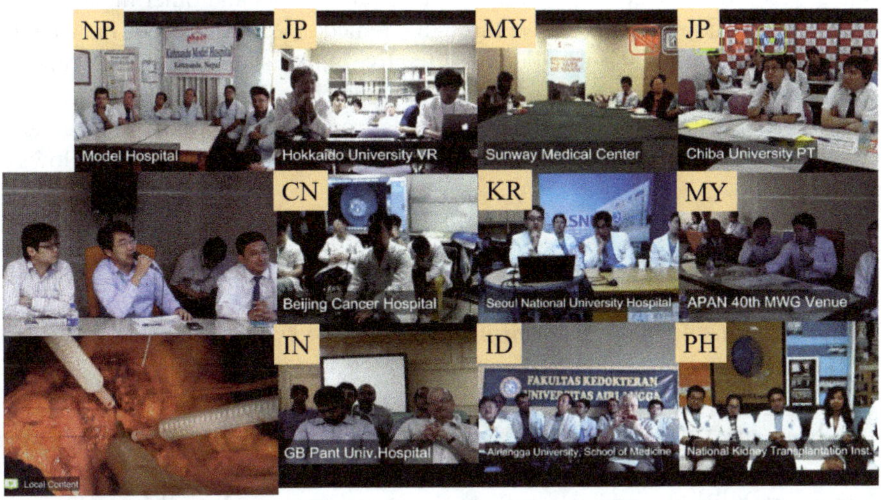

Figure 11.2 Surgical teleconferences connecting multiple countries in Asia. CN; China, ID; Indonesia, IN; India, JP; Japan, KR; Korea, MY; Malaysia, NP; Nepal, PH; Philippines

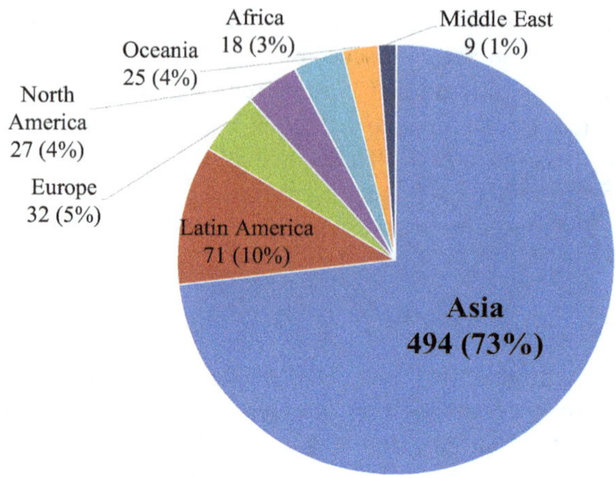

Figure 11.3 International telemedicine activities by continent

As of March 2019, our hospital has organised 1,010 telemedicine programmes with 685 collaborating institutions in 70 countries.

11.2.4 Three key factors for success

More than 15 years of experience has revealed three key factors for success in telemedicine, namely access, needs and skills. Access refers to a good internet connection, which ensures that teleconference quality will meet medical standard in terms of resolution. Needs refer to the demands of doctors and other medical staff regarding what they want to achieve through telemedicine. These needs must be the starting point to make the programme attractive and sustainable. Skills refer to those of engineers that need to support telemedicine. Because telemedicine is relatively new, many technical staff in hospitals are not yet familiar with the related technology. These three key factors are explained in more detail in the following sections.

11.3 Access

11.3.1 Academic versus commercial networks

An advanced network for academic purposes, called a research and education network (REN), was a requirement when we started telemedicine with the DVTS. Because the DVTS required a bandwidth of up to 30 Mbps, regular commercial internet was unsuitable at the time. For hospitals and medical colleges that were members of a REN, medical staff could use the network without additional cost [11].

Table 11.1 lists the major RENs in Asian countries. Most countries have RENs to facilitate academic activities using digital devices. Myanmar, a new member,

Table 11.1 Research and Education Network in Asia

Country	REN*	URL
Japan	SINET5	https://www.sinet.ad.jp/en/top-en
Korea	KREONET	https://www.kreonet.net/eng/
China	CERNET	https://www.edu.cn/english/
Thailand	ThaiREN	http://www.thairen.net.th/
Vietnam	VinaREN	http://www.vista.gov.vn/
Malaysia	MYREN	https://myren.net.my/
Philippines	ASTI	https://asti.dost.gov.ph/
Indonesia	IDREN	https://idren.id/
India	NKN	http://nkn.gov.in/
Bangladesh	BdREN	https://www.bdren.net.bd/
Sri Lanka	LEARN	https://www.ac.lk/
Nepal	NREN	https://www.nren.net.np/
Bhutan	DrukREN	https://drukren.bt/
Kyrgyzstan	KRENA	http://www.krena.kg/index.php/en

*REN; research and education network

formally announced the international connection of its REN in December 2018 with the Trans-Eurasia Information Network (TEIN).

With the development of videoconferencing systems that can provide excellent image quality even with compression and improvement in commercial networks in terms of bandwidth and stability, RENs are no longer prerequisite for telemedicine. This is important because RENs connect large institutions (e.g., universities), but not small hospitals in rural areas, where demand for telemedicine is growing. The number of our collaborating members who use commercial networks has thus grown (i.e., the ratio of REN users has decreased) [12]. The availability of new videoconferencing systems and fast commercial internet has accelerated telemedicine adoption in rural hospitals.

11.4 Needs

11.4.1 Medical needs

Our policy is that medical needs come first and engineering support follows. When engineering staff initiate a telemedicine programme, the programme seldom continues because it often becomes a technology showcase and attracts few medical participants.

Our first live surgery was organised based on a proposal from a Korean doctor who visited Japanese hospitals several times to watch a new surgery developed in Japan for gastric cancer. When this doctor found out about telemedicine, he set up a system to learn more about the surgery at lower cost. After participating in several remote education programmes, he established this new surgery in Korea. This has become a milestone for various programmes [2].

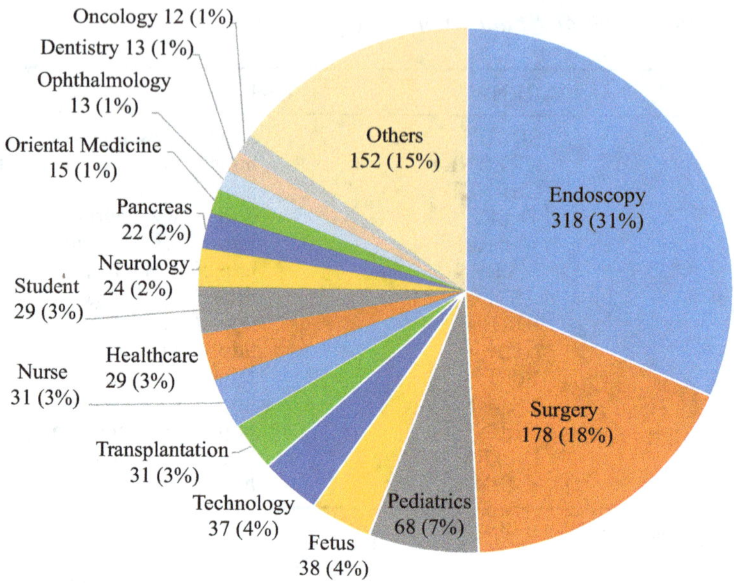

Figure 11.4 Content of telemedicine programmes

11.4.2 Medical content

We started the first telemedicine programme in February 2003. As of March 2019, we have organised over 1,000 programmes. As shown in Figure 11.4, endoscopy and surgery account for about half of all programmes (31% and 18%, respectively). The remaining programmes include paediatrics, transplantation, heart disease and infection, reflecting the spread of telemedicine. Of note, in addition to medical doctors, dentists, nurses and medical students have used our programmes.

11.5 Skills

11.5.1 Systems

Videoconferencing equipment has changed dramatically over the last few decades. When we stated, DVTS and a REN were required for telemedicine to satisfy doctors in terms of quality and cost. The situation greatly changed after 2010, as shown in Figure 11.5, with the introduction of H.323 with high-definition video (Polycom Co., Santa Cruz, CA), Vidyo (Hackensack, NJ) and most recently Zoom (San Jose, CA). Remote participants can now choose the best available option according to their conditions.

11.5.2 Training programmes

We regularly organise two types of training programme, namely a week-long programme for beginners twice a year during Asia–Pacific Advanced Network

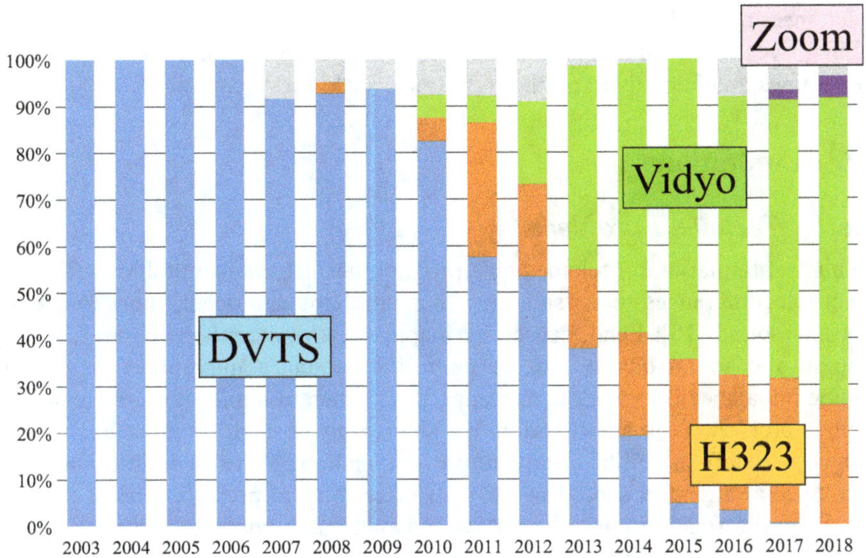

Figure 11.5 Change in videoconference systems over time

meetings and a month-long programme for potential trainers in our centre in Japan. The programmes have been positively evaluated by the participants as they increase skills and knowledge [13]. A technical manual has been published and is freely downloadable [14].

11.5.3 Interdisciplinary meetings

We organise an annual interdisciplinary meeting in Asia where doctors and engineers get together to share information regarding doctors' needs, new technologies and troubleshooting. The introduction of new members and the exploration of new areas of medicine are also important topics.

In addition to this international meeting, we started national meetings in several countries to further develop telemedicine. These meetings allow participants from all over a given country to discuss telemedicine in their native language [15]. This has worked very well, particularly in Indonesia. In 2016, a workshop was first organised and a doctor and an engineer from 11 major university hospitals were invited. After sharing information regarding current medical needs and technical problems, they decided to start a monthly teleconference for endoscopy. With leadership by a doctor and technical staff, this teleconference was implemented in only 2 months and has become a very educational programme.

These national meetings also allow participants who usually interact remotely to meet each other in person. These in-person exchanges contribute to the success of telemedicine. Although remote education is a useful tool, the addition of in-person meetings makes programmes more attractive because it deepens friendships and improves understanding. An annual local workshop is a good idea to facilitate programmes and keep them on the right track.

11.6 Limitations

11.6.1 Technical problems

The biggest limitation for telemedicine programmes is technical problems. Doctors expect teleconferences to go smoothly, but problems can occur, most frequently regarding sound [16]. Echo, caused by inappropriate microphone control, is very common and sound quality can be poor if low-quality microphones are used. Volume imbalance is another common problem when multiple sites are connected. Another problem is image deterioration due to an unstable internet connection. Engineering staff should take steps to prevent such problems in addition to fixing them. Special attention should be devoted to security to preserve patient privacy. All private information must be masked and encrypted when necessary.

11.6.2 Programme organisation

Organisers, support engineers and coordinators are needed to organise a successful programme. Organisers of the programme, usually doctors and medical staff, make decisions regarding the topics, connecting sites, presenters and other issues. The support engineers make the technical preparations. In a multi-party teleconference, the chief engineer at the main site has the most difficult job [13]. The coordinators, or secretariat, communicate with all other staff to make things run smoothly. Sometimes not all required staff are available. In such cases, there are often problems with the preparations, leading to delays or improper settings.

11.6.3 Time differences

Time differences should be considered for international activities. This is usually not a serious problem for activities where all participants are from the same continent. However, when the time difference is large (e.g., 12 h), one party must get up early and the other must stay up late to participate.

11.7 Future

Telemedicine will become increasingly common and spread to various settings such as clinics. The supporting technology will become even more user-friendly and cost-effective.

The United Nations announced 17 sustainable development goals. Among them, our main goal is Good Health and Well-being, but telemedicine can also contribute to the goals Quality Education and Reducing Inequality. We sincerely hope that telemedicine will be globally adopted to help people synergistically with local support.

References

[1] Marescaux J., Leroy J., Gagner M., *et al.* 'Transatlantic robot-assisted tele-surgery'. *Nature.* 2001;413(6854):379–80.

[2] Shimizu S., Nakashima N., Okamura K., *et al.* 'International transmission of uncompressed endoscopic surgery images via super-fast broadband Internet connections'. *Surg. Endosc.* 2006;20(1):167–70.

[3] Shimizu S., Kudo K., Antoku Y., Hu M., Okamura K., and Nakashima N. 'Ten-year experience of remote medical education in Asia'. *Telemed J. E. Health.* 2014;20(11):1021–26.

[4] Ho S.H., Rerknimitr R., Kudo K., *et al.* 'Telemedicine for gastrointestinal endoscopy: The Endoscopic Club E-conference in the Asia Pacific Region'. *Endosc. Int. Open.* 2017;5(4):E244–52.

[5] Eto M., Lee T.Y., Gill I.S., *et al.* 'Broadcast of live endoscopic surgery from Korea to Japan using the digital video transport system'. *J. Endourol.* 2007;21(12):1517–20.

[6] Moriyama T., Han H.S., Kudo K., *et al.* 'Role of international tele-education with live surgery for pre-clinical medical students' early exposure to surgery'. In *Proceedings of the APAN – Research Workshop 2019.* 2019;48–53.

[7] Huang K.J., Cen G., Qiu Z.J., Jiang T., Cao J., and Fu C.Y. 'Application of international videoconferences for continuing medical education programs related to laparoscopic surgery'. *Telemed J. E. Health.* 2014;20(2):157–60.

[8] Shimizu S., Ohtsuka T., Takahata S., Nagai E., Nakashima N., and Tanaka M. 'Remote transmission of live endoscopy over the Internet: Report from the 87th Congress of the Japan Gastroenterological Endoscopy Society'. *Dig. Endosc.* 2016;28(1):92–7.

[9] Kudo K., Tomimatsu S., Moriyama T., Tannimoto M., Jalife S.L.V., and Shimizu S. 'Remote medical education in Latin America'. *TICAL.* 2017:267–76.

[10] Shimizu S., Tomimatsu S., Doyle G., *et al.* 'Live surgery broadcast from Japan to South Africa: High-quality image transmission over a high-speed academic network'. *J. Int. Soc. Telemed eHealth.* 2013;1(3):80–85.

[11] Shimizu S., Han H.S., Okamura K., Nakashima N., Kitamura Y., and Tanaka M. 'Technologic developments in telemedicine: State-of-the-art academic interactions'. *Surgery.* 2010;147(5):597–601.

[12] Kudo K., Tomimatsu S., Houkabe Y., Moriyama T., Nakashima N., and Shimizu S. 'Five-year progress of technological changes in remote medical education'. *J. Int. Soc. Telemed eHealth.* 2017;5:e10.

[13] Kudo K., Moriyama T., Tomimatsu S., Ueda S., and Shimizu S. 'A train-the-trainers (TtT) program for engineers for hosting multiparty international clinical teleconferences'. *J. Int. Soc. Telemed eHealth.* 2019;7:e16.

[14] Kudo K., and Antoku Y. 'Telemedicine Conferencing: An Introductory Guide for Engineers' [online]. Tokyo: National University Hospital Council

of Japan; 2017. Available from http://www.univ-hosp.net/english/internationalization/teleconference/. [Accessed July 2019]
[15] Domestic Telemedicine Workshop, Telemedicine Development Center of Asia http://www.temdec.med.kyushu-u.ac.jp/eng/our_domestic.html. [Accessed July 2019]
[16] Tomimatsu S., Kudo K., Moriyama T., Moriyama T., Taguchi T., and Shimizu S. 'Technical troubles and how to prevent them in regular medical videoconference'. *J. Int. Soc. Telemed eHealth*. 2018;6:e10.

Section III

Sustainable and resilient mHealth services

Chapter 12

Generic disaster information model for message delivery triage in disaster response

Teuku Aulia Geumpana[1] *and Fethi Rabhi*[2]

Massive amounts of data during disaster situations require timely collection and analysis for the emergency team to mitigate the impact of the disaster under challenging social-technical conditions. The absence of the Internet or its intermittent and bandwidth-constraint connection in disaster areas may exacerbate and disrupt the data-collection process during the emergency response, and may cause delays for vital information to reach the control room in time. Instead of solving the problem at a network level, the chapter provides an alternative solution at the software design level.

Our solution is called the priority over cloudlet terminal (POCkET) Framework, which consists of two components. The first one, called GIMo, is a generic disaster information model that defines dataset attributes and how each attribute is structured and customized. The second one, called AMMo, adapts GIMo structure and customization into a cloudlet implementation by assigning priority value for each dataset attribute and aggregates the attribute values into new priority level of a dataset. This mechanism ensures that a dataset with a higher priority value receives special treatment over a limited network situation.

In this chapter, we will only focus our discussion on how we create GIMo as a part of POCkET Framework solution. Later, GIMo and AMMo are evaluated by observing the accuracy of the assigned priority compared to predefined scenarios using a distance measure technique. A scenario from bushfire case study was created and tested using different contexts. Eventually, the experiments have shown a better result in the customized context. For that reason, POCkET Framework has provided a potential alternative solution to the network problem in disaster environments by modifying the emergency response system requirements.

12.1 Introduction

In disaster response, the emergency response teams are required to provide rapid and real-time communication using any readily available tools to collect important

[1]School of Electrical Engineering and Computing, The University of Newcastle, Newcastle, Australia
[2]School of Computer Science Engineering, University of New South Wales, Sydney, Australia

information from disaster site, regardless of the infrastructure breakdown. There are many recommendations about which a tool can be used to facilitate communication from disaster ground to the control room. Choosing the right communication tool is a matter of getting the right information to the right people at the right time so that they can make the right decisions. Recent advancement of wireless mobile service communication and spatial information services has brought up an alternative option as an essential solution to provide a quick support in difficult circumstances. This is important especially in reaching remote areas or when used in emergencies. Both of these services may offer portability, flexibility, and digital data processing in informing accurate location positioning of certain information around the disaster location or any other early disaster information required by the emergency response team.

The existence of mobile ad-hoc network (MANET) in the area may begin transmitting information within a matter of hours, much faster than the time it takes to repair or replace existing network infrastructure equipment. With these technologies, the team can quickly supply important data to the control room for crucial decision-makings. Irrespective of the benefits it may offer, the wireless mobile service will not provide its best-intended services upon the absence, neither the unstable internet network within the disaster area.

The speed of getting accurate information from disaster ground to the control room can be compromised especially when communication infrastructures are damaged or functioning in a slow rate. With such a vulnerable situation, while most of the solutions to the problem are proposing hardware setting–based solutions, the chapter investigates solutions related to how to design software that can make a more effective use of an ad-hoc network given that information can have different values for different stakeholders. It is just like using triage assessment approach in medical emergency procedure in which, the triage is required to determine the priority of patients' treatments based on the severity of their condition [1]. As in information delivery, we want to establish procedure to classify information based on their important level with respect to disaster situation.

Thus, the chapter will be focusing on addressing multi-contexts solutions. Knowing the value of information, certain types of information can be treated differently during transmission to allow appropriate response from the control room. For example, during the bushfire disaster situation, knowing the wind direction that blows toward a residential area could trigger an immediate evacuation warning even though the fire points are still in a far distance.

This chapter is structured into seven sections. In Section 12.1, we introduce the potential problem in designing a software system for the disaster emergency response. Then, the chapter shows some related works to our solution Section 12.2. Next in Section 12.3, the chapter discusses the POCkET Framework that is composed of GIMo and AMMo. As our focus is on GIMo, more discussion on GIMo is done in Section 12.4. In Section 12.5, we presented case study and evaluation result. Meanwhile in Section 12.6, we discuss our observation of the result. Finally, Section 12.7 concludes the limitation and future works.

12.2 Related works

Opting software, as an alternative solution to solve the network problem, can be challenging for the following problems: how to design information model that can adequately represent information items related to disaster management (DM) and their importance in different contexts? How to enable users to define, implement, and test an information model in DM? In order to solve these problems, the present study proposes that the emergency response system (ERS) should be robust in solving the network problem and applicable to run in different disaster context. The following surveys are conducted to look into existing work that specifically related to creating information model that accommodates different disaster contexts.

The design work in [2] prioritizes information for resource allocation in the reconstruction phase. This work focused on identifying key information elements to better allocate resources for construction project using an analytic hierarchical process (AHP). The procedure used in this solution generally involves dividing information based on its categories, splitting information into different phases of construction project, and classifying information with cross-combination of the above-mentioned two steps. This work is indirectly related to disaster response, as it demonstrates a priority mechanism for classifying important information at the software design level.

Other works such in [3–5] address the process of modeling information during the emergency response. The work in [3] is a dynamic emergency response management information system (DERMIS) framework. The framework incorporates thinking about the value of insights and information from communities of geographically dispersed experts and suggests how that such expertise can be brought to bear on crisis decision-making. The DERMIS framework has four major design components: design premises, conceptual design, general design principles, and supporting design considerations prior to developing functionality requirements that the software needs for planning and executing the emergency response management functions. The framework can be used as a basis for the initial information model but lacks elaboration of how it is going to be implemented in different disaster contexts.

Authors in [4] implicitly claim that their framework may be implemented in different disaster contexts from the way dimensions are defined. The general context is left for users to define to suit different situations. However, no prioritization has been considered with regard to network problems in a disaster area. Meanwhile, the work in [5] proposed a framework that contains one of the five basic elements of the emergency response coordination life cycle. An information element is observed from three phases of response: pre-incident, during incident, and recovery. None of these works has considered information exchange failures that may happen during transmission and not dedicated to be implemented in multi-context disasters.

After looking into surveys related to frameworks for designing and developing the ERS, it is essential to see the related works on existing information models for the ERS. As defined, an information model is a representation of concepts, relationships, rules, constraints, and operations to specify data semantics for a particular domain of discourse. An information model provides a formal description of a problem domain without constraining how that description is mapped to an actual implementation in software. There are many mapping techniques of the information model including data flow diagrams (DFD), entity-relationship diagrams (ERD), and others. The works in [2,6–8] are identified related to this research.

Information prioritization is an important part of design system to allocate resources in the construction field. The AHP prioritization technique that is used decomposes an unstructured problem into a decision hierarchy. The problem in a decomposed form may help inducing an iterative process to solve inconsistent responses during the construction period. This is a direct example of how information prioritization is useful in creating more efficient resource allocation. Almost similar goals are set during disaster response operations; minimizing operation times, speeding up the recovery process, saving lives, and preventing more casualties [9–11] are benefits to be gained from efficient resource allocation.

Another work used W4H approach to create classification. The W4H is a way to question 'who', 'where', 'when', 'what' and 'how' of a process. The work in [6], presented a context information model for disaster response which adopted the *W4H* classification for the context data consisting a set of general classes, properties and relations. This model exploited five semantics dimensions: identity (*who*), location (*where*), time (*when*), activity (*what*) and device profiles (*how*). The work in [7] proposes an information model to examine the mechanism by which social capital contributes to information exchange in virtual communities in the context of a major natural disaster. This solution claims to provide timely access to comprehensive, relevant, and reliable information that are critical for DM.

DM is a challenging domain to model because of the variety of dynamic characteristics attached to the domain. One way to overcome multi-characteristics domain information is by grouping this information into classes using metamodeling technique. The metamodeling collection of classes describes domain concepts, which represent domain entities, actions, or states [12]. Examples of metamodeling information design built for different contexts are described in [13].

Kirillov *et al.* (2012) created a metamodel of shared situation awareness for resilient management in the built environment [13]. Then, the authors developed a conceptual framework for a Russian nation-wide multi-hazard crisis management by proposing two-time-scale adaptive architecture to cope with the problem of delayed response in high-consequence buildings and structures.

Other work by Othman *et al.* proposed disaster management metamodel (DMM) to generically represent a unified view of common concepts and actions that apply in various disasters [14]. This metamodeling work studies the characteristics of the response in a disaster area through evaluating DM documents like reports, manuals, and standard operating procedures from different resources [15,16]. The DMM is developed by applying the meta object facility (MOF) framework [17] to represent the DM domain using several modeling layers. The MOF framework represents DM knowledge domain in three abstraction layers: M0, M1, and M2. M0 represents the real-world object, which describes how knowledge related to tactical activities is structured. Meanwhile, M1 describes the model for policy and planning context and M2 is the metamodel itself in which the knowledge is abstracted in the conceptual model. This abstraction is later to be instantiated as real objects. In the data modeling domain, instantiation is the process of making abstract object into real (data-filled) object [18]. In the DMM, the lower layer of the MOF is an instance of the higher layer. This means that a model in a higher abstraction layer will represent the language to be expressed for the model in the lower layer.

The DMM was developed based on existing literature and domain-specific disaster models based on a comprehensive study on disaster reports and manuals. The DMM provides a foundation for creating a generic information model. For instance, in [14] the DMM is validated using a specific disaster of a devastating bushfire disaster, which hits the state of Victoria in Australia and led to a catastrophic loss of life, nearly 200 in 2008. The DMM analysis was then generated at M2 level, basing its work on model guidelines developed by the government, which were set at M1 level, which in turn were set on the actual DM application for bushfire at M0 level. The DMM is not the only model that tries to accommodate multi-contexts. The work in [19] by Dick *et al.* (2017) also creates information model in different contexts. The process it took to generate a generic information model includes two types of information: requirements and qualification strategies.

Although the work in [19] has introduced a generic information model, the implementation did not include disaster-response-test scenarios. Therefore, it is unproven that the model can be implemented in a disaster emergency context. Currently, we have not found any works that propose disaster information system to run on ad-hoc network using metamodel approach to collect and deliver disaster information response.

Hence, the contribution of this chapter is to create an information-model-design process that accommodates different context of disaster response. Later, as the continuation of this chapter, we will discuss how we create priority functions and adaption-mechanism-design process for simulation design-time and simulation runtime in cloudlet environment.

12.3 POCkET Framework

POCkET is an abbreviation of priority over cloudlet emergency terminal. The framework name itself reflects a direct analogy toward the limitation of the real pocket function. Usually, a shirt's pocket is small and can contain limited items that are important or portable within the pocket size. In response to the network problem in disaster context, the analogy indirectly reminds the designer that urgency levels should be given accordingly to fit the limited available bandwidth in the temporal network.

1. POCkET GIMo—GIMo stands for generic information model. POCkET GIMo refers to the proposed generic information model that can be used in multiple disaster emergency response contexts. It encapsulates important datasets that are used to enable effective communication in emergency response.

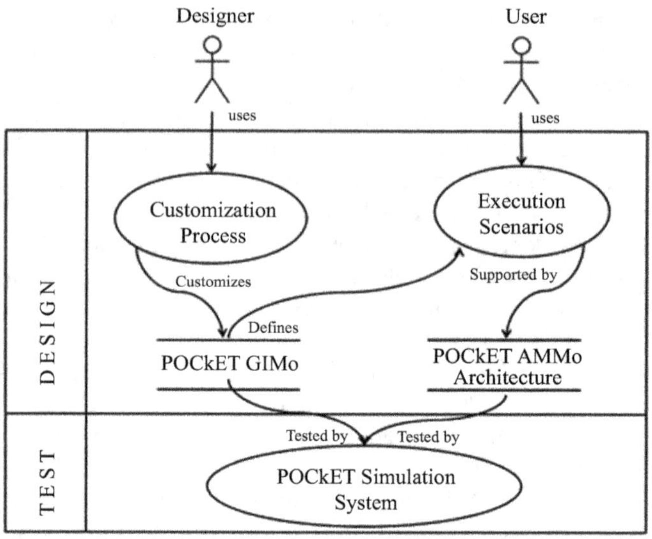

Figure 12.1 POCkET framework

2. POCkET AMMo Architecture—AMMo stands for adaptive mechanism model. POCkET AMMo refers to the architecture that supports the execution scenarios that adapt GIMo into the ERS.

Figure 12.1 depicts the overall view of the POCkET framework. The POCkET framework proposes two artifacts to help designers and users creating a robust ERS. Each of them is named as follows.

12.4 GIMo

As a generic information model, GIMo should demonstrate universal applicability in different disaster contexts. Hence, it has to satisfy certain criteria. More specifically, GIMo should demonstrate:

Generic scope: The model must not describe a particular disaster context, or use concepts that are specific only to a particular type of disaster.

Completeness: The model should capture the core information entities, namely the information resource stakeholders, information, information resources, associated technology, emergency response tasks, and critical success factors. To gain the full advantage of multiple sources, a designer/developer must query all available sources and integrate the results. Even if automated, this is a tedious and often expensive task. Some measure is needed to determine which sources are to be preferred over others. This measure must take into account both the number of objects provided by the source and the amount of information per object it provides.

Extensibility and reusability: The model should be easily applied in different disaster contexts and used by the developers so that it could be reused and extended, according to the emergency needs. To achieve this, each of the core classes must be self-contained; bearing attributes which do not depend on any other class. Moreover, attributes that exist in different classes and could hold the same information, as well as excessive or meaningless associations between classes, must be eliminated.

GIMo has a dataset that is defined as a collection of data elements that correspond to information being collected during the emergency response operation. It will be regularly collected by a source device and sent to the cloudlet when new information becomes available. GIMo dataset has the following attributes: dataset ID (DsID), dataset source location information (DsLOC), dataset creation time (DsCT), dataset arrival time (DsAT), dataset category (DC), dataset type (DT), dataset size (DS), dataset frequency (DF), dataset recency (DR), distance to cloudlet (D2C), hubs to hop (H2H), and dataset priority value (DPV).

The priority level associated with a dataset is calculated on arrival at the cloudlet by applying an aggregate function on the following attributes: DC, DT, DS, DF, DR, D2C, and H2H. To do so, a weight value is also defined for each of these attributes.

Figure 12.2 shows the resulting POCkET GIMo using a class diagram. The diagram shows how a dataset is related to all of its attributes. It also shows the entities that store information about default attribute value ranges, priority ranges, and weights. These default attribute values can be customized by designers. The attributes representing priority ranges are labeled _PR for each attribute variable, i.e., for attribute category (DC) the attribute for priority range is DC_PR.

A weight in this model is the value that is given to store dataset attributes based on user analysis. A weight is assigned in a numerical value from 1 to 10, with 1 being the least important information and 10 being the most important information. At run time, an aggregate function is applied to the values of these attributes to generate the priority level value for a particular dataset. Each dataset attribute that has a weight attribute has the suffix _W added after each attribute variable name, i.e., for attribute category (DC), the label for weight is DC_W.

In addition, an attribute priority function (_PF) is stored with the same dataset attributes. This priority function is generated from a training dataset by observing how well a model fits the data of a particular attribute. The priority function is labeled with a _PF extension, i.e., for attribute dataset category (DC), the label for priority function is DC_PF.

12.4.1 Overall process of customizing pocket GIMo for a specific context

POCkET GIMo is a generic information model that enables users to modify information values according to different contexts. A developer still needs to adjust POCkET GIMo to suit a specific disaster context. A developer should

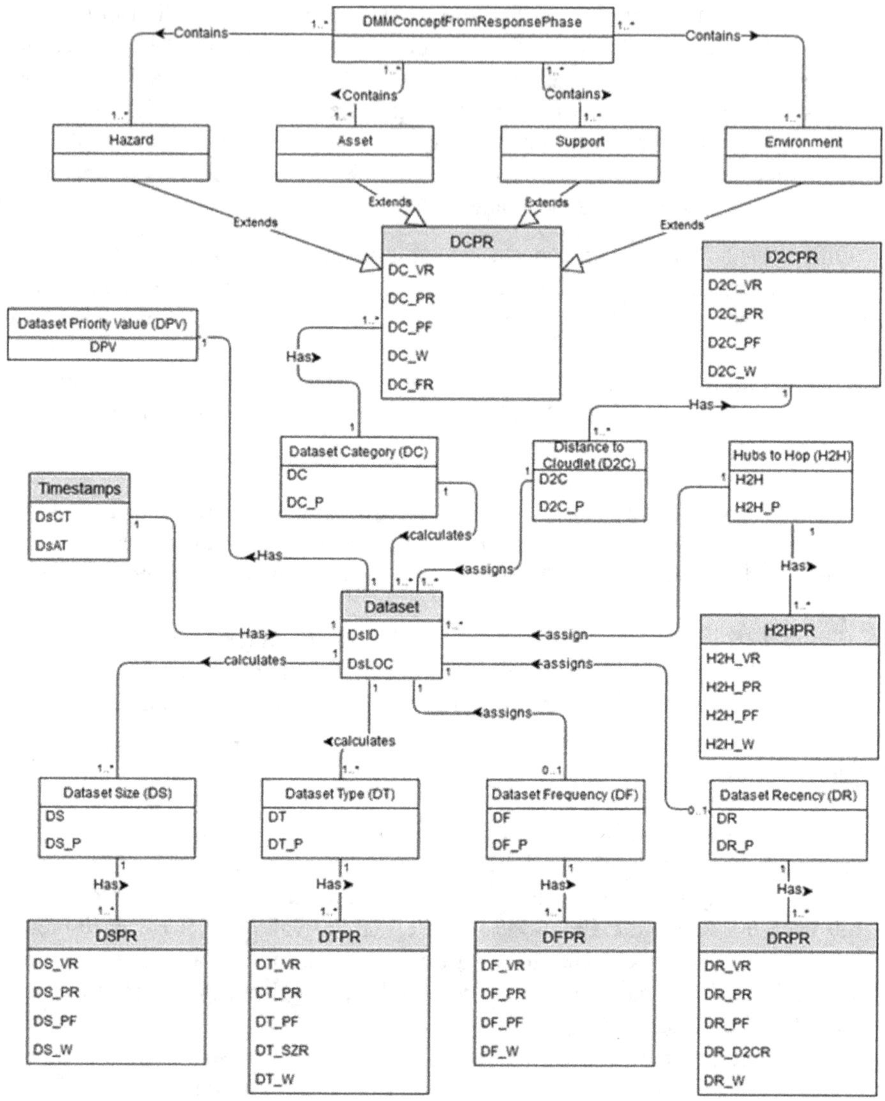

Figure 12.2 POCkET GIMo

consider three steps prior to customizing the POCkET GIMo for a specific context: reviewing categories of DMM concepts, reviewing the default values of the relevant dataset attributes, and defining a priority function for these dataset attributes.

Upon reviewing categories of DMM concepts, the developer first needs to study response guidelines of a particular disaster. Then, a GIMo template is accessed to review frequency terms that have been assigned. If default values are not relevant, the developer can modify them accordingly. The developer may create a new category or assign different priority range values to existing DMM concepts. Then, to reviewing default values, the developer reviews default values of selected attributes along with their ranges. After defining the range of priority values for each attribute, a weight is assigned to each attribute by the POCkET application user. The weight is described as a value from 1 to 10 that is given based on user analysis for each attribute. Last, in defining priority functions, each priority function is constructed by observing the best model that fits a training dataset that is composed of 11 selected dataset attributes.

Once the training dataset has been generated, we run an estimation function on each dataset attribute to calculate an equation that minimizes the distance between the fitted line and all of the data points on the model. A model fits the data well if the differences between the observed values and the model's predicted values are small and unbiased. There are many ways to statistically measure for goodness-of-fit of a model. In the implementation described in Section 12.5, we will apply the framework to a case study; a regression function will be used as an estimator. For this function, the most common used measure to find goodness-of-fit of a model is the R-squared (R^2) observation. In general, the higher the R^2, the better the model fits the data. In the process of finding the fitted model of each attribute, much iterations are performed on each model and the _PF is selected based on the best fit for each attribute model.

12.5 Case study

12.5.1 Case study description

We created a case study that generates potential datasets of an emergency response (Dsj-u). Each of information carries details from different categories and attributes based on bushfire scenario. We then defined a predetermined priority value (PPV) for each dataset that is based on user analysis and literature reviews to create a baseline data. For a given PPV, we also assign expected numbers of order (ENO) accordingly (Highest PPV is assigned ENO = 1).

Table 12.1 shows the PPV and the ENO of each dataset.

Datasets wind speed (Dso) and fire spread rate (Dsu) are the first two datasets with the highest priority of 9. So, bushfire status (Dsr) dataset with priority value of 8 comes as the next high-priority dataset. Smoke density (Dst) and estimated nearby suburban population (Dsp) datasets come after bushfire status (Dsr) with priority number of 7. Based on Table 12.1, victims' conditions and treatments (Dsm) dataset comes last with lowest priority of 2.

12.5.2 Context setting

Based on information available for the case study, the designers customize GIMo in different ranges. The customization outputs from this process are sets of contexts, which are used in the experiments.

Table 12.1 PPV and ENO of bushfire scenario

Dataset arrival order	Ds_n	PPV	ENO
Safe evacuation route options	j	6	6
Nuclear plant	k	5	9
Victims' general information	l	3	10
Victims' conditions & treatments	m	2	12
Victims' locations	n	3	11
Wind speed	o	9	1
Estimated nearby suburban population	p	7	5
Military base	q	5	8
Bushfire status	r	8	3
Safe place for evacuation	s	6	7
Smoke density	t	7	4
Fire spread rate	u	9	2

To begin setting up the context, we follow the guideline of three steps of GIMo customization: review categories and DMM concepts of the case study, review default values and priorities of the case study, and generating training dataset and its priority functions.

Default values for dataset categories of are hazard, asset, support, and environment. To customize GIMo for the case study, a designer may modify the default values. For example, in the case study, the groups that compose an emergency team, one of them is responsible in collecting specific information about the victims. For this reason, new category of "Victim" is added and category "Others" is removed. By changing the default values of dataset category attributes, the designer also needs to define new priority value ranges of the newly created value. To define the new priority value ranges, the designer can either reuse the previous priority values ranges or create new priority value ranges for victim. These activities are conducted in the next GIMo customization step.

After adding new value of "Victim" under dataset category, the designer then defines priority value ranges, and weights for "Victim" and reviews the default values of other datasets attributes. Using a priority ranges customization control in POCkET simulator, a designer can change the priority value ranges by moving the slider provided in the panel. For this example, newly added category of "Victim" is assigned priority range of seven and eight. "Victim" as the newly created value under dataset category will be the second highly important datasets after hazard if no other values in the categories and dataset values are changed.

The adding of "Victim" into dataset category and the definition of its priority range values create a new context variation for Scenario 1. Therefore, additional changes on other dataset attribute values and priority range values of Scenario 1 will create more contexts for testing.

Priority function is then generated from each training dataset as guided earlier.

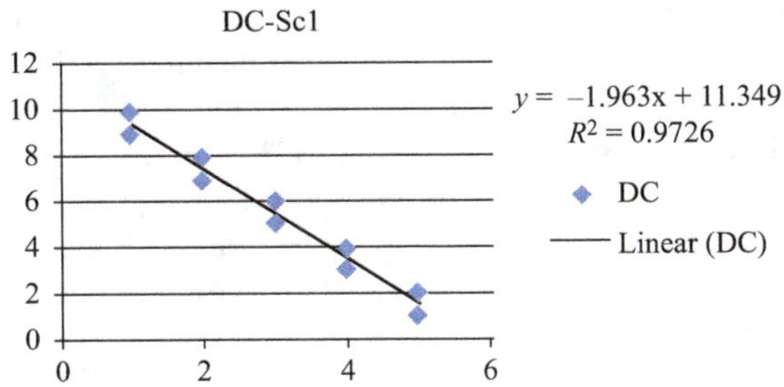

Figure 12.3 DC regression model for C1V1

From the case study, we train the dataset by assigning values to each dataset attribute and observe the best-fitted line model from the regression function. For example, to generate a priority function for dataset category (DC) attribute in C1V1, we first convert the DC value into numbers (Hazard = 1, Victim = 2, Asset = 3, and so on). Then, we assign priority value for DCj (PV_DC) by randomizing priority range values based on the dataset category attribute value (DC_VR). We repeat the process to all DCn. Once PV_DC is completed, we can now apply the regression measure to plot the model. The following scatter plot shows the result of regression performed on DC.

From Figure 12.3, we observe the R^2 value to identify the best-fitted line for DC (Hint: the closer the number to 1 gives better function). For C1V1, we select the y function with the R^2 value of 0.9726, which defines the priority function for DC (PFDC):

$$y = -1.963x + 11.349 \tag{12.1}$$

We repeat the process for other dataset attributes until all priority functions are completely acquired.

12.5.3 Simulation result of scenario 1

Scenario 1 is then tested through different contexts: the first context is called C0, which is composed of the default values and followed by other variations of bushfire contexts. To set the comparison baseline, we look at the results with No Priority Context (NPC) in which no priority functions are applied on the datasets. The total distance in the NPC is 66. Using the baseline result, we also compute how significant does a solution improve in other experiment results by comparing the baseline result with other results.

C0 is simulated in Scenario 1. This is done by applying GIMo default setting on Scenario 1. The result has shown a promising value of total distance of 32. This means that when tested using default GIMo values, the result of Experiment 1 has improved 52% than the result in the NPC. The first context variation (C1V1) gives the total distance of 26. This result has improved 60% compared to the baseline result. Next, we had another context variation (C1V2) and acquired the total distance of 28. This result has also shown an improvement of 57% better than the baseline result. The third context variation (C1V3) has a distance of 34, which is 48% improvement. Last context variation has total distance result of 28 (57% improvement).

Overall, best context from Experiment 1 is C1V1 that gained 60% improvement from the NPC. This is because in C1V1, we assigned victim priority value to be the second highest priority in DC attributes. This setting pushes down all other priority attribute values.

12.6 Discussion

Using a predefined scenario, we can expect the worst performance (highest distance) should come from the NPC when no priority is assigned. This means, at Cloudlet, datasets are forwarded to the remote server in the same order as they are received from mobile devices. A better result should be acquired when C0 context (default GIMo values) is applied on the datasets. This is because C0 calculates and assigns priority to each dataset based on its default values. Therefore, C0 result should be better than the NPC. However, C0 may not be the best result for every context.

In all the results, customized contexts were appearing better or equal to the default context. For example, in Experiment 1 the best result is gained from C1V1 and in Experiment 2 the best result is gained from C2V2. In terms of relating the experimental results to the assessment criteria (i.e., the framework meets the criteria of genericity, completeness, extensibility, and reusability) the following conclusion can be made.

12.6.1 Genericity

The POCkET GIMo model has successfully been applied in bushfire disaster scenario. However, just the bushfire scenario is not sufficient to demonstrate that POCkET GIMo can model other types of disasters such as earthquake or tsunami.

12.6.2 Completeness

GIMo has defined 12 dataset attributes, which were sufficient to represent datasets used in two disaster contexts. However, the dataset themselves were created via simulation and the better way of checking the completeness would have been to use real datasets.

12.6.3 Extensibility and reusability

The experimental results from bushfire have shown that POCkET GIMo was extensible and reusable to some extent. In the first example shown in Scenario 1, the default GIMo context was extended to match the bushfire context. “Victim” was added to DC attribute that caused the priority range values to be readjusted as a variation from the default context. Despite the attribute being extended, most of the attributes were reused. These results have proved that GIMos were extensible and reusable in the Scenario 1.

Based on information available for the case study, the designers customize GIMo in different ranges. The customization outputs from this process are sets of contexts, which are used in experiments.

12.7 Conclusion and future woks

This work was motivated by the need of creating adequate infrastructures for dealing with information overload during emergency response. While most of related work is concerned with hardware and networking solutions, this research has focused on software challenges faced by software engineers in dealing with design requirements that can adapt to multiple disaster contexts.

We have presented a solution that helps addressed these questions in the form of the POCkET framework and its realization. The main contribution of this chapter is GIMo, a generic information model acquired from an existing metamodel (DMM), which allows the main dataset attributes to be modeled. GIMo also allows the designer customization of dataset attributes' priority values and ranges according to different contexts. The generic information model also allows the use of training datasets to configure priority functions according to available datasets.

12.7.1 GIMo limitations

Although based on an existing metamodel, the proposed GIMo is strongly influenced by the documentation that has been used in the case studies (bushfire). There could be many additional information concepts that have not been represented.

In addition, GIMo customization still requires a significant effort from the designer in analyzing disaster-related information and translating available guidelines into the information required. In particular, generating the training datasets and priority functions is still a labor-intensive process in the existing customization process.

12.7.2 Validation limitations

Validation techniques used relied on predefined scenarios, which are very time consuming to construct, and therefore there were fewer experiments performed due to the difficulty in creating realistic datasets. Obtaining datasets related to disaster has also proved to be very costly and file formats were inconsistent due to different standards that were used in different countries. In addition, there were limitations in the way different configurations were evaluated. For example, the proposed distance measure used to compare between effectiveness of different prioritization schemes is a very basic measure of comparison. Finally, not all the customization possibilities offered by GIMo have been tested for time restrictions. Therefore, it was not possible to test how all the concepts defined in GIMo contributed to changes in the observed priorities except for few ones.

12.7.3 Validity threats

The first limitation relates the research methodology adopted. The Software Development Life Cycle (SDLC) research process only allows for a restricted number of requirements to be addressed for time limitations. In this research, the focus was on the prioritization of the datasets at the cloudlet level but many other requirements have not been addressed. A realistic implementation would have provided a much better way of validating the proposed framework.

All of these limitations are to be improved in the future works, which will be discussed in Section 12.7.4.

12.7.4 Future work

Although this research has offered a potential alternative to solve the network problem in disaster environment, further works are still required to improve the proposed solution. These improvements can be performed by addressing GIMo limitations, expanding the options for validation, and addressing the limitation of the research methodology.

The first area of future work should focus on assessing the completeness of GIMo. A publication in [20] describes a complete framework for dealing with the specification and integration of the quality of information provided by a single data source or a set of data sources. One approach to ensure completeness is by considering the intentional character of information quality (called density) and the extensional character of information quality (called coverage). The combination of the two aspects will ensure completeness criterion, which assesses the quality of data sources and leads to various applications such as source selection, query optimization, bounding result sizes, etc.

Future work should also concentrate on improving validation methods used in this research. Firstly, some mechanism to assist users in generating datasets for scenarios must be investigated. For instance, some general goals can be specified and datasets generated accordingly instead of users being required to specify various datasets' attributes separately. Secondly, more disaster contexts need to be considered to determine a wider range of attribute values and priorities. Thirdly, assessing the suitability of a context for a particular scenario needs to be done using improved measures than the one used in this research.

Finally, in term of improving the research methodology, the analysis of information guidelines could be conducted in a more systematic way. The use of text-mining techniques could help in extracting information categories and determining priorities based on text metrics such as frequencies. In addition, the use of a more realistic simulation environment of the different activities performed during emergency response could be an important avenue of future work. For example, providing an adequate representation of the timings between different events during information exchanges between mobile devices and cloudlet can be investigated. A realistic small-scale implementation may be a more effective validation technique than simulation.

References

[1] Noda, I., K. Egawa, H. Shimora, and I. Yoda, *Process simulation of triage for emergency medicine under huge disaster*. In *SICE Annual Conference (SICE)*, 2011 Proceedings of. 2011.

[2] Moore, H. *Out-of-control Sydney bush fire spreads towards nuclear reactor and army ammunition warehouse as residents in surrounding suburbs are told 'it's too late to leave'*. 2018 15 April 2018 [cited 2018, 16 April]; Available from: http://www.dailymail.co.uk/news/article-5617263/Sydney-bushfire-spreads-nuclear-reactor-army-base-residents-nearby-evacuated.html#ixzz5Co2FauAh

[3] Turoff, M., M. Chumer, B. Walle, and X. Yao, *The design of a dynamic emergency response management information system (DERMIS)*. JITTA: Journal of Information Technology Theory and Application, 2004. 5(4): p. 1.

[4] Chen, R., R. Sharman, H. Rao, and S. Upadhyaya, *Design principles for critical incident response systems*. Information Systems and E-Business Management, 2007. 5(3): p. 201–227.

[5] Cheng, E.W.L., and H. Li, *Information priority-setting for better resource allocation using analytic hierarchy process (AHP)*. 2001. p. 61–70.

[6] Chen, R., R. Sharman, H. Rao, and S. Upadhyaya, *Coordination in emergency response management*. Communications ACM, 2008. 51(5): p. 66–73.

[7] Truong, H.-L., A. Manzoor, and S. Dustdar, *On modeling, collecting and utilizing context information for disaster responses in pervasive environments*. In *Proceedings of the first international workshop on Context-aware software technology and applications*. 2009, ACM: Amsterdam, The Netherlands. p. 25–28.

[8] Lu, Y., and D. Yang, *Information exchange in virtual communities under extreme disaster conditions*. Decision Support Systems, 2011. 50(2): p. 529–538.

[9] Zuo, P., Y. Hua, X. Liu, *et al. BEES: Bandwidth-and energy-efficient image sharing for real-time situation awareness*. In *Distributed Computing Systems (ICDCS)*, 2017 *IEEE 37th International Conference on*. 2017. IEEE.

[10] Fiedrich, F., F. Gehbauer, and U. Rickers, *Optimized resource allocation for emergency response after earthquake disasters*. Safety Science, 2000. 35(1): p. 41–57.

[11] Kusumasari, B., Q. Alam, and K. Siddiqui, *Resource capability for local government in managing disaster*. Disaster Prevention and Management: An International Journal, 2010. 19(4): p. 438–451.

[12] Li, Y., Y. Liu, H. Zhang, J. Xiao, Y. Zhao, and W. Guan, *Study of emergency resource distribution model based on genetic algorithm*. In *Information and Automation (ICIA), 2010 IEEE International Conference on*. 2010.

[13] Kirillov, I.A., S.A. Metcherin, and S.V. Klimenko. *Metamodel of shared situation awareness for resilience management of built environment*. In *Cyberworlds (CW), 2012 International Conference on*. 2012.

[14] Othman, S.H., G. Beydoun, and V. Sugumaran. *Development and validation of a Disaster Management Metamodel (DMM)*. Information Processing & Management, 2014. 50(2): p. 235–271.

[15] Barrantes, S.A., M. Rodriguez, and R. Pérez, *Information management and communication in emergencies and disasters*. Pan American Health Organization, 2009.

[16] Kusumasari, W., *Technical guidelines for health crisis responses on disaster*. In *Guidelines for health workers involved in health crisis responses on disaster in Indonesia*. 2011, The Ministry of Health of Republic of Indonesia: Jakarta. p. 228.

[17] Inan, D.I., G. Beydoun, and S. Opper, *Agent-based knowledge analysis framework in disaster management*. Information Systems Frontiers, 2017: p. 1–20.

[18] Rouse, M. *Instantiation*. 2005 [cited 2018]; Available from https://whatis.techtarget.com/definition/instantiation.

[19] Dick, J., E. Hull, and K. Jackson, *Requirements engineering*. 2017: Springer.

[20] Naumann, F., J.-C. Freytag, and U. Leser, *Completeness of information sources*. 2003.

Chapter 13
Application and development of drones for health services in developing countries

Ruchi Saxena[1,2,3]

Unmanned aerial vehicles or drones are all set to transform the healthcare supply chain, to enable last-mile deliveries, not only in remote inaccessible regions but also for the urban communities. From blood packets, vaccines, sputum samples, and to emergency medical supplies, drones are being looked at as an option that can complement existing methodologies for reducing the accessibility gap in healthcare.

This chapter shares the work done in healthcare drones across the world. As more demonstrations and experiments are being conducted, national-level policies are being drafted and funds have been directed toward this futuristic technology.

13.1 Introduction

According to the World Health Organization [1], at least half of the world's population still does not have full coverage of essential health services. All UN member states have agreed to try to achieve universal health coverage (UHC) by 2030, as a part of the sustainable development goals.

The Declaration of Astana, observed at Global Conference on Primary Health Care, 2018, was committed to by ministers, health workers, academics, partners, and civil society for making primary healthcare as the cornerstone of universal health coverage. It was acknowledged that in spite of remarkable progress over last 40 years, people in all parts of the world still have unaddressed health needs and health is still a challenge for many people, particularly the poor and people in vulnerable situations. It was declared that primary healthcare will be accessible, equitable, safe, of high quality, comprehensive, efficient, acceptable, available and affordable, and will deliver continuous, integrated services that are people-centered and gender-sensitive.

[1]Caerobotics Healthcare Solutions, London, UK
[2]Caerobotics Consultancy Pvt. Ltd., Mumbai, India
[3]India Flying Labs, Mumbai, India

It was declared that a variety of technologies should be used to improve access to healthcare, enrich health service delivery, improve the quality of service and patient safety, and increase the efficiency and coordination of care. Individuals and communities shall be enabled to identify their health needs, participate in the planning and delivery of services, and play an active role in maintaining their own health and well-being through digital and other technologies.

Technologies that can help in reducing the accessibility gap in global healthcare scenario have made strides especially in digital space where telecommunication tools have helped people connect rural health facilities to their urban counterparts. However, the distance and the sparseness that separate health facilities in remote inaccessible regions call for the next layer of technologies to take over the responsibility of reducing this gap.

Mountainous terrains such as the Himalayas that cover all of Bhutan, most of Nepal, and the northern and north-eastern parts of India have one such example where the existing road network is not dependable due to erratic weather conditions. Landslides, floods, and torrential rains cause large-scale damage and make the resources even more inaccessible. If roads and land are not the option we can consider, we need to look at the aerial routes. Expensive manned aircraft will soon give way to unmanned aerial vehicles or UAVs or more colloquially, drones to reach all those places where it is either too expensive or risky for manned aircraft to reach. Drones shall replace man with machines for the routine and tedious activity of delivering healthcare to the remotest populations. This technology is gradually evolving and we would like to give a glimpse of what is happening and what is possible in the application of drones in healthcare.

13.2 Challenges

Imagine you are out on a trek with your friends in Nepal. One of your friends has an asthma attack and she realizes she has left her inhaler back home. The altitude is making it worse and her health is deteriorating. Where you are, there is nothing but forest around you and the nearest village is about 15 km away. You only have a basic telecommunication signal and that is enough to send an SMS or a basic call to ask for help. You explain the coordinator where you are and what is the medical need like. Mostly, you will be asked to bring your friend to the nearest motorable road where an ambulance may arrive if you are lucky, and the ambulance is available.

More often than not, you will struggle to reach the nearest village; hope there will be a clinic there or at least a drug store from where you can buy the inhaler that she needs.

In an alternate reality, not very far into the future, as soon as you ring in to ask for help, the coordinator will locate you on a map, command an attendant to load a drone with the needed drugs, and order a dispatch. It will reach you sooner than any other help that you can hope for; in some cases, it can be a serious lifesaver.

Any of us could be in such a situation. But for many, this is a routine challenge.

For the rural areas, healthcare facilities continue to be poorly resourced in many locations. The road network may not be available in many places or may not be in a good condition. In Nepal, people still walk for days to get to the nearest motorable road in many regions. Many populations living in remote islands still depend on boats for transport; during rough weathers, this option is almost cutoff. Similarly, tribal populations living closer to or inside a forest are nearly detached from mainstream healthcare developments and the challenge continues to remain for hilly regions and deserts. Health workers often have a hard time reaching the communities and are forced to trek for days to deliver even basic healthcare.

Not just rural, even urban populations that have sufficient well-resourced healthcare facilities face challenges due to heavy traffic and overcrowding. Aiming for better efficiency and effectiveness, cutting down time it takes to transport essential medical supply, urban hospitals in Europe [2] and North America [3] are taking the lead in implementing drone-based delivery solutions to connect to their satellite clinics, labs, and blood banks.

13.3 Unmanned aerial vehicles

Drones are remotely piloted UAVs. Drones can be loaded with anything – and that adds to the weight of the aircraft costing the efficiency and range, hence are called "payloads." These payloads can be different kinds of cameras, sensors, GPS systems, boxes, or audiovisual equipment. As the industry gets more creative and enthusiastic about these handy unmanned aircraft, drones have evolved and are now much more advanced than a decade ago.

They are popularly used as a hobby tool for racing, photography, and videography. They became unpopular when they were used to drop bombs in Middle East and viewed as tools for destruction. However, lately better uses of drones have been explored. They are also being considered for operations where human life can be at risk or where human labor can be replaced. They have mainly evolved as tools for photogrammetry, mapping, and aerial imagery data collection, and are also being considered for carrying packages.

While defense continues be the biggest consumer of drone technology [4], the applications are now being explored for social-good projects and humanitarian aid. Healthcare, disaster response and management, nature conservation, and sustainable agriculture are the major activities taken up by the global Flying Labs network through knowledge and technology transfer to empower local experts who use drones and data for social good applications.

Depending upon the applications, drones can be of various shapes and sizes and come with variable features and functions.

Fixed-wing drones appear like planes and even take off and land like planes. Like planes, they either need special take-off and landing systems – in the form of runways, propulsion and catching systems such as catapults and nets, or are pushed in the air like a kite and land on a flat ground. They can travel longer distances with better add-on weight of payloads but are considered less resistant to rough weathers [5].

Improved designs are now making these fixed-wings sturdier and safe. Service providers using these designs tend to carry parcels from point A to point B and para-drop supplies instead of landing at point B. They are hence best used there is just one-way supply needed like blood packets (Photo 13.1).

Multicopters are like choppers – they have rotating propellers on a frame – and depending on the number of propellers, they can be tricopters, quadcopters, hexacopters, and octocopters. They take off and land vertically (VTOL or vertical take-off and landing), just like a helicopter and do not need special runways, landing sites, or take-off and landing mechanisms. Although they are more stable and sturdy compared to fixed wings, they cannot travel longer distances. Hence, they are used for flying over small areas within visual line of sight; however, in many situations they serve well for beyond visual line of sight over small distances. Although they have been popularly used for surveillance, mapping, and photogrammetry, modified multicopters have also been used for delivering medical cargo over short distances, spraying insecticides on crops, and as disaster-response tools (Photo 13.2).

A third variety that is being explored are termed as "hybrid" drones as they combine features of both fixed-wing drones and multicopters. They vertically take off and land (hence, called hybrid VTOL) like a helicopter, thus needing less space and infrastructure at take-off and landing sites, and fly like a plane, thus covering larger distances efficiently. This design is considered the best for healthcare needs especially when we have to deliver packets from point A to point B and also carry something back from point B to point A or move further from point B to point C (Photo 13.3).

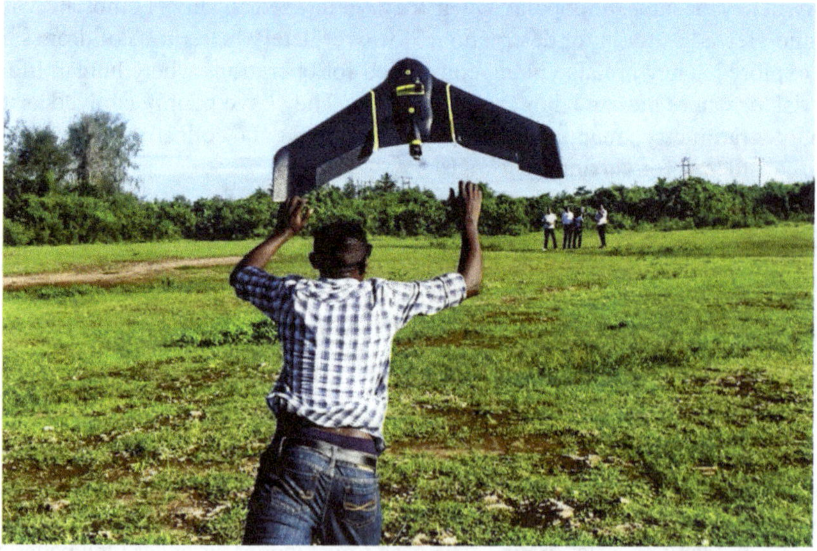

Photo 13.1 Fixed-wing drones being tested in Tanzania. Source: WeRobotics

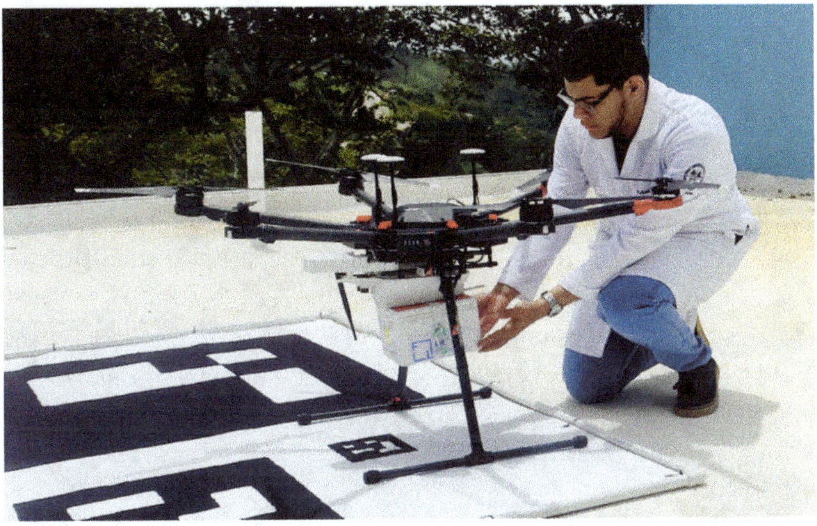

Photo 13.2 A multicoptor being tested in Dominican Republic. Source: WeRobotics

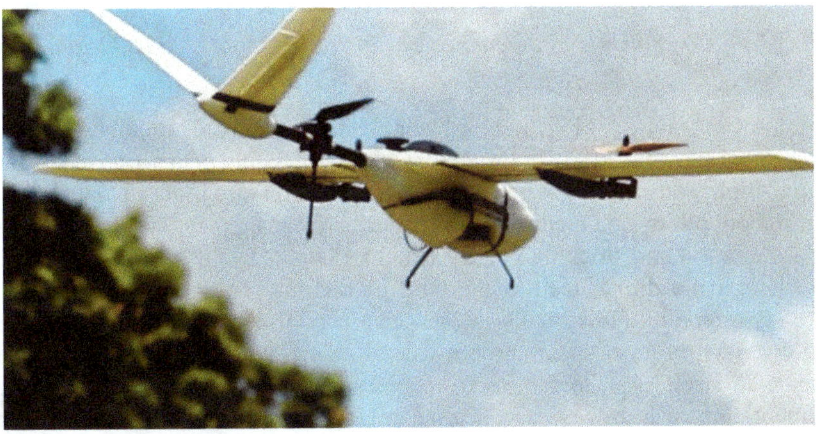

Photo 13.3 Hybrid VTOL being tested in Papua New Guinea. Source: WeRobotics

13.4 Drone ecosystem

Drones need a robust control and implementation system. Drones by themselves are just hardware. But together with other back-end and front-end controls and monitoring tools, they are a part of unmanned aerial systems. In case of operating drones for healthcare, we would need as a minimum, well-tested drones with in-built fail-safe systems such as obstacle avoidance, efficient ground control systems,

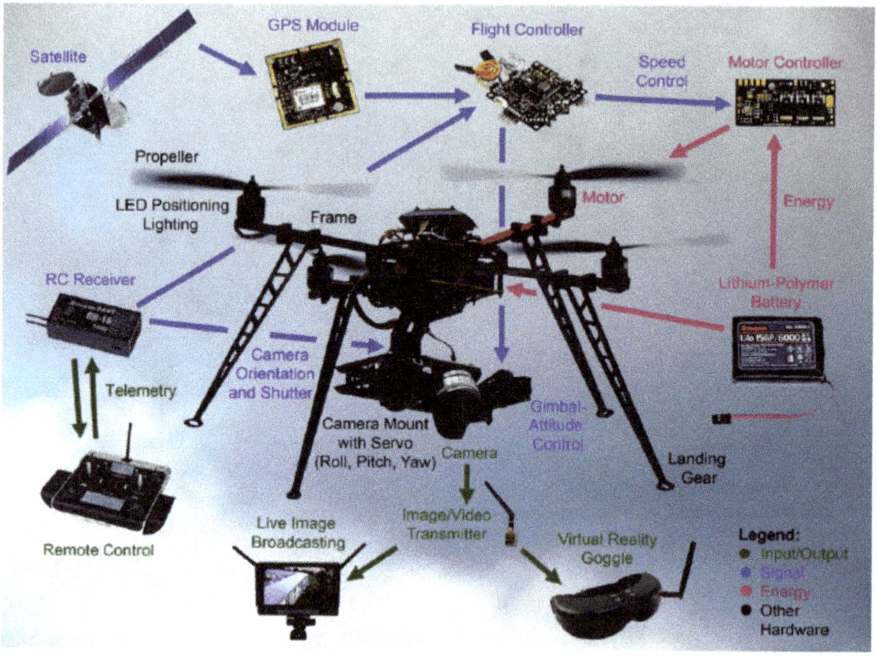

Photo 13.4 Components of unmanned aerial system. Source: Mechlectures.com

communication and tracking systems, command-control-coordination center and personnel, unmanned traffic management system – equivalent to air-traffic controls, pre-flight and post-flight maintenance systems, on-site flight maintenance and repair, remote pilots, and medical cargo inventory management system, to ensure a seamless rotation and stock movement (Photo 13.4).

Although the drone itself is the hero of the show, it needs all components seamlessly operating individually as well as a part of a whole system. Ensuring a robust ecosystem for healthcare drones with all components synchronized is a huge challenge in itself. As the felt need becomes more demanding of a large-scale implementation of a drone-based healthcare service, strengthening these systems will be equally, if not more important than just manufacturing, the best quality drones.

Besides drone technology and control and command system, a robust policy framework that allows and encourages drones for social good will remain to be the most important factor to ensure large-scale drone implementation globally. Drone policies vary from country to country and range from total ban to selective permissions to easy online permission systems. While this is good for hobby flyers and other mapping industries, for delivery drones used in healthcare, significantly stringent rules apply. While ensuring the public safety in case of a drone crash and ensuring that the drones themselves have enough fail-safe measures in place, to preventing the bio-hazard in case of a drone crash carrying potentially infected materials, healthcare drones have to cross many more hurdles to be fully accepted by the public healthcare systems and policies.

We also do not have to ignore the role the community engagement plays in ultimate success of a drone delivery project. At the end of the day, it is the community that will be driving these projects forward; in addition, if they are involved right when the drone ecosystems are being designed, they will be in a more acceptable frame of mind to appreciate the impact these technologies shall bring to them. WeRobotics and Flying Labs have been particularly serious when it comes to community engagement, and ensure that local engineers, health workers, and local representatives from the communities are directly and completely involved in the healthcare cargo drone projects right from the beginning, from the stage of ideation to the stage of implementation, thus becoming essential contributors to the whole design. This ensures greater success of the whole project [6].

13.5 Drones for healthcare

For healthcare, long-range drones that can fly several kilometers of aerial distance are being experimented in various projects across the globe. Drones are now getting evolved as an essential medical cargo logistics tools for carrying small-to-medium-sized packets across short or long distances in medical emergencies as well as non-emergency routine medical cargo deliveries. The research and applications have been so far mainly for blood and blood products, vaccines and emergency drugs, and medical supplies.

The promise of these drone-based healthcare services is of improving accessibility by reducing the time taken to deliver a medical product to communities generally located in remote and inaccessible regions. The rural and tribal populations in these locations generally have poor access to mainstream healthcare, which leads to imbalance and inequality. It takes a long time to deliver the medical supplies to these locations and the last-mile delivery is an even bigger challenge, which is often done on foot or motor bikes. The underdeveloped road infrastructure in these resource-poor countries across difficult terrains and unreliability of existing infrastructure due to disasters such as heavy rains, floods, landslides, and earthquakes make it necessary to have an aerial delivery system to bridge the accessibility gap.

Although aerial routes using manned aircraft is an option, they cannot be depended upon in emergencies, as they tend to be expensive, many times unavailable, and even risky to operate in harsh weather conditions. During routine transports, they can serve as a good option for large cargos; but for last-mile delivery of small packets, drones still appear to be a good option.

Drones have showed promising results in all the successful as well as unsuccessful experiments conducted so far. The technology is still maturing and we will have to wait and watch how these machines are able to fulfill their promise. Points that give us reasons to be optimistic are that there are documented cases, which have directly benefited from the timely delivery aided by drones.

13.5.1 Blood deliveries

Stocking adequate quantities of different types of blood and blood products in every health facility is tricky since each blood packet has a limited shelf life. If unused within a couple of months, they need to be discarded. In a small community setting, it is almost impossible to predict what blood or blood component would be needed in what quantity. So, even if all primary and secondary health facilities do have a blood bank or even a blood storage facility, it will still not solve the problem of having timely access to adequate amount of specific blood type or its component.

The health department of Rwanda has adopted a unique drone ecosystem that has centralized blood processing and storage that responds to request for blood or its component by just-in-time delivery using long-distance fixed-wing drones. The blood packet is packed in a paper box and dropped at the specific health facility using disposable parachute. The drone drops the packet, returns to its home facility, and is ready for the next delivery. This helps in maintaining no infrastructure at drop site except a mobile-based request system. Highly advanced technologies and systems are maintained at the central facilities. A steady demand and just-in-time supply have made drones for blood deliveries an effective, efficient, sustainable, and replicable model [7,8].

As an alternative design, South Africa National Blood Service recently declared that they would be introducing national scale drone blood-delivery system using hybrid VTOL drones that will land at the health facility with the box containing the blood component, while also taking back samples for cross-matching. [9]

13.5.2 Vaccine deliveries

Last-mile delivery of vaccines in remote inaccessible regions is still a challenge, which organizations like UNICEF are trying to champion. Malawi, Tanzania, Vanuatu, and recently Democratic Republic of Congo are the countries where UNICEF has been actively experimenting with various drone solutions and test the efficacy of the system in terms of maintaining the cold chain and potency of vaccines [10].

WeRobotics had also recently experimented with drones for vaccines in association with the Government of Papua New Guinea and Papua New Guinea Flying Labs. A full-scale vaccine-delivery program is yet to be established as a service [11].

13.5.3 Emergency medications and snake anti-venoms

Saving life in critical emergencies such as poisonous snake bites would definitely be a very important use case for drones, understanding that poisonous snakes put the rural tribal populations at high risk. WeRobotics and Dominican Republic Flying Labs had used an indigenously made drone to fly snake venoms across Amazon rainforest over a distance of 30 km. DRC Flying Labs also recently used a short-distance caged drone to fly essential medical supplies to demonstrate the public safety aspect of using such a drone to deliver last-mile medical needs over short distances [12,13] (Photo 13.5).

13.5.4 Laboratory samples

Drones are being used for transferring sputum samples in Nepal from health centers in Pyuthan to an advanced diagnostic laboratory with GenExpert kit as the part of tuberculosis case-detection program promoted by Britain Nepal Medical Trust and executed by Nepal Flying Labs and WeRobotics. The Nepal Drone Observed Therapy System (DrOTS) project, The DrOTS project, aims to improve TB case detection through active case finding (ACF) of tuberculosis (TB), drone transport of specimens and supplies, and rapid molecular diagnostics, and thus improve treatment completion through electronic reminders and video curriculums. The project is funded by Stony Brook University and will work in Pyuthan in partnership with National TB Center [14] (Photo 13.6).

13.5.5 Vector control

South Pacific Flying Labs is working in Fiji on a pilot project with World Mosquito Program (WMP) to disperse mosquitoes infected with Woubachia bacteria that make them naturally resistant to mosquito-borne diseases such as malaria using a specially modified drone system. Till now, the WMP used jars of mosquitoes and went door to door, engaging with the community requesting them to release it in their backyard (Photo 13.7).

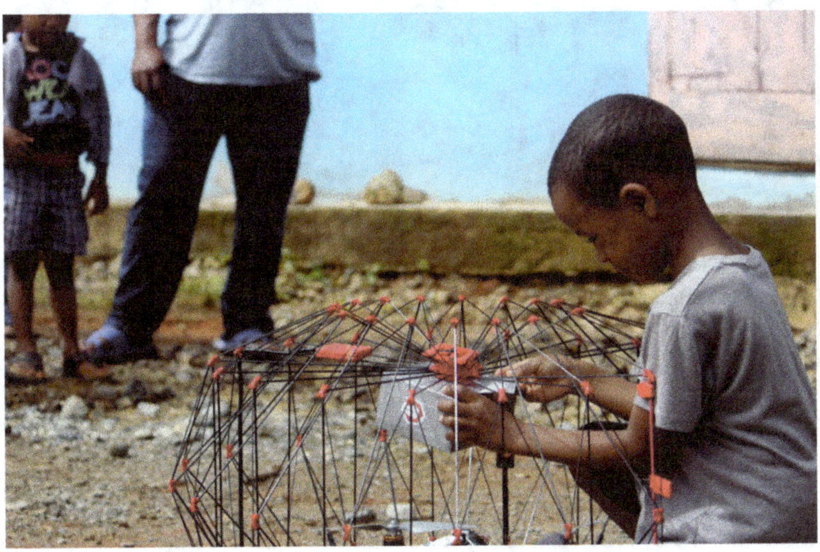

Photo 13.5 A caged drone being tested in Dominican Republic. Source: WeRobotics

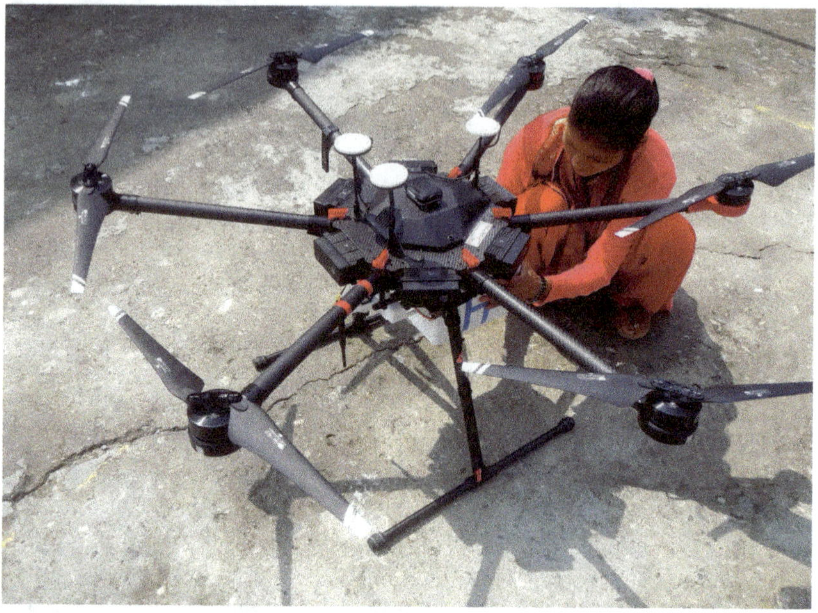

Photo 13.6 A drone used to carry blood samples in Nepal. Source: Nepal Flying Labs/WeRobotics

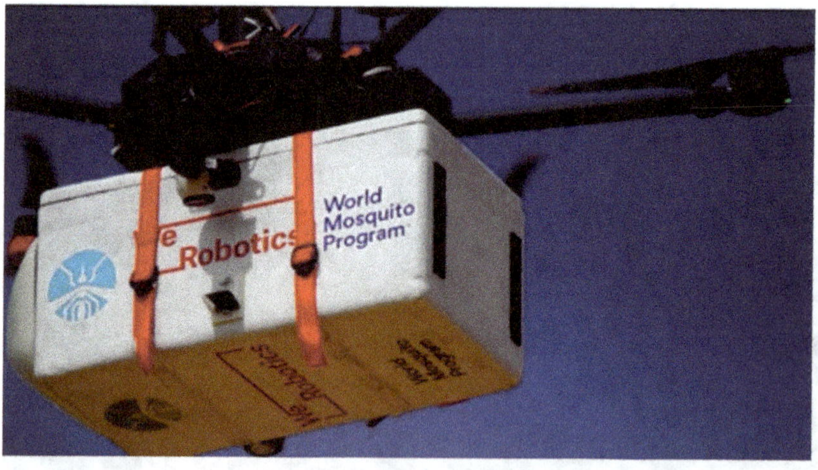

Photo 13.7 World Mosquito Program trial project in Fiji. Source: WeRobotics

With this new drone-based system, they are able to do this task much quicker, aiming for more uniform and widespread distribution of the modified mosquitoes [15].

13.5.6 Organ deliveries

Organ transplant is a time-bound activity and the donated organs have to be delivered safely and as soon as possible to the recipients. Aerial route is a promising way of delivering organs, and choppers are frequently used for this. However, that adds to the cost and not all hospitals have access to helicopters and helipads. Using drones along dedicated green corridors between hospitals can be an efficient way of delivering organs quickly. Efficiency of this method has to be tested. In one such test, a kidney was successfully transferred to University of Maryland [16]. India has declared that its Drone Policy 2.0 will have special consideration for such green corridors, have accelerated the discussions to allow drone companies to experiment BVLOS flights, and invited Expression of Interest to do the same [17].

13.6 Way ahead

While drones, or for that matter any technology or futuristic intervention, is great, there is only so much that they can do to ensure sustainable development of a society. Technology should go hand in hand with baseline development. Drones will be great to watch when they cut down time to reach remote communities, but that must not be an excuse to delay development of roads, bridges, and airports in these place.

We also do not want that drones that deliver medical supply to a villager directly at his doorstep become an excuse to not have a health facility in his neighborhood or for doctors to avoid visiting these places or a reason for cutting down budgets for ambulances or improving the hospital facilities. We do not want healthcare to become easy while the overall livelihoods remain difficult. That can lead to patchy development and will lead to questioning the whole investment in drone technology. We want that drones continue to improve the life of people and efficiency of the health systems. Drones can be a major contributor to the next evolution in healthcare, but should not be treated as a crutch.

As we write this chapter, newer drones are being tested in more places and the technology continues to evolve. We are about to witness a revolution together!

References

[1] World Health Organization, *Universal health coverage fact sheet*. 2019. Available from https://www.who.int/en/news-room/fact-sheets/detail/universal-health-coverage-(uhc). Accessed 10 October 2019.

[2] Swiss Post, *Drones: A vision has become reality*. 2019. Available from https://www.post.ch/en/about-us/innovation/innovations-in-development/drones. Accessed on 10 October 2019.

[3] UPS, *Press releases*. 01 October 2019. Available from https://pressroom.ups.com/pressroom/ContentDetailsViewer.page?ConceptType=PressReleases&id=1569933965476-404. Accessed on 10 October 2019.
[4] Goldman Sachs, *Drones reporting for work*. https://www.goldmansachs.com/insights/technology-driving-innovation/drones/. Accessed on 10 October 2019.
[5] Boon M.A., 'Comparison of a fixed-wing and multi-rotor UAV for environmental mapping applications: A case study'. The International Archives of the Photogrammetry, Remote Sensing and Spatial Information Sciences, Volume Xlii-2/W6, 2017.
[6] *Humanitarian UAV guidelines on community engagement*. Available from https://uavcode.org/further-guidance/136-2/. Accessed on 10 October 2019.
[7] World Health Organisation. *Drones take Rwanda's national blood service to new heights*. June 2019. Available from https://www.who.int/news-room/feature-stories/detail/drones-take-rwandas-national-blood-service-to-new-heights. Accessed on 10 October 2019.
[8] World Economic Forum. *In Rwanda, high-speed drones are delivering blood to remote communities*. December 2018. Available from https://www.weforum.org/agenda/2018/12/in-rwanda-drones-are-delivering-blood-to-remote-communities/. Accessed on 10 October 2019.
[9] The South African National Blood Service Press Release. *SA Blood service unveils its new delivery drone*. May 2019. Available on https://sanbs.org.za/uncategorized/18765/. Accessed on 10 October 2019.
[10] UNICEF, Programme Report. *Drones, addressing transport, connectivity and better emergency preparedness*. Available on https://www.unicef.org/innovation/drones. Accessed on 10 October 2019.
[11] WeRobotics. *Building cargo drone capabilities in Papua New Guinea*. February 2019. Available from https://blog.werobotics.org/2019/02/25/building-cargo-drone-expertise-in-papua-new-guinea. Accessed on 10 October 2019.
[12] WeRobotics. *Field testing cargo drones in Amazon Rainforest*. July 2017. Available on https://blog.werobotics.org/2017/07/24/field-testing-cargo-drones-in-amazon-rainforest. Accessed on 10 October 2019.
[13] WeRobotics. *Testing agile cargo drone delivery to improve healthcare in the Dominican Republic*. June 2019. Available from https://blog.werobotics.org/2019/06/03/testing-agile-cargo-drone-delivery-to-improve-healthcare-in-the-dominican-republic/. Accessed on 10 October 2019.
[14] Liverpool School of Tropical Medicine. *Drones trialed to assist in TB diagnosis in Nepal*. June 2019. Available from https://www.lstmed.ac.uk/news-events/news/drones-trialled-to-assist-in-tb-diagnosis-in-nepal
[15] WeRobotics. *How local drone pilots are helping to reduce dengue in Fiji*. December 2018. Available from https://blog.werobotics.org/2018/12/13/how-local-drone-pilots-are-helping-to-reduce-dengue-in-fiji. Accessed on 10 October 2019.
[16] University of Maryland Medical Center. *University of Maryland's Schools of Medicine and Engineering first to use unmanned aircraft to successfully deliver kidney for transplant at University of Maryland Medical Center*.

April 2019. Available from https://www.nytimes.com/2019/04/30/health/drone-delivers-kidney.html. Accessed on 10 October 2019.
[17] Ministry of Civil Aviation, Government of India. *Drone ecosystem policy roadmap*, January 2019.

Further reading

[1] Michelle Sing Yee Hii, Patrick Courtney, and Paul G. Royal. *An Evaluation of the delivery of medicines using drones*. June 2019. Institute of Pharmaceutical Science, Kings College, London.
[2] World Economic Forum. *Advanced drone operations toolkit: Accelerating the drone revolution*, December 2018.

Chapter 14

Build back better in the drone application by the Nepal Flying Labs

Uttam Pudasaini[1], *Darpan Pudasaini*[2] *and Yasuhiro Soshino*[3]

14.1 Introduction

Nepal is a landlocked country sandwiched between two of the largest economic centres of the world, India and China, and pervades a rich diversity in geography with its inclusion of the world's highest peak (Mt. Everest) at 8,848 m to as low as 60 m (Kechana in Jhapa). In addition, the cultural, climatic and biological diversity in a country this small is remarkable, establishing Nepal as one of the finest tourist destinations in the world. In Nepal, amongst its 29 million population, 8 per cent of total population live in the Himalayan, 45 per cent of them live in the Hilly areas and 47 per cent in the Terai region [1]. Whilst the rich geographic diversity makes Nepal one of the most beautiful countries in the world, it also causes two different types of challenges. The first challenge is natural disasters that results in 'the social emergencies' in Nepal. Nepal is highly prone to disasters, and hence has been ranked as the fourth most vulnerable country against climate change, the 11th against earthquakes and the 13th against floods. Furthermore, the second challenge is the limited access to rural healthcare facilities, which could be termed as 'the individual challenged'. Historically, Nepal suffered from various natural disasters. From 1900 to 2005, over 13,000 disasters caused a total 7,400,000 human casualties in Nepal [2]. In this century, a lot of human lives were lost by the natural disasters such as the 2014 avalanche in Mt. Everest, the 2014 floods and landslides at Sunkoshi River, the 2015 Nepal earthquake and the 2019 South Asia floods. The geographical diversity has increased the complexity and difficulty of the relief efforts by humanitarian organisations in cases of emergencies. Evident from the 2015 Nepal earthquake, due to lack of updated maps of vast majority of areas in Nepal, humanitarian responders could not efficiently plan and respond. In terms of access to health

[1]Nepal Flying Labs
[2]DroNepal
[3]Japanese Red Cross Kumamoto Hospital

services, the major hindrance to healthcare services is attributed by the topography of the country. In Nepal, insufficient drugs, long walking distance to health facilities and unavailability of adequate healthcare personnel are the important factors for the deprivation of quality public health facilities [3]. A large number of local healthcare facilities in rural Nepal are not accessible by vehicles. The majority of people in rural areas are forced to access the existing health infrastructures on foot. In addition, the means to deliver medicines which are usually stored at the nearest urban hospital rely on the earthen roads that are completely flooded during the monsoon season. Advanced healthcare facilities and diagnostic laboratories are not present in most primary health facilities in rural areas and they are concentrated only in urban areas. The access to healthcare facilities is hence still a huge challenge mostly in rural villages and hilly areas of Nepal.

The applications of drones provide the cost effective and efficient solutions to improve the access to health facilities and to ensure the link between the skilled healthcare personnel and the patients. For example, drones deliver the medicines and testing samples such as blood, urine and stool for diagnosis between the healthcare facilities and the patients in the hard-to-reach areas. Drones can reduce the time and obstacles in accessing the hard-to-reach areas, which increases the resilience against natural disasters. In this way, to cope with the social and individual emergencies in Nepal, drone technology is a key solution that aids in overcoming the geographic challenges in the rural areas. Nowadays, drones are well known for their effectiveness in the rapid damage assessment in the disaster-affected areas, and in the transportation of medical items both during disasters and at normal times. In fact, the catastrophic 2015 Nepal earthquake became a kickstarter of the application of drones in the country. Therefore, this study discusses the application of drones in the healthcare sector and the disaster management sector in Nepal. In addition, this study presents the role of the Nepal Flying Labs, which was established after the 2015 Nepal earthquake, to foster the proper technology transfer by capacity building of local drone stakeholders.

This study is structured as follows. Section 14.2 reviews the development of the drone applications in Nepal. Section 14.3 introduces the formulation of Nepal Flying Labs. Section 14.4 presents the drone applications in the healthcare and disaster management sectors. The section also describes the capacity building of the local drone stakeholders. Discussion will be shown in Section 14.5 and Section 14.6 concludes this study.

14.2 Review of the drone applications in Nepal

14.2.1 Initial stage of drone applications

Antecedent to the influx of post-earthquake drone usages, a selected group of research organisations, hobbyists and university students had been making use of the technology in Nepal, whilst little publications were available. Amongst the recorded cases, in June 2012, WWF Nepal carried out a pilot test of two fixed-wing UAVs for wildlife conservation and to combat against illegal poaching and logging. Since then, they have implemented the technology alongside government and local communities [4]. In co-ordination with Utrecht University of the Netherlands, ICIMOD carried out first-ever UAV-based glacier studies in Lirung Glacier of Nepal [5]. Student groups from Kathmandu University also had done a comparative study of different image-processing tools for feasibility of use of drones in surveying and mapping sector [6] and biomass estimation [7]. In this way, the major purpose of the drone applications was for the academic and research purpose whilst its implementation for disaster responses and medical purposes before the 2015 Nepal earthquake was not popular.

14.2.2 The drone applications in the 2015 Nepal earthquake

The 2015 Nepal earthquake, which caused widespread damage throughout the country, urged the humanitarian communities, journalism and research communities to introduce drones in the rescue, relief and recovery operations. In the acute emergency phase, Canadian drone-maker Aeryon Labs, partner company Monadrone of Monaco, and the Canadian humanitarian aid organisation, GlobalMedic, used drones for capturing images of quake-stricken regions before aid workers were deployed [8]. One of their significant uses of drones was in the search and rescue operation for a missing US Marines' helicopter that was carrying six Marines and two Nepali soldiers [9]. A drone footage captured by a local amateur drone pilot was published by the BBC [10]. Various news and media agencies and humanitarian organisations used drones for ground situation reporting purposes and drones-based footages were also used for studies on construction of 3D models in the disaster-affected areas [11]. In addition, drones were also deployed to assess the geotechnical damage assessment in the disaster-affected areas by the research communities [12].

UAVs were widely introduced to the public and the government agencies in Nepal in the aftermath of the 2015 Nepal earthquake. Although the significance of drones was realised, the applications of the drones were still limited, possibly due to two major reasons. Firstly, drones were still not popular technology in Nepal, which resulted in the limited drone operators and equipment in the country. Secondly, the humanitarian organisations mostly relied on traditional approaches and tools for their operations in Nepal. Hence, in order to formalise and implement drone technology for better disaster preparedness and increased healthcare accessibility in Nepal, the need for local capacity building for sustainably contextualising drone technology and empowering local drones-based businesses became evidently clear.

14.2.3 Capacity building of drone communities in Nepal

In September 2015, the first-ever drones for crisis mapping training in Nepal, titled 'Professional UAV training for Disaster Preparedness and Recovery', was organised by UAViators, an international humanitarian network, in association with

Kathmandu University (hereafter, the KU), Kathmandu Living Labs, DJI and PIX4D [13]. A group of 30 Nepalese individuals from different sectors were trained on the use of drones for post-disaster mapping and data processing. This marked an epoch in the brewing of many local professionals using drones for various purposes in Nepal. Furthermore, the organisers handed over ten drones and smartphones with the software (PIX4D) to the KU and Kathmandu Living Labs for training local drone professionals for the future expansion of drone applications. After the completion of 2 days training, the team together with Community Disaster Management Committee (CDMC) Panga (Kirtipur) also did a drone-based survey of the affected community in Panga-Kirtipur. The team printed a flex map and shared it with the CDMC. The community members easily identified the damaged buildings and new locations for temporary settlements using the high-resolution aerial base map of the community. The printed high-quality map catalysed a community-wide discussion and it also set a baseline for a model of participatory mapping and GIS (PPGIS).

14.3 The Nepal Flying Labs

14.3.1 The Flying Labs initiative and the Nepal Flying Labs

Following the first drone training in the KU, a significant milestone achieved was the establishment of a local entity to take forth similar activities and create a favourable ecosystem around the use of drones and robotics in Nepal. In December 2015, Dr Patrick Meier and his colleagues established an international non-profit-organisation titled 'WeRobotics', which focuses on robotics for social good and humanitarian purposes. As one of the main activities of WeRobotics, Flying Labs were established in developing and prone-to-disasters countries. The mission of the Flying Labs is to localise suitable robotics solutions by the capacity building of local experts who use the solutions for humanitarian and social good activities in a sustainable way. The Nepal Flying Labs is a social enterprise aiming to serve the vulnerable and underprivileged regions of Nepal by capacity building of local stakeholders to bridge the technology gap between the socio-economic development needs in the regions and the emerging technology solutions such as drones, robotics, artificial intelligence. The Nepal Flying Labs is one of the members of the Global Flying Labs Network [14], which now exists in more than 20 countries. The Flying Labs are established in disaster-prone and low-income countries with the aim of local intervention in accelerating and scaling the use of technologies in a sustainable manner by localisation of robotics solutions. The Flying labs are always co-created with local expert centres, universities, local companies, local authorities, research institutes and private companies focusing on technological solutions. As the first NPO (Not-For-Profit Organisation) in Nepal focusing on drones and robotics for humanitarian purposes, the Nepal Flying Labs has a strong rapport with the government and other drone stakeholders such as Civil Aviation Authority of Nepal, Local government, local universities, robotics association of Nepal, hospitals and private research institutions.

14.3.2 Localisation of drone technology by the Flying Labs

> *'If Drone operators aren't already on site by the time disaster strikes, they probably will not arrive in time to be useful*'. [15]

As this quote points out, both the technology and the capacity to use that technology need to be locally available so that the local people themselves can use it whenever there is a need. The Nepal Flying Labs mainly focuses on localising the technology according to a framework shown in the Figure 14.1. The framework designed by WeRobotics for all the flying labs consists of the following four steps.

1. Identify local need: Through partnerships with local institutions, organisations and communities, the Nepal Flying Labs first identifies appropriate technology for local problems and brings international expertise as partners in helping make the solutions accessible to the local stakeholders.
2. Build local skills: The Nepal Flying Labs organises various trainings, (Figure 14.2) workshops and interaction programmes to provide the local stakeholders with the required skills and technologies to use the solutions themselves sustainably in the future. It's usually done through technical partnerships in ensuring effective and immediate impacts, collaborating on local projects.
3. Increase local impact: Once the local partners are self-dependent in their areas of work, the Nepal Flying Labs continually works with them in globally sharing experiences and lessons learned, and hence improving and expanding the positive impact of the local works. The Nepal Flying Labs also provides drones-based consulting support, rental support availing necessary additional technologies to the local partners and helping them grow.
4. Catalyse local business: With local partners capable of carrying projects on their own, the Nepal Flying Labs then provides 'Robotics as a Service'

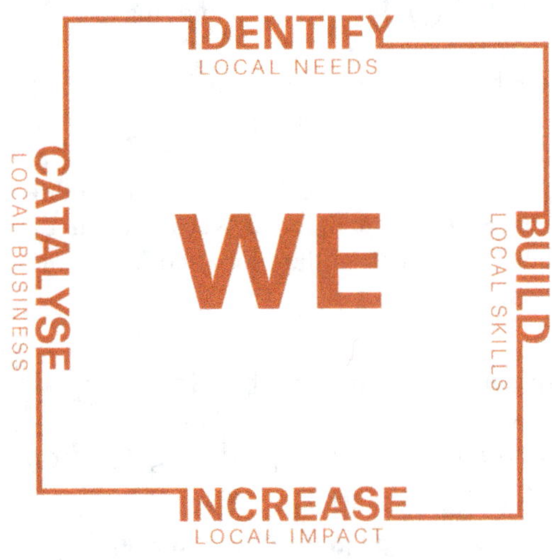

Figure 14.1 The Flying Labs

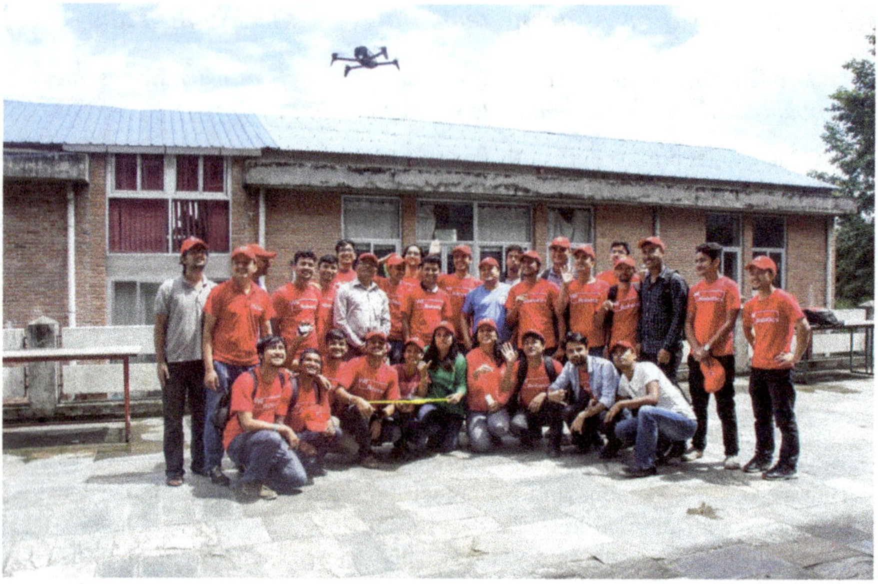

Figure 14.2 Drone training

business incubation programmes, where seed funds mentorships and required trainings are provided to help the local partners start their own robotics as a service businesses.

In these four steps, a newer local need is identified and ultimately new local businesses are helped to establish. In any of the above steps, whenever and wherever required, the Nepal Flying Labs also creates data products and services for local organisations in helping them assess and make effective use of UAV-generated data.

In addition, through interactions programmes and meetups, the Nepal Flying Labs sensitises the local partners to the social good aspects and benefits of the drone technology. For example, the Nepal Flying Labs advocates the policy changes for the better localisation of technologies and building the proper drone ecosystem in the country. In particular, the Nepal Flying Labs disseminates the UAV code of conduct [16], which is the global code of conduct for the humanitarian drone operations.

14.4 The drone applications by the Nepal Flying Labs

14.4.1 Post-disaster resettlement planning by drones

14.4.1.1 The project background

The 2015 Nepal earthquake highlighted the vulnerability of the houses in the mountainous areas. Since most of the rural villages of Nepal are located in the hills and mountains, a number of houses are exposed to the risks of landslides caused by the floods and earthquakes. In addition, in rural areas of Nepal where majority of the houses are scattered in random clusters, the lack of building construction standards and community planning increases the vulnerability to natural disasters. In fact, following the 2015 earthquake, the houses in rural areas tend to be rebuilt at the exact same location where the damaged houses used to be before the earthquake struck. To avoid the future recurrence of the calamities, it is imperative in the resettlement process that the houses are rebuilt according to the proper construction plan based on the critical assessment and analysis of the suitable locations. However, limited efforts are seen in proper resettlement planning due to the rough topography in rural areas of Nepal. In addition, the proper resettlement planning has been hindered due to the lack of updated maps and topographic data for depicting the possible relocation and rehabilitation places. Following the devastating aftermaths of the Nepal earthquake 2015, rebuilding efforts are still seen ongoing in the fifth consecutive year, and still an estimated 100,000 plus people are living in emergency stopgap shelters [17]. If drones could be used for intervening resettlement planning in other earthquake affected areas as well, a much efficient and sustainable settlement plans could be made ensuring more resilient infrastructures and beautiful villages.

14.4.1.2 Implementation

In March 2019, the Nepal Flying Labs in conjunction with a drone service company 'DroNepal' carried out a detailed topographical mapping of a possible relocation site in a rural village of Bijaykharka in Khotang district. This drone-assessment activity was a part of the resettlement project lead by Rupakot-Majuwagadi Municipality in Khotang district. Before this project started, the local government had already identified some of the possible sites for the relocation of more than 20 houses in a village. However, due to the lack of sufficient topographical data, their decision-making was hindred, which resulted in delaying the effective master plan for the resettlement. In particular, the data for verifying the feasibility of the location of the housing sites and the spaces for roads, water supply and drainage were crucially needed.

The project aimed to present a drone application model for encouraging the data-driven resettlement and infrastructure planning in the disaster-affected areas of Nepal.

In this project, drones captured the high-resolution aerial images of the possible relocation site. These images were utilised to generate an accurate topographical map. The high-resolution orthophoto maps were much appreciated by the local government since it provided them with the visual overview of the entire site with the accurate geographical information. The maps and data products generated also contained height information along the contours of the land, which was significantly useful in finding suitable construction areas and groundwork planning.

In this way, the drones were effectively deployed for capturing the high-resolution aerial images and topographical data to design the evidence-based master plans for the resettlement (Figure 14.3). The master plan was presented in an

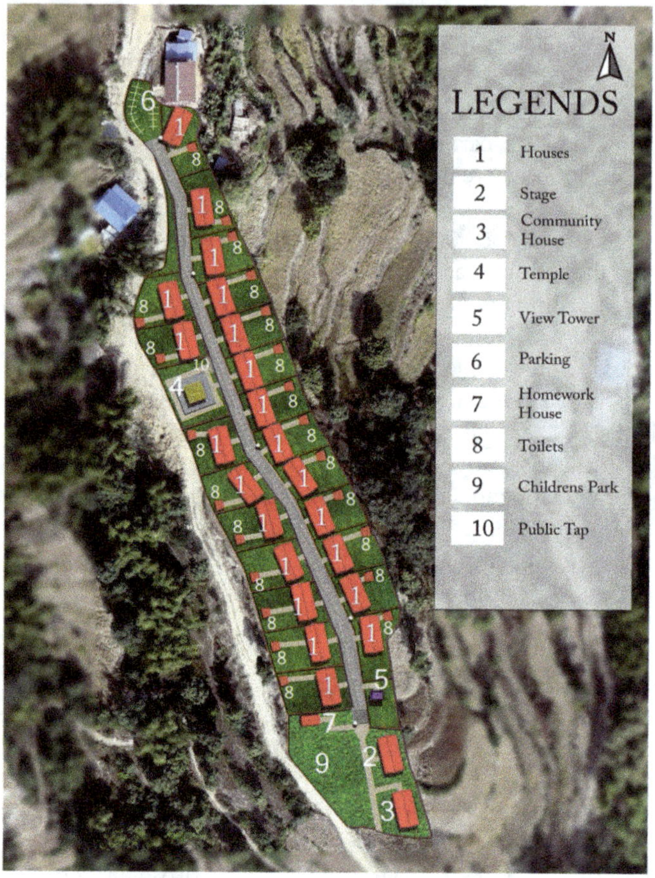

Figure 14.3 Resettlement master plan

interactive workshop in which the representatives of the local government, the affected communities and the drone experts participated to discuss the relocation plan. The highly detailed and visual master plan was useful to the local stakeholders in sharing a clear vision of the resettlement plan, which contributed in greatly reducing the time for the controversial discussions amongst stakeholders.

14.4.2 Drones for rural health in Nepal

14.4.2.1 The project background

In Nepal, there are annually 44,000 tuberculosis infections, which kill approximately 6,000–7,000 lives and 12,000–13,000 undiagnosed TB cases are left undiagnosed [18]. The government of Nepal recognised the need to intensify efforts to identify the missing TB cases in the community. The Strategic Plan for 2016–2021 of the National Tuberculosis Centre (hereafter, 'NTC') aims to find an additional 20,000 TB cases relative to the baseline in 2015. Innovative means are required to achieve this goal, since the access to healthcare facilities is always challenging in the rural areas of Nepal. Therefore, this pilot project called 'Drones Optimized Therapy System' (DrOTS Nepal) aims to improve case finding by linking community health workers with state-of-the-art diagnostic tools (hereafter, 'GeneXpert') by using drones (Figure 14.2). The pilot project also aims to become a model of the rural healthcare services that can be scaled nationwide. The overall goal of this project is to establish an 'on-demand' drone service in Pyuthan and Swargadwari in Pyuthan district. This overall goal will be achieved by clearing some sub-steps, which are (1) remote TB diagnosis, (2) remote observation of TB therapy and (3) empowerment of local health staff to assume the whole services in a sustainable way.

14.4.2.2 Implementation

This pilot project has been implemented since October 2018 in the Municipality of Pyuthan and Swargadwari in Pyuthan district as a year long pilot project. The project is led by Birat Nepal Medical Trust and DroNepal and the Nepal Flying Labs, under the technical guidance by WeRobotics, has been working as technical partner together with the NTC, Stony Brook University, Liverpool School of Tropical Medicine and Nick Simons Institute. In Pyuthan and Bhingri Municipalities, there are 14 health facilities including 12 rural health posts, one district hospital and one public healthcare centre. Amongst them, eight health facilities are connected by the drone service. In this project (Figure 14.4), a user-

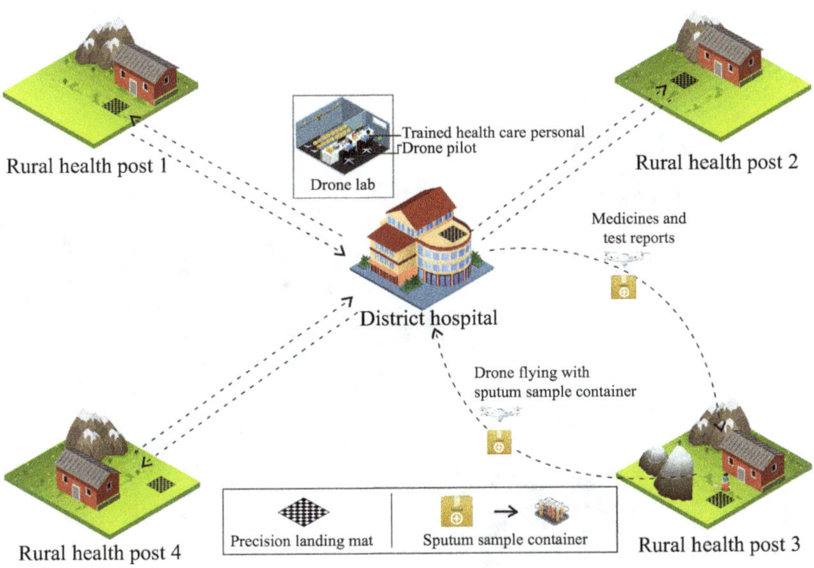

Figure 14.4 The DrOTS project

friendly autonomous hexacopter drone dispatches from district hospital to the health centres in the remote villages (Figure 14.5) and returns with a box of the sputum samples to the referral hospital (Figure 14.6) in a scheduled process. The collected sputum samples are examined at the hospital laboratory using the GeneXpert Machine. The drone's control system has been customised to make it

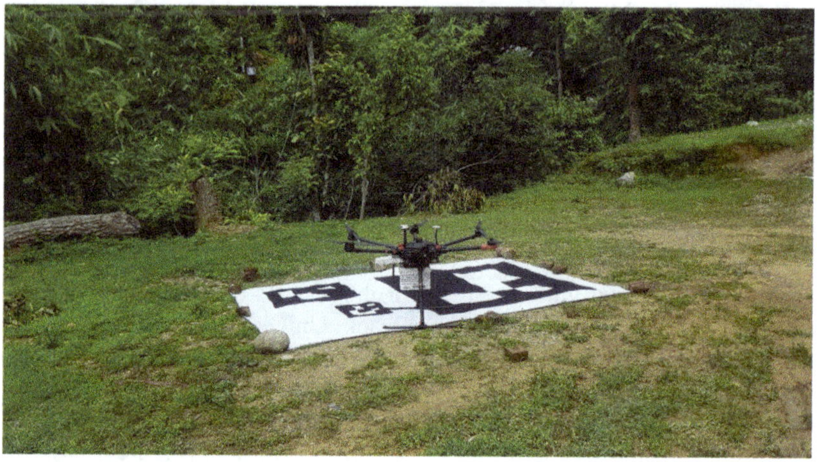

Figure 14.5 The medical cargo drone

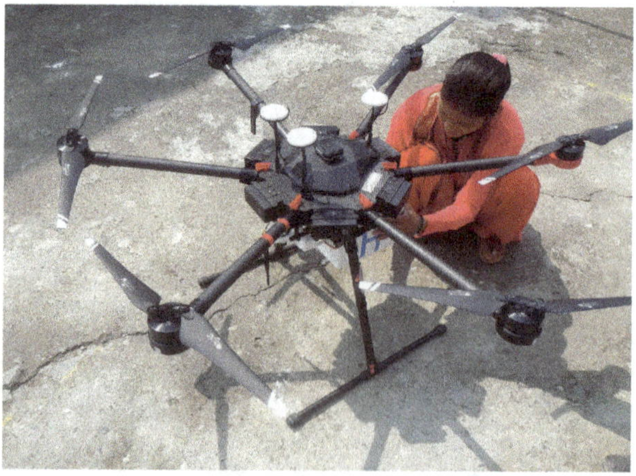

Figure 14.6 Arrival in the hospital

Table 14.1 The finalists of the incubation project

Name	Services
DroNepal	Customised drones and data services provider in surveying and mapping
Map Hub	Drone services provider in surveying and mapping
Airlift	Medical cargo drone service provider
Kalpavriksha	Drones for crowd management in various events

much easier for anyone to operate with automatic precision landing feature at health centres and easy-to-use tablet interfaces for drone control.

In this way, this drone service proposes the solution for the geographic challenges in access to health services in hard-to-reach areas. In addition, by capacity building of local health staff, this project also aims to ensure the sustainability of the project.

14.4.3 Sustainable localisation of drone technology

For the sustainable drone applications in Nepal, it is imperative to have a variety of dedicated drone service providers in various sectors. To ensure the establishment and sustainability of drone service providers, the business incubation is of great significance. Therefore, the Nepal Flying Labs, WeRobotics, the Nepal Engineers' Association and the Robotics Association of Nepal organised a 4-month business incubation programme called 'Drones as a service business incubation' from February to May 2017. The purpose of this programme was to help establish 'drones as a service' businesses in Nepal. The incubated business teams learnt necessary business skills that are essential for their growth and sustainability through a multi-stage incubation process [19].

The initial ideation stage received the submissions of drones-related business ideas from 110 local teams and individuals. Amongst the applicants, four of the groups (Table 14.1), who had strong interests and potential for pushing applications of drones in Nepal, were selected by a jury consisting of local domain experts for the final stage, where the four teams competed for a seed investment for jump-starting their business.

14.5 Discussions

14.5.1 The role of the drone ecosystem

The influx of drone applications in Nepal after the 2015 Nepal earthquake clearly showcased the great potential of drones in developing countries. Drones are valuable tools to overcome the logistical and accessibility challenges in accessing the health services and rapid disaster response during emergencies. The applications of drones aid in improving the access to healthcare services and disaster management in other developing countries, in particular rural areas with geographical challenges. However, the rapid increase in use of drones post Nepal Earthquake also resulted in unexpected cases of privacy infringement and many other misuses of drones, particularly in emergencies. Therefore, for the proper dissemination of drone technologies in developing countries, the establishment of a drone ecosystem is crucial, and the Nepal Flying Labs is ideally placed to help create and facilitate this ecosystem. It is very much important to understand the local culture, local knowledge and how things work locally. So, a local entity must be established prior to disasters for better preparedness since the networking and formulation of such ecosystem in a developing country takes a long time. Furthermore, for the public sector in developing countries, it requires certain time and resources to get accustomed to the advanced technologies, including drones as acceptable technology. In this sense, the drone ecosystem can play an important role in filling the gap between the advanced technologies and the public, private and non-profit sector in developing countries, whilst at the same time facilitating local as well as international humanitarian responders to effectively operate at the time of need.

14.5.2 Rural areas for reverse innovation

This study presented a field study on the transportation of medical items by drones in rural areas of Nepal. Such 'medical cargo drones' are effective tools to improve the access to healthcare services in rural areas of developing countries. The regular use of medical cargo drones builds up the drone operating capacity to prepare for future emergencies. In addition, the medical cargo drones will be the effective tools to sustain the healthcare services in developed countries such as Japan, where the population is rapidly decreasing and aging in rural areas. However, Japan in particular, as a developed country, where the existing laws and regulations hinder the rapid application of new technologies, there is a limited testing field for advanced and challenging technologies including medical cargo drones. On the contrary, in developing countries, where it is relatively flexible for the introduction of new technologies, there are suitable places for creating, and fine-tuning new technologies and services. In this sense, it is effective that the drone stakeholders in developing countries such as the Nepal Flying Labs establish an open innovation hub with the testing field for advanced technologies. Such innovation hubs can also create the opportunities for 'reverse innovation', and open new doors for cross-country collaborations; for example, the Nepal Flying Labs and the Japan Flying Labs collaborating in a knowledge and skills-exchange programme.

14.5.3 Challenges in the drone applications

Drone technology is a most rapidly growing technology all over the world with newer use cases emerging, specially in the developing countries. In addition, the circumstances of drone operations are dramatically different in each country. In Nepal, (1) technical challenges, (2) legal challenges and (3) stakeholder-engagement challenges are the typical challenges to be solved towards the effective operations of drones. Firstly, technical challenges contain the adaptation of drones to the geographic characteristics in Nepal. For example, the drones should be operable in the high altitude in mountainous areas. In addition, whilst the needs for the fixed-wing drones clearly exist, due to the complex topography, limited flat surfaces are available for launching and landing of the fixed-wing drones. Furthermore, establishing proper repair and maintenance systems is a serious challenge in Nepal where there are no official service centres of drone manufacturers. Secondly, the legal challenges have been identified after the 2015 Nepal earthquake, which had triggered the influx of the drone use cases in the country. For example, drones and other related communication equipments are only allowed to use specific communication frequencies in the current regulations. In addition, the time-consuming application processes are counter intuitive to the idea of drone operations which are meant to be rapid. In fact, in the DrOTS project, the import of drones with lithium-ion batteries by air, which is the only feasible way for receiving drones in this landlocked country, required several months for the administration processes and permissions. Finally, the third challenge is the mindset of the people on the use of drones. Since the majority of people in Nepal are just beginning to familiarize with drone technologies, drones are not properly recognised as solutions for social challenges, rather they are recognised as the military technologies used in spying and destruction.

14.6 Conclusion

This chapter discussed the localisation and the practical applications of drone technologies by the Nepal Flying Labs after the 2015 Nepal earthquake. As a Build Back Better approach, stated in Sendai Framework [20], building a drone ecosystem in post-disaster settings is expected to be applied to the future recovery programme in other developing countries. In addition, such an ecosystem in developing countries could act as use cases of new technologies to be later implemented as innovative solutions in developed countries, with the concept of 'reverse innovation'.

References

[1] *Geography of Nepal* [online]. Available from http://web.gps.caltech.edu/~avouac/nepal_trip/geography.htm

[2] Komal Raj Aryal, *The History of Disaster Incidents and Impacts in Nepal*, Int. J. Disaster Risk Sci. 2012, 3(3): pp. 147–154

[3] Rajan Paudel, Tirthalal Upadhyaya, and Durga Prasad Pahari, *People's Perspective on Access to Health Care Services in a Rural District of Nepal*, J. Nepal Med. Asso. 2011, 52(185): pp. 20–24

[4] WWF Nepal, *Unmanned Aerial Vehicle to aid Nepal's Conservation Efforts* [online]. Available from https://wwf.panda.org/?205266/Unmanned-Aerial-Vehicle-to-aid-Nepals-Conservation-Efforts

[5] Immerzeel, W. W., P. D. A. Kraaijenbrink, J. M. Shea *et al.*, *High-Resolution Monitoring of Himalayan Glacier Dynamics Using Unmanned Aerial Vehicles*, Remote Sens. Environ., 1994, 150: pp. 93–103. https://www.sciencedirect.com/science/article/abs/pii/S003442571400176X

[6] Biplov Bhandari, Upendra Oli, Niroz Panta, and Uttam Pudasaini, *Generation of High Resolution DSM Using UAV Images (7439)*; FIG Working Week 2015 From the Wisdom of the Ages to the Challenges of the Modern World Sofia, Bulgaria, May 17–21, 2015.

[7] UAV for biomass estimation [online]. 2015. Available from https://geospatiallab.wordpress.com/2015/07/15/uav-for-biomass-estimation/

[8] Leo King, *Nepal Earthquake Relief And The Urgent Boost From Drones* [online]. Forbes; Apr. 30, 2015. Available from https://www.forbes.com/sites/leoking/2015/04/30/nepal-earthquake-drones-relief-aid/#191ec84a600e

[9] Reuters, Choppers, drone hunt for missing US Huey in Nepal [online]. May 14, 2015. Available from https://www.news24.com/World/News/Choppers-drone-hunt-for-missing-US-Huey-in-Nepal-20150514

[10] *Nepal earthquake: Drone footage of Kathmandu devastation* [online]. BBC; Apr. 27, 2015. Available from https://www.bbc.com/news/av/world-asia-32481945/nepal-earthquake-drone-footage-of-kathmandu-devastation

[11] F. Yamazaki, T. Matsuda, S. Denda, and W. Liu, 'Construction of 3D models of buildings damaged by earthquakes using UAV aerial images', Proceedings of the Tenth Pacific Conference on Earthquake Engineering Building an Earthquake-Resilient Pacific; Sydney, Australia, Nov. 6–8, 2015.

[12] *Geotechnical Extreme Events Reconnaissance GEER Association*. Report No. GEER-040, Version 1.1, Aug. 7, 2015.

[13] Denise Soesilo, and Patrick Meier, *Drones in Humanitarian Action, Case Study No.3: Mapping- Small-scale Mapping with Consumer Drones in Nepal*, Mar. 26, 2016.

[14] *Global flying labs network* [online]. Available from http://www.flyinglabs.org/

[15] WeRobotics, Localizing Humanitarian Drones: Robotics & Disaster Response [online]. 2018. Available from https://blog.werobotics.org/2018/02/01/localizinghumanitarian-drones/

[16] UAViator, Humanitarian UAV Code of Conduct, *2014* [online]. Available from https://uavcode.org/code-of-conduct/

[17] *Nepal earthquake recovery enters 5th year* [online]. Available from https://reliefweb.int/report/nepal/nepal-earthquake-recovery-enters-5th-year
[18] Nepal Tuberculosis Program Nepal, Annual Report *(2017)* [online]. Available from https://nepalntp.gov.np/wp-content/uploads/2018/03/Final-Annual-Report-NTPN-2018.pdf
[19] *Incubating Robotics Businesses in Nepal* [online]. Available from https://blog.werobotics.org/2017/04/26/incubating-robotics-businesses-in-nepal/
[20] *Sendai Framework for Disaster Risk Reduction* [online]. Available from https://www.unisdr.org/we/coordinate/sendai-framework

Chapter 15

Sustainable and resilient community development by drones

Yasuhiro Soshino[1], Takahiro Oohata[2] and Yuuki Inada[3]

15.1 Introduction

In the twenty-first century, Japan has been facing two different types of disasters. The first one is 'silent disasters', which includes the super-ageing society, the population reduction society and the ageing infrastructure in Japan. According to the Ministry of Health, Labour and Welfare, the average life expectancy in Japan is 80.98 years for a male and 87.14 years for a female as of 2016 [1]. The National Institute of Population and Social Security Research reports that the population in Japan is expected to decrease from 127,090,000, in 2015, to 110,920,000, in 2040 [2]. The number of live birth also declined from 2,091,983, in 1973, to 976,978, in 2016 [3]. The challenges in the number of the live birth and super-ageing society, and the population reduction society cause significant impact on local authorities in Japan. In fact, by 2040, more than half of the adult female population will decrease in 896 local authorities, which occupies 49.8 per cent of the total number (1,799) in Japan. Amongst these 896 local authorities, 523 local authorities will have less than 10,000 population by 2040 [4]. In addition to these population challenges, the ageing of infrastructure has become a serious social challenge. In 2012, the deteriorated ceiling of the Sasago Tunnel was collapsed by 130 m and killed nine people. As of 2016, there are approximately 10,000 tunnels in Japan and the most of them were constructed during the period of rapid economic growth from 1955 to 1973. Japan has approximately 720,000 bridges and in 2016, 40 per cent of their in-service period have exceeded 50 years [5]. The challenges in ageing infrastructure suppress the administration of public finance in local authorities, which have been shrinking their size due to the low birth rate and longevity, and population movement of younger generations to urban cities. In this way, the local authorities in rural areas have been facing difficult challenges in maintaining and renewing the deteriorated infrastructures.

[1] International Medical Relief Department, Japanese Red Cross Kumamoto Hospital, Kumamoto, Japan
[2] Realglobe Inc., Tokyo, Japan
[3] Emergency medical and Disaster coping Automated drones support system utilisation promotion Council (EDAC), Tokyo, Japan

Whilst the impact of 'silent disasters' has been affecting the entire parts of the country, there has been a growing concern about the sudden onset mega-disasters such as Nankai Trough Earthquake and Tsunami (hereafter, the NTET) and Tokyo Inland Earthquake (hereafter, the TIE) in Japan. The NTET is expected to kill more than 300,000 people in the western part of Japan [6]. In the NTET, approximately 60 million people in 700 local authorities will experience more than intensity six tremor. In other words, half of total population in Japan will be affected and the Japanese Disaster Relief Act will be applied to 700 affected local authorities by this super widespread mega disaster. The NTET is expected to force approximately 900 to 1,900 agricultural rural communities and 300–400 fishing rural communities to be isolated by the impact of disaster [7]. The TIE is also a catastrophic disaster, which kills more than 20,000 people and causes the long-term paralyse in the capital function of Japan [8]. In addition to these earthquakes, the impacts of the climate change will cause serious weather-related disasters in Japan. For example, the super typhoons, which are expected to cause long-term flooding in Tokyo, Nagoya and Osaka, are also the serious concerns [9]. In fact, the fierce rainfall caused the severe floods and landslides in the northern Kyushu in the July 2017, and in the western part of Japan in the July 2018.

In this way, Japan is obliged to prepare for the future sudden onset national crisis, whilst it has been struggling with the silent disasters. Therefore, positive utilisation of innovative technologies is the key to cope with these two types of disasters. The Disaster Management Basic Plan in Japan, which is the supreme and the most fundamental plan in the disaster management by the Japanese government, states the utilisation of the late Information and Communication Technology (ICT) technologies in the disaster management [10]. In the second periods of cross-ministerial Strategic Innovation Promotion (SIP) programme, which spreads from 2018 to 2022, 'National Resilience' is set as one of the main research goals. To accomplish this purpose, various innovative research projects have been conducted such as rapid damage estimation technology by drones and satellites, and using the big data for supporting the decision-making in evacuation by local authorities. In this way, various efforts have been made to build up the resilient societies by the effective use of innovative technologies. However, towards the effective emergency uses of the advanced technologies such as mobile, satellites, drones, big data and Artificial Intelligence (AI), these technologies should be commonly used amongst the local communities before disasters strike. In this point, the small local communities in rural areas, which have been experiencing the rapid progress of super-ageing and population reduction, have two challenges. Firstly, a large number of such communities have difficulty in financial conditions to invest the sufficient budget for introducing the ICT only for disaster management. In this sense, the introduction of advanced technology should be designed for both daily uses and disaster management. Secondly, rural communities lack the ICT specialists due to the population movement of younger generation from rural to urban. Thus, in rural communities, the introduction of advanced technologies requires the collaboration with the private companies, social businesses and non-profit organisations.

Therefore, this chapter discusses the design and development of the drone-operating platform and its application in rural communities in Japan. This chapter also introduces the collaboration between a non-profit organisation, a private company and local rural community in Japan towards the sustainable solution for social challenges by advanced technology. Following the introduction, Section 15.2 explains the development of the advanced drone-operating platform by a non-profit organisation and a private company. Section 15.3 presents the field application of the drone-operating platform for a disaster drill in rural coastal community. Section 15.4 introduces the case study on the practical applications of the drone-operating platform for solving the various social problems in both the daily life and emergencies. The discussion will be shown in Section 15.5 and Section 15.6 concludes this study.

15.2 Design and development of the drone-operating platform

15.2.1 Backgrounds

This section introduces the development of the drone-operating platform by a non-profit organisation and a private venture company. In 2016, 'Emergency medical and Disaster coping Automated drones support system utilisation promotion Council' (hereafter, the EDAC) was established to foster the application of the advanced technology such as drones, the Internet of Things (IOT) and the ICT in the areas of the emergency medicine and the disaster response. The EDAC organised various seminars and trainings to promote the drone, which was the new technology in the society of Japan. In 2016, Japanese Red Cross Kumamoto Hospital and the EDAC started the collaboration towards the effective use of drones in disaster management. In a discussion between the Red Cross hospital and the EDAC, the brief concept of a drone-operating platform for emergency use was formulated. The concept of the platform is to enable multiple drone pilots to upload the images on a map that can be accessed by the relief agencies. In April 2016, magnitude 6.5 and 7.3 earthquakes struck in Kumamoto Japan. These earthquakes killed 50 people and caused the serious damages in Kumamoto City and its suburb town of Mashiki, and other rural areas in Kumamoto and Oita prefectures. In this disaster response, the EDAC immediately mobilised a drone team for the rapid assessment of the disaster-affected areas. The drone team also operated drones in various places in Nishihara village and showed the images and movies to the evacuees in the refugee centre. Even in 2019, in the recovery period, the EDAC continues aerial filming by drones in the town of Mashiki where its scenery has been rapidly changing. In the Kumamoto earthquake disaster response, the EDAC identified two challenges in operating drones in emergencies. Firstly, there was a technical need of a drone-operating platform. The EDAC reconfirmed the need and effectiveness of the drone-operating platform, which could share the images and movies taken by drones with the simple system structure. Secondly, the drone should have been used as a common tool in the community before the sudden onset disaster struck. In the Kumamoto earthquake response, drones and drone pilots were available; however, the official requests from local authorities were required for operating drones in the disaster-affected areas, which was quite challenging for the disaster-affected local authorities. To solve these two challenges, the EDAC accelerated its activities in collaboration with the Red Cross hospital, a number of local authorities including their fire departments and the academia.

15.2.2 Field test in the search and rescue

In January 2017, the EDAC conducted a field test of the prototype of the drone-operating platform in the search and rescue operation. In this test, the comparative tests were conducted between the search and rescue with and without a drone. The tests compared the time until the search and rescue team found the injured person after the command post received the rescue request from the mobile app of the simulated injured person in the mountains. In the search and rescue with the drone (Figure 15.1), the GPS information, which was sent by the mobile app, was shared with the command post and the drone pilot. The image and movie taken by the drone were shared with the command post and the rescue team with the smart glasses. In this case, the drone itself worked as an 'advertising balloon' by floating the drone above the injured person, which resulted in the rapid contact between the rescue team and the injured person. The search and rescue operation with the drone required only a half period compared to the rescue operation without the drone.

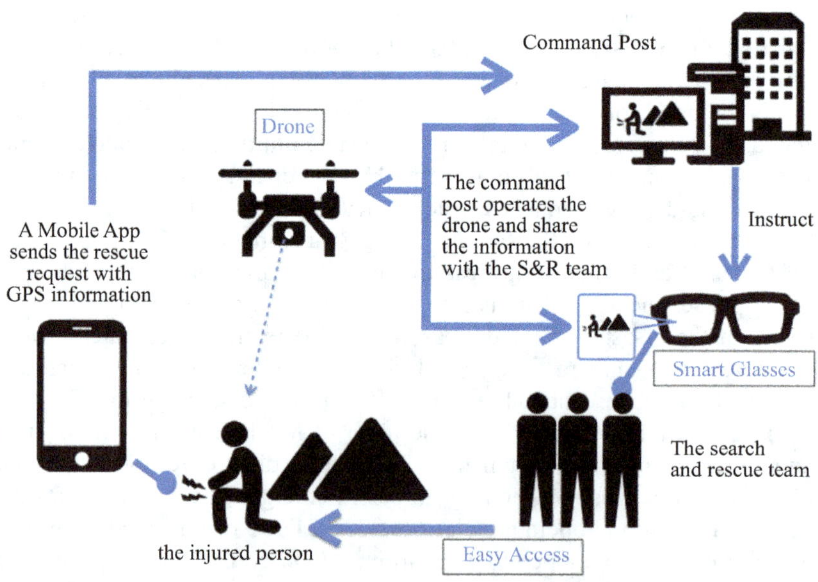

Figure 15.1 The overview of the field test

15.2.3 Development of Hec-Eye system

In the autumn of 2017, the EDAC and a venture company Realglobe Inc. successfully completed the drone-operating platform called 'Hec-Eye'. Figure 15.2 shows the brief overview of the platform. Hec-Eye is the real-time information-sharing system, which can upload the images and movies, which are taken by drones and smartphones, on a cloud-based map. This platform consists of a drone and a smartphone attached with a drone controller for the drone pilot. The key functions of this system are the real-time information sharing, marking of the position of the drones on a cloud-based map, and displaying the images and movies taken by drones and smartphones on a cloud-based map. These key functions enable the drone pilot and the command post to share the same information in a real time. In addition, the staff of the command post can give the drone pilot the exact position and areas by pointing the locations on a cloud-based map and chatting with the drone pilot. This system has the high-vision movie mode (24 images per s), the normal-vision movie mode (12 images per s) and the photo mode. For example, in case the telecommunication is not stable in the operation areas, the drone pilot can choose the photo mode for ensuring the minimum information sharing with the command post.

15.3 Field test of the drone-operating platform

15.3.1 Background of the field test

This section discusses the effectiveness of the key functions of the Hec-Eye by testing the system in the emergency rapid assessment drill in rural areas of Saiki, Oita prefecture. Saiki city is expected to become the tsunami-affected area in the NTET of which likelihood of occurrence is 70 per cent in 30 years. In the NTET, the tsunami with the maximum height of 13.5 m high arrives after 34 min, after the

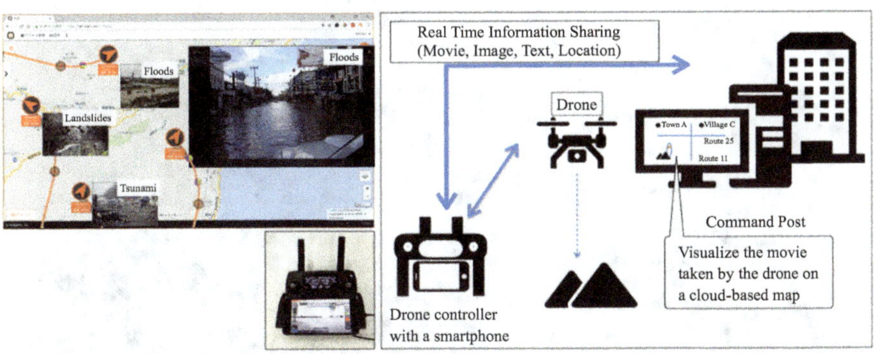

Figure 15.2 The overview of Hec-Eye system

maximum seismic intensity of six plus earthquake strikes Saiki. If the tsunami hits Saiki, some areas of this city will be isolated by flooding and landslides. In this case, the emergency centre of Saiki will need to grasp the overall situation, identify the needs and allocate the resources for lifesaving relief activities, whilst the situation dramatically changes as the time advances. Therefore, Saiki city fire department and the EDAC jointly organised the tsunami rapid-assessment drill using the multiple drones operated on Hec-Eye system.

15.3.2 Method of the field test

This field test was conducted based on the scenario in which the arrival of tsunami in the coastal areas of Saiki after the strong earthquake caused landslides in the various parts of the city. In the drill, the command post was established at the Oita prefectural office. Two drone-assessment teams were mobilised. One team assessed the coastal areas of the city whilst another team assessed the mountainous part of the city by drones. The communication between the two drone teams and the command post were established by the radio communication and Hec-Eye system. The drill was held in August 2018 and approximately 40 participants from the local authorities, fire departments and media observed the drill. This study received the feedbacks and suggestions from the seven staff of the local authorities.

15.3.3 Results

The drone-assessment teams successfully uploaded the movies on a cloud-based map and shared the information with the command post (Photo 15.1). The instruction from the command post was sent to the drone teams by the official radio

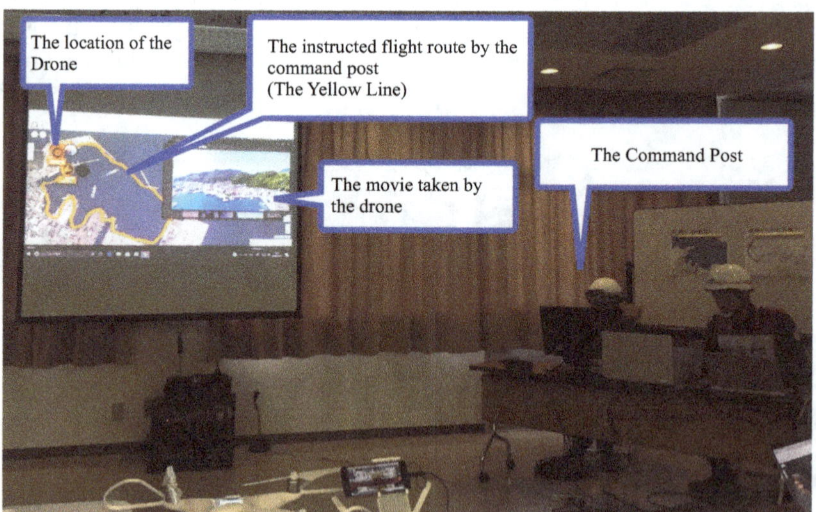

Photo 15.1 The command post in the field test

communication and the chatting function of the Hec-Eye system. The command post also instructed the assessment areas to the drone team by pointing the areas on a map.

15.3.4 Summary of the field test

Table 15.1 summarises the feedback and the suggestions by seven observers from the local authorities including Saiki city. In general, amongst the key functions of the Hec-Eye system, the real-time information sharing and uploading the movie taken by drones were positively evaluated. One participant from the fire department pointed out that the quality of the movie was better than the present system of the fire department. In the rapid assessment in tsunami disasters, the command post will have a difficulty in grasping the situation in the wide geographic areas, whilst the situation dramatically changes. Therefore, the key functions of the real-time information sharing and the high-quality movie received the positive feedback.

The limitation of this field study is that the Hec-EYE system is based on the availability of the data communication network. As the Great East Japan Earthquake and Tsunami in 2011 destroyed the Internet connections in the disaster-affected areas, it is expected that the NTET causes the catastrophic damage to the Internet connection. Since the Hec-Eye system is strongly relying on the Internet connection, the availability of the Internet connection becomes a critical issue in emergencies. In addition to the Internet connectivity, one of the observers pointed out the financial effectiveness of the drone-operating system. As the participant suggests, local authorities in rural areas may not have afford to invest the advanced technologies only for disaster response. In this way, this field test revealed the needs for the new drone-use model, which is effective in both peacetime and emergencies, in rural areas.

15.4 Sustainable community development by drones

15.4.1 Backgrounds

This section presents the community development by the effective use of drones as a solution for various social problems in Minami-Oguni of Kumamoto prefecture.

Table 15.1 The feedbacks from the observers

Functions	Feedbacks
Real-time information sharing	Higher resolution is preferable if the stable telecommunication is available.
	Better than the present information system in the fire department.
	The transmission of images was smooth and clear.
	Real-time viewer helps the command post to grasp the situations of multiple locations.
Pointing on the map	Positioning data are useful in emergencies.
Visualise the movie on the map	Higher resolution is preferable if the stable telecommunication is available.
	The quality of the images and movies was very clear.

Kumamoto prefecture is the neighbouring prefecture of Oita and Minami-Oguni is located in the mountainous areas, which are 100 km away from Saiki city. Approximately, 85 per cent of the lands in Minami-Oguni is covered by the beautiful forests and the grassland. Miami-Oguni is quite famous for the natural hot spring 'Kurokawa Onsen'. Main industries of Minami-Oguni are tourism, agriculture and forestry.

15.4.2 Social challenges in Minami-Oguni

As most of the local authorities in Japan, the super-ageing and the population reduction have been proceeding in Minami-Oguni. The total population of this town has been decreasing from 7,761, in 1955, to approximately 4,000, in 2019. The National Institute of Population and Social Security Research estimates that the population of this town will decrease to 2,422 in 2060. The working-age population in the town also has been decreasing from 55.8 per cent, in 2010, to 51 per cent, in 2016. The population-ageing rate became to 38 per cent. In addition, the population movement of young generation to urban resulted in the lack of the workforce in agriculture and forestry. The scarcity of manpower in the primary industry is one of the main causes for the damage to the agriculture by the wildlife and illegal waste dumping in the forest. In addition to these social challenges in daily life, Minami-Oguni experienced the 2016 Kumamoto earthquake and the Northern Kyushu flash floods in 2017. During the floods in 2017, the town had a difficulty in accessing the flooded areas and understand the situation in the disaster-affected areas.

15.4.3 Community development using drones

In August 2017, Minami-Oguni, the EDAC and Realglobe Inc. reached to the cooperation agreement on the community development by using the drones. This agreement aims to solve the community problems such as tourism, agriculture, forestry, illegal dumping and disaster management by using the advanced technologies including drones. Based on this agreement, the town purchased six community drones and trained its staff as the drone pilots. The trained drone pilots were assigned to all the departments in the town office. In 2018, these three organisations tried to use drones for the promotion of tourism, the surveillance of illegal waste dumping, monitoring of the wildlife that damages the vegetables, monitoring of the livestock and drawing the hazard maps. In this way, by using the drones as a solution for the social problems in peacetime, the drones are recognised as a daily tool for the community. This common recognition on the community drones enables the community members to use the drones in the sudden onset disasters.

15.4.4 Drone applications in the community

15.4.4.1 Dissemination of the drone in the community

In January 2019, the EDAC organised a training seminar on the drone operation and the introduction on the Hec-Eye system. The participants from the tourism committee, the hunters' association, the chambers of commerce, the fire brigade, the forest union, the board of education and the hotel association joined the seminar. The participants learned the basic knowledge on drones, the relevant laws and regulations, key points in the drone operations, the case studies on the application of drones in other areas of Japan and the practical operation of drones. In addition, the EDAC organised the active learning courses in the elementary and the junior high schools in the town (Photo 15.2).

15.4.4.2 Tourism promotion by drones

In October 2018, the Minami-Oguni tourist association and a private drone venture company launched the drone-free zone service called 'Minami-Oguni Drone Rally Pass'. This service allows the drone pilots to operate the drones at the five main tourism spots in the town (Photo 15.3). The users reserve the service in the Internet and pay the cost at the designated spots in the town. The users receive the 'Drone Rally Pass' made of the oak tree 'Oguni-Sugi', which is the famous main product in the town. The drone pass costs 1,000 Japanese Yen (approximately, 9 USDs) for the inhabitants of the town and 3,000 Japanese Yen for the visitors. This service also contains the drone insurance and the rental mobile batteries. In Japan, limited places are available for the beginner drone pilots so the rally pass service encourages the trainings of the drone pilots. In addition, the drone-free spots are the main scenic areas of the town, which are very attractive for the matured drone service providers who distribute the photos and movies for the commercial uses. For Minami-Oguni town, this service attracts the visitors who see the photos and

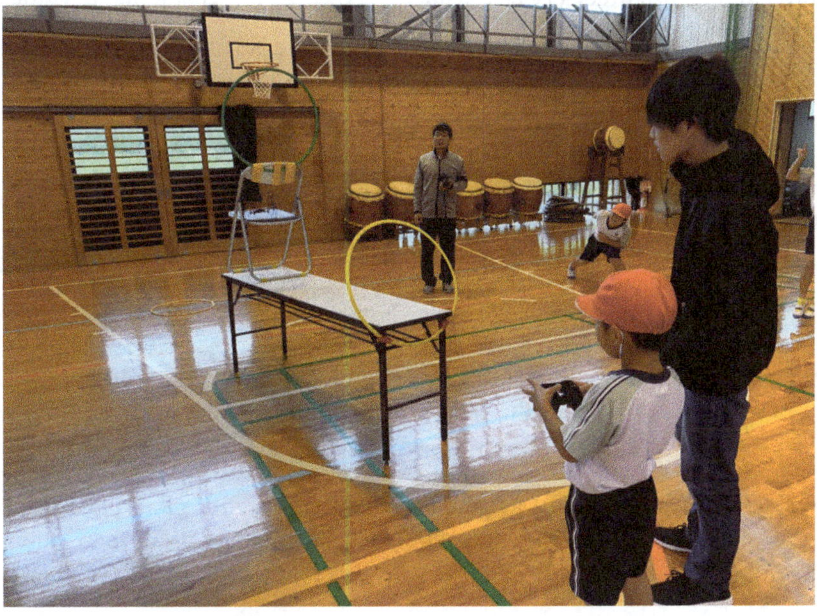

Photo 15.2 Drone learning course

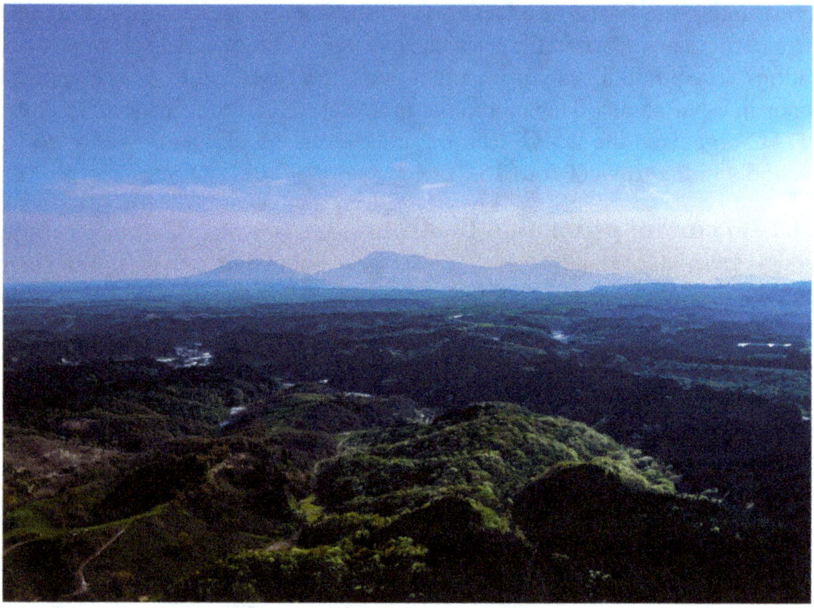

Photo 15.3 The tourist spot

the movies uploaded by the other service users. As of June 2019, approximately 100 drone pilots used the services, which is expected to become the new tourism service in the town.

15.4.4.3 Surveillance of the illegal waste dumping

The drone and the Hec-Eye system were used by the EDAC and the staff of the town office for the surveillance of the several places where illegal waste dumping cases were seen in the past. In the surveillance of the illegal dumping, there had been a difficulty in accessing the places in the valley, the forests and the mountains. The aerial access by using the drones the staff of the town office can grasp the overview of the situation in the inaccessible places. According to the aerial survey, the illegal dumping cases at the five places were found. Amongst the five cases, two cases were in the deep valley where only drones were accessible. The photos of the other three places were taken by the smartphones of the staff. The photos and movies taken by the drone or the smartphones were uploaded with the GPS positioning data by using the Hec-Eye system (Photo 15.4). The challenges in this surveillance were the gaps between the GPS positioning data, the position on a map in the Hec-Eye system and the actual location. To reduce the gaps, the drone pilot should record the exact positioning data before uploading in the system.

15.4.4.4 Monitoring the wildlife

In January 2019, the EDAC and the hunters' association conducted the field study on the monitoring the wildlife by drones. The hunters' association designated two

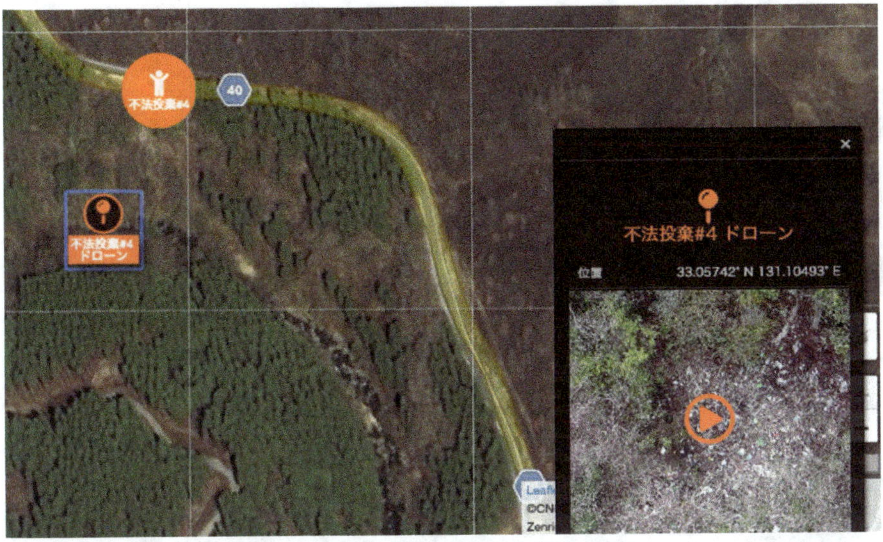

Photo 15.4 Surveillance of the illegal waste dumping by Hec-Eye system

possible lairs of the boars and the deer. On January 21, the surveillance was conducted by using a drone with a high-vision camera. The drone found the vision of a deer and chased the deer for nine mittens from the grassland to the woods. According to the hunters' association, by identifying the trace of the deer, it will be easy to chase them by the hunting dogs. Therefore, a collaborative field test by drones and hunting dogs was proposed by the member of the hunters' association.

15.4.4.5 Monitoring the livestock

Also areas, where Minami-Oguni is located, are famous for the cattle breeding. The breeders need to grasp the condition of the particular cow, whilst the breeders are getting aged. Therefore, the EDAC used a drone with a high-vision camera and an infrared camera for monitoring the cows. The temperature was 7°C at 2 p.m. and 5°C at 5 p.m. in the field test. In both the cases, the drone clearly captured the cows from 300 m away from them. The infrared camera was able to distinguish the temperature gap between the cows and the grass field (Photo 15.5).

15.4.4.6 Disaster preparedness

Minami-Oguni experienced the 2016 Kumamoto earthquake and the 2017 Kyushu flash floods. In both the disasters, the town had two technical challenges. Firstly, there was a difficulty in the rapid assessment in the disaster-affected areas. Secondly, the need for the analysis by comparing the disaster-affected place before and after the disaster. Therefore, in January 2019, by using the drone and the Hec-Eye system, the EDAC and the town office jointly assessed the possible places of sediment disasters in the future. The drone took the photos of the sediment disaster alert areas and uploaded the photos on a cloud-based map (Photo 15.6). The photos

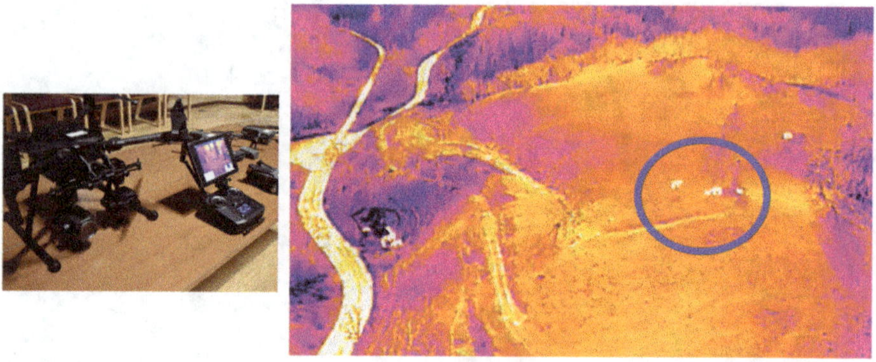

Photo 15.5 The drone with infrared camera and the cattle in the field

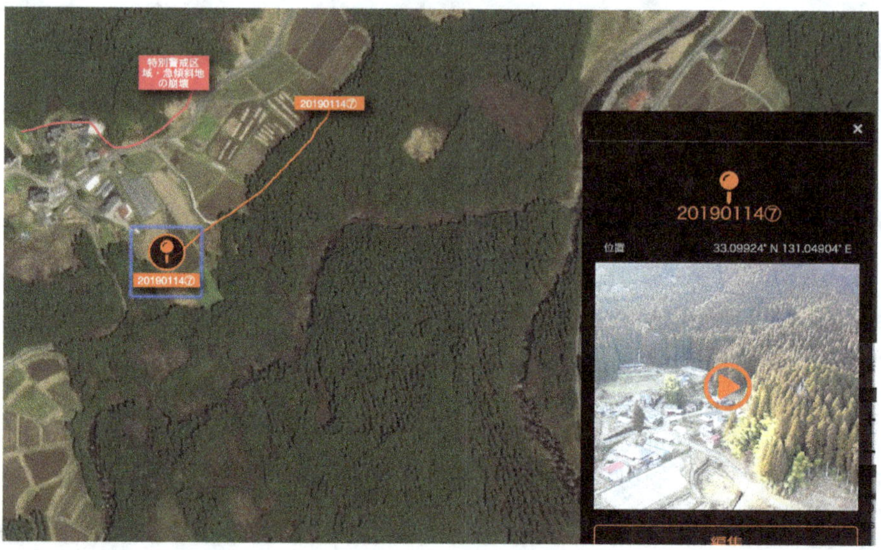

Photo 15.6 Aerial assessment by the drone for making the hazard map

on the map were shared with the town office and the fire department. The technical challenge in this field test was establishing the link between the documented hazard maps and the cloud-based map in the system. Since the official hazard map was not shown on the cloud-based map, it was difficult to identify the exact place for the aerial assessment by using the cloud-based map. One more challenge in this field test was how to make a balance between the privacy and the disaster preparedness. In some target places for the assessment, the drone had to fly above the private houses and the public roads, where the drone operation was restricted. If the assessment by the drone is necessary for the disaster preparedness, the public

Table 15.2 Functions and applications of the drone-operating system

Functions and applications	Real-time info. sharing	Positioning on the map	Movie on the map
Tourism	(b) Live transmission for attracting visitors	(a) Attract visitors by sharing beautiful photos/movies	(b) Information sharing of the local hotels and restaurants
Illegal dumping		(a) Recording the positions (b) Information sharing	(a) Recording the positions (b) Information sharing
Wildlife	(b) Collaboration with hunting dogs	(a) Tracing wildlife (b) Recording the location of the traps	(b) Recording the location of the traps
Livestock	(a) Monitoring the location of the livestock	–	–
Hazard map	(b) Location of the landslides	(a),(b) Recording the hazardous areas before disasters	(a),(b) Recording the hazardous areas before disasters
Others	(b) Location of the traffic jams	(b) Plot the paces of traffic accidents	(b) Location of the traffic jams

authority and the community need to discuss how to issue an official permission for the drone pilots in both the peacetime and emergencies.

15.4.5 The community challenges and the Hec-Eye system

Table 15.2 presents the problems in Minami-Oguni and the function of the Hec-Eye system. The comments in each box were categorised into (a) the effective function in the field tests and (b) the suggestions from the people in Minami-Oguni. As a solution for the social challenges in the town, the system was useful. In particular, amongst the key functions of the system, uploading the GPS positioning data and the images were considered effective in the practical uses. For example, in the surveillance of the illegal dumping, the same information should be shared with the different organisations such as the town office and the police station. In the disaster response, the information sharing between the fire department, the police and the town office is quite important. Therefore, these two functions are considered to be the fundamental functions in information sharing. The real-time information sharing was useful in targeting the dynamic subject such as livestock and wildlife in peacetime and the ongoing emergency events. In terms of the daily uses of drones, a staff of the fire department pointed out the effectiveness of the recording the scenery in the sediment disaster alert areas before the occurrences of disasters. The comparative analysis of two different photos of before and after the sedimental disaster, it will be easy to identify how the floods and landslides fly the houses. This information is critical in the decision-making on where to start the search and rescue activities. For this purpose, at least in the places where the sedimental disasters are expected, the pre-disaster assessment should be done by the daily use of drones including the community-shared drone-operating platform as the Hec-Eye system. In this way, using the drones as the solution for the various problems in the community, the community gradually accepts and recognises the drones as a common tool. This positive recognition of the drone in the community is quite important in the rapid deployment of the drones in emergencies (Figure 15.3).

15.5 Discussions

15.5.1 Drone use as a community drone

By collaborating with the Non Profit Organization (NPO), the private sector and other stakeholders in the community, the town office of Minami-Oguni plays a key role in building the platform for using the drone as a daily tool for solving the various daily problems in the community. In this way, the drone is recognised as ‘the Community Drone’, which is mobilised for solving the social problems in both daily lives and emergencies. In fact, the drone seminar that was organised by the town office and the EDAC, a participant expressed his interest in introducing the drone for the agricultural use. Therefore, in the town, the private farmer also will introduce the drone for the private use. This means, if the community members introduce their own drones as the daily tools, and the

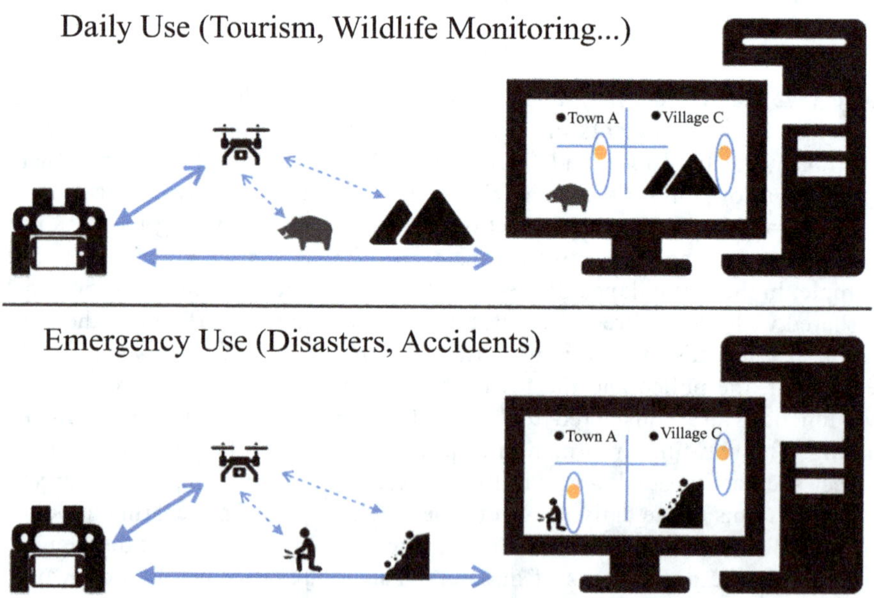

Figure 15.3 Daily and emergency use of the drone-operating system

members upload the images and movies in emergencies, the town office and the other emergency responders will easily grasp the situations in the affected areas. In this way, the community drone can be belong to the local authorities, and to the members in the community. The important thing, there should be the common platform, which at least is open to every community member in emergencies, as the Hec-Eye system aims.

15.5.2 Common drone-operating platform for rural communities

The field tests in Saiki for the emergency assessment, and Minami-Oguni for the daily uses, demonstrated the effectiveness of the drone-operating system in both daily life and emergencies. In rural areas, where the community members scatter in the wide geographic areas, limited human resources are available for grasping the overviews of the whole areas. Therefore, it would be ideal that there is a common drone platform for uploading and sharing the information collected by the drones. In addition, this platform for the community drone should be open to the community drone stakeholders, particularly in emergencies. In this study, all the field tests were only for the information sharing. However, in rural areas of Japan, there are a lot of places that have the logistic difficulties in shopping and accessing the health services. Nowadays, several groups consisting of the telecommunication providers and the commercial companies are trying to use the drones for transport the small amount of the commercial items and the medicines by drones. In the future, the common drone platform in the community can serve not only for information sharing but also for transportation and health services by drones to sustain the daily services in the rural areas of Japan. In addition, the ideas of the community drone and its common operating platform can be applied for the rural areas of developing countries. However, in that case, the operating system should be affordable, accessible and based on the simple technology, which can function even though the capacity and speed of the telecommunication are limited in rural settings.

15.6 Conclusion

This chapter discussed the sustainable drone uses in the rural areas of Japan. The field tests on the drone-operating platform, which can upload the data taken by drones, were conducted to examine its effectiveness in both the daily life and emergencies. The results of the both tests were positive. In particular, in Minami-Oguni, where the town office takes a lead to operate the drones for solving the problems in the community, the community build up the common understanding and acceptance for operating the community drone as a solution for the various problems in the community by collaborating the NPO, the private sector and other community stakeholders. This common recognition and understanding on the drone uses in the community also contribute to enhance the resilience against disasters in the community.

References

[1] Ministry of Health, Labour and Welfare (Japan). Annual Health, Labour and Welfare Report; 2017

[2] National Institute of Population and Social Security Research (Japan). Population Projections for Japan; 2017

[3] Cabinet Office (Japan). A 2018 Declining Birthrate White Paper (summary), Chapter 1. Current Status of Declining Birthrate; 2018

[4] Hiroya Masuda, Future Land and Transport Strategy toward the Era of Regional Extinction, National Institute of Land and Transport Policy Research Institute (Japan), Policy Task Study Session; 2014

[5] Japan Society of Civil Engineering, Infrastructure Health Report, Road Sector Trial Version; 2016

[6] Central Disaster Preparedness Council (Japan). Nankai Trough Mega Earthquake Preparedness Working Group, Report on the Damage Estimation in the Nankai Trough Earthquake, First Version; 2012

[7] Central Disaster Preparedness Council (Japan). Nankai Trough Mega Earthquake Preparedness Working Group, Report on the Damage Estimation in the Nankai Trough Earthquake, Second Version; 2013

[8] Cabinet Office (Japan). Tokyo Inland Earthquake Preparedness Working Group, Report; 2013

[9] Japan Society of Civil Engineering, Technical Report on the Preparedness for the Mega Disasters Causing National Crisis; 2018

[10] Cabinet Office (Japan). Disaster Management Basic Plan; 2018

Section IV

mHealth for the elderly

Chapter 16

Mitigating isolation and loneliness with technology through emotional care by social robots in remote

Roger Andre Søraa[1,2], Eduard Fosch-Villaronga[4], João Quintas[5], Jorge Dias[6], Gunhild Tøndel[3], Jon Sørgaard[1], Pernille Nyvoll[1], Henk Herman Nap[7] and J. Artur Serrano[1,8]

16.1 Being "social" with "others"

The idea of being social firmly interlinks with the idea of humans relating to other humans as social beings. The adjective "social" is defined as "relating to society or its organization" and the noun as being "an informal social gathering, especially one organized by the members of a particular club or group" [1]. The renowned feminist techno-philosopher, Donna Haraway, suggests an extended multi-species approach. In her 2016 book *Staying with the Trouble: Making Kin in the Chthulucene* [2], she urges us to transcend this understanding of "social" and form social relations with other species and entities in addition to the human interrelations. This understanding builds upon her earlier "Cyborg Manifesto" [3], where the term "cyborg" is used to discuss the merging of humans and technology.

In a Scandinavian context, being social strongly interlinks with its antonym, *being lonely*, which seems on the rise in modern societies. It is also a condition that strikes the

[1]Department of Neuromedicine and Movement Science, NTNU Norwegian University of Science and Technology, Trondheim, Norway
[2]Department of Interdisciplinary Studies of Culture, NTNU Norwegian University of Science and Technology, Trondheim, Norway
[3]Department of Sociology and Political Science, NTNU Norwegian University of Science and Technology, Trondheim, Norway
[4]eLaw Center for Law and Digital Technologies, Leiden University, Leiden, The Netherlands
[5]Laboratory for Automation and Systems, Instituto Pedro Nunes, Coimbra, Portugal
[6]Department of Electrical and Computer Engineering, Coimbra University, Coimbra, Portugal
[7]Vilans – National Expertise Centre on Long-Term Care, Team eHealth; Department of Human-Technology Interaction, Eindhoven University of Technology, Eindhoven, The Netherlands
[8]Norwegian Centre for eHealth Research, University Hospital of North Norway, Tromsø, Norway

population unevenly, as it is the oldest and youngest members of society who are experiencing loneliness the most. Loneliness is not dangerous, but persons can experience it as a personally disastrous situation. It can also be a barrier for social participation and, therefore, a barrier for getting informal assistance from one's social network. These barriers may escalate loneliness into a societal problem: its prevalence places a strain on public service resources that could be eased if societal loneliness were mitigated. Consequently, there have been conversations in the public policy arena, especially concerning elderly care, about how to tackle loneliness. Addressing these problems offers a threefold benefit: advancing future welfare policy, supporting the growing welfare technology industry, and improving the quality of life of users.

In this book chapter, we explore how social robot's emotional care could mitigate experiences of isolation and loneliness in remote areas. We first map loneliness in different European regions, which are characterized by having vast geographical distances between cities, public services, and people's homes. We then introduce the concept of *welfare technology* and explain how technology is currently used to bridge the gap technology poses. As a possible solution, we propose the use and development of social robots equipped with emotional care. We review different European projects directed toward developing robots to assist older adults and persons with disabilities socially and explain their characteristics. We close the article with reflections on the consequences of such a sensible choice.

16.2 Being lonely in remote areas

16.2.1 Being lonely in the North

The Norwegian poet Inger Hagerup captured the essence of loneliness in her poetic work:

> *Tonight I'll close the door and only think about you.*
> *I wonder if the loneliness still finds me [4].*

In Scandinavian languages, "loneliness" – and its more positive English-language cousin "solitude" – share the same wording. Thus, self-chosen solitude does not have its term in the languages. Norway, covering 13° latitude, from 58° to 71° North (with the island archipelago Svalbard being 81°N), is located in the northernmost part of continental Europe. It is projected that by 2040, it will be one of the key destinations of the Arctic Road and Belt Silk Road that will become available when the Northwest Passage becomes ice-free due to climate change. This will allow for faster trade, travel, and contact with Asian countries. Norway's total land area is 385,170 km^2, making it just a bit smaller than Japan – but with a population of only 5.3 million people. This small population density creates an intense and noticeable solitude and the settlements are quite dispersed when venturing outside of the largest cities. As the country is so stretched, this often leads to people living far away from their families, as well as people with no families and a lack of social network resources.

Loneliness is not a secluded feeling but is often interlinked with depression, loss of social status, and networks and despair. Research has shown that loneliness is mainly present within the older population [5] and that it is particularly pertinent in people with few or no friends or family to provide emotional support [6]. Unlike other geographical settings of this book, which often focus on areas where it is common for families to live together in the same household for extended periods, northern societies are much more individual-based. It is not common for parents to live with their children after they become adults. Further, the democratic welfare state model allows for high female workforce participation for individuals that otherwise might have been operating in caregiving roles. A high degree of caring activities are outsourced from the family to public care facilities, e.g., nursing homes and home care services. However, despite being climatologically cold and geographically dispersed – and being perceived as socially cold – Norway ranked as the number one country in the Human Development Index for 2017 [7] had the second highest Gross National Product per capita in 2018 (ranking behind Switzerland and not counting microstates) [8] and ranked number three in the 2019 World Happiness Report (ranking behind Finland and Denmark) [9]. Norway is one of the happiest and most affluent countries in the world. Yet, even here loneliness can creep in.

16.2.2 Being lonely in the South

In order to contextualize loneliness in a broader geographical setting, we can look at other remote areas like the Portuguese Centro region. The Centro region is the second-largest national region and contains 22 percent of the total population in Portugal. In terms of demographic characterization, 25 percent of the Centro Region's population is older adults (65+), and the region has negative demographic growth. Most of the region is rural. This feature justifies the importance of designing interventions concerning aging, digital literacy, and access to health and social care (e.g., preventing loneliness, social exclusion, and isolation). The problem of aging and geographic isolation is especially prevalent in the innermost municipalities of the region, making them exceptionally high priorities for such interventions.

To overcome such challenges, the Centro Regional Coordination and Development Commission has incorporated a specific thematic objective into the Smart Specialization Strategy (RIS3) that addresses the topic of Information and Communications Technologies for improving health and quality of life. This thematic objective includes three specific sub-topics: Digital Future, Health Innovation and Active, and Healthy Ageing. Additionally, in line with the concerns raised by demographic changes and associated consequences, the Centro Region hosts a reference site of the European Innovation Partnership on Active and Healthy Ageing. The region has also developed an individual initiative – Ageing@Coimbra [10] – a unique ecosystem that is developing best practices in healthcare-associated with active and healthy aging.

16.3 Living well with "welfare technology"

Scandinavian research and policy often use the term "welfare technology" to describe the "new technologies in municipal- and specialist services [...] tested out and implemented at a large scale within a health and care context" [11, p. 4]. In an international context, this often falls under the terms "Gerontechnologies" or "Active Assisted Living (AAL) technologies," or even medical technology or E-health technology. Welfare technologies are a large group of often digital devices with integrated platforms that public services use to promote welfare among patients and caregivers. Thus, they perform in a welfare state context, thereby giving them their distinct identity.

One of the chief goals of welfare technology is to allow people to better cope with their health impairments and improve their quality of life by increasing their autonomy [12]. The term has instrumental features, but it also points directly to an emotional aspect, i.e., the individual perception or experience of a kind of well-being. Lay associations to welfare technology are often related to elderly care. Governmental initiatives to develop the welfare technology industry were primarily grounded in arguments for the need for technology to solve challenges related to aging populations. However, the technology is now being used and developed to assist individual needs independent of age. Importantly, in the Scandinavian context, it is not one's functional or cognitive function level, medical diagnosis or age that defines the inclusion into the user group, but whether one is granted a health and care service through the public health and care service system.

Welfare technologies are further thought to contribute to support people's self-reliance, personal monitorization, and enhanced knowledge about one's health status, while also encouraging social contact with caregivers, friends, and loved ones [13]. They also have the potential to extend the work of doctors in medical interventions [14]. These goals are often complementary, but different technology traditions within the healthcare field have different terminology and emphasis. One example of this is the use of active lower-limb exoskeletons for rehabilitation and training of patients with reduced gait function [15]. Although exoskeletons belong to rehabilitative medical technology, they are also tools that increase patients' independence in their daily life by allowing them to participate more easily in social activities.

The policy also frames welfare technology as a tool for re-skilling healthcare work and supplementing the increasing shortage of healthcare workers. The World Health Organization (WHO) [16] has estimated that the global population over 60 will double by 2050, implying a looming shortage of healthcare workers. Innovative approaches of care-through-technology are often thought of as a way to mitigate against the lack of workers, which results in a need for knowledge on how humans and machines may provide care together while simultaneously ensuring adequate working conditions. One example of this potential future trend is the recent use of "virtual nurse visits" in Finland [17]. Virtual lunch groups offer the opportunity for older adults to have some company while preparing and eating their lunches with a nurse. The virtual care delivery is part of the strategic shift in Finland toward managing the consequences of aging, increased care demands, a decreasing birth rate, and lower tax revenues [18].

One area of growing importance within the field of welfare technology is the use of robotics and artificial intelligence. The Finnish Ministry of Social Affairs and Health proclaims that such novel technologies can provide a more refined well-being coaching and rehabilitation program and that they are crucial for prolonging living at home and ensuring effective and efficient care delivery services [19]. These advancements illustrate an essential challenge for welfare technology that must be solved at both an international and national policy level; they require policies that can ensure a balance between innovation and the protection of users' rights. As of 2019, the Future of Life Institute has identified national Artificial Intelligence (AI) strategies for more than half of the OECD countries, including Denmark, Finland, and Sweden, as having national AI strategies. However, Norway is not on that list, even though the need for such policies is evident [20]. At the European level, the latest robot and AI regulatory initiatives have scarcely dealt with healthcare, educational, or therapeutic robot technologies [21,22]. Because of the potential benefits that AI and robotics have in the caregiving sector are increasingly being recognized; however, it seems to be a growing priority area for Europe [23].

16.4 Social robots against loneliness

Because the scientific community generally acknowledges the boundaries of what constitutes a robot as being difficult to pinpoint, the current state of the field is challenging to evaluate. The only consensus seems to lie on the role context plays in defining what robot technology is. Any robot that performs, with varying degrees of autonomy, useful services to humans are considered *service robots*. Manufacturing operations are relegated to traditional industrial robotics [24,25]. Social robots are service robots and, as the name implies, they are primarily created to interact with humans socially. Social robots express and perceive emotions, communicate through high-level dialogue, learn and recognize models of other agents, establish and maintain social relationships, and use natural cues such as gaze or gestures [26]. Robots that use these social abilities specifically to assist or support humans socially are called *socially assistive robots* [27].

Since the domestication of wildlife into pets, social interaction between humans and animals have played a significant role in society. Because humans tend to anthropomorphize [28], these social interactions can be replicated with robots, even though they are not biologically alive. These anthropomorphizations direct at zoomorphic robotic companions such as the dog AIBO, the seal robot PARO, and the dinosaur PLEO; humanoid social robots such as Pepper and Asimo; and more object-shaped robots such as pot-plant robot Tessa and the spherical Roomba vacuum cleaner.

Loneliness is one of the key areas where social robots can be particularly useful. We will here describe some detailed case studies of how robots have been used to solve or mitigate problems concerning loneliness, drawn from projects we have conducted with a specific focus on welfare technologies.

16.4.1 Examples of European and national projects on welfare technology

In recent years, there has been significant investment on research and innovation on social robots and welfare technologies both on a European and a national level.

Below, we show some examples of projects that we have been involved with, and how they have focused on this topology.

SocialRobot (2011–2015) was a FP7 (EU's 7th Framework Programme for Research and Technological Development) project aimed to provide assistive services and companionship robots for elderly people – the project primarily geared toward assisting in navigation indoors and unstructured environments and providing affective and empathetic interactions. In its work, it ensured that it took into account the capabilities of and acceptance by elderly users. The project made an outstanding contribution in terms of identifying individual needs and requirements related to aging (e.g., physical mobility limitations or/and cognitive decline) that social robotic interventions should take into account. It also emphasized the provision of support through timely involvement of care teams – including family members, neighbors, and friends – that would collaborate dynamically and virtually at different times and without regards to their physical location. It included behavior analysis to adapt to changing social relationships and contexts of older adults as they age.

VictoryaHome (2013–2015): For those in the later years of their life, living alone can be challenging and unsafe. It often places a heavy burden on friends and family who routinely offer informal care. As the population ages, this burden will increase, placing an unsustainable demand on public care systems. VictoryaHome was a project co-funded by the AAL – European Active and Assisted Living Joint Programme, which addressed the needs of the elderly living alone at home (Figure 16.1). It included partners in Norway, the Netherlands, Sweden, and Portugal.

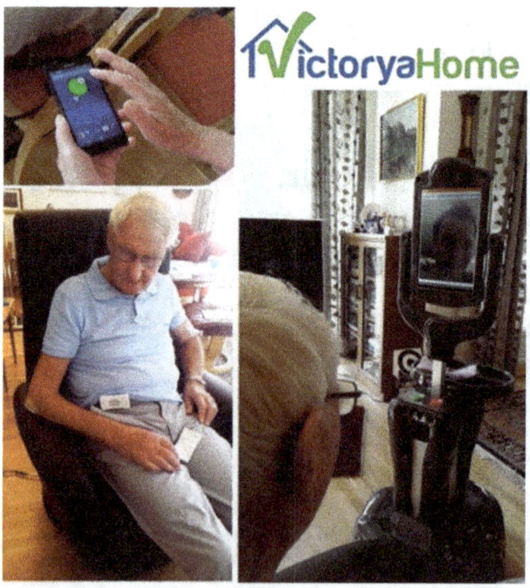

Figure 16.1 VictoryaHome. Source: Picture from the VictoryaHome Consortium in 2005

VictoryaHome offers an open platform able to integrate the following services: activity monitoring, fall detection, medication adherence, and telepresence visits. The main scenario of using VictoryaHome builds on the following scenario:

> Imagine old Irene with a robot that knew her schedule, circumstances, and could share this knowledge with her caregivers in case there is a problem. The caregiver could teleoperate the robot and see what happened and take action. Having the possibility to check on the patient via the robot would improve the reaction time of caregivers while reducing the costs of rushed or unnecessary interventions. [29]

The robot used in the VictoryaHome system was the Giraff, a telepresence robot that allows one person to enter or visit another person in a remote place virtually. The robot may be remotely controlled using a personal computer, via the Internet, using an accessible user graphical interface. The user – normally a caregiver – can move freely about the remote place simply by moving the computer mouse and interact with the residents there via videoconferencing. Access is secured via login and password, and the communication is fully encrypted. On September 24, 2015, VictoryaHome received the award for the best project in the EU AAL program.

GrowMeUp (2015–2018), a Horizon 2020 project, built on the SocialRobot project's results and extended them with novel concepts and features including context-awareness – which allows it to learn the older persons needs and habits over time and adapt its functionality, compensating for as the older person' capabilities degrade over time – and cloud robotics, which enables the sharing and distribution of knowledge with multiple robots performing a similar job.

eWare (2017–2020): The European AAL eWare project provides people with dementia and their (in)formal caregivers a novel and user-friendly solution that can support independent living by combining social robotics and lifestyle monitoring. Lifestyle monitoring is a technology that was developed specifically to support caring for people with dementia. This technology involves monitoring for the person with dementia to perform specific, desired activities, such as going to bed, getting a meal, or watering the plants. These activities can be defined, including the timeframes the patient should perform the actions, by the (in)formal caregiver via an eWare mobile application. The technology then monitors for signs that an activity is taking place, e.g., activity in the kitchen when it is time to eat. The eWare program integrated a social robot – *Tessa* – to allow for bidirectional communication. The robot looks like a jar with a plant in it and has blinking eyes.

The caregiver can program specific verbal reminders that the Tessa will speak in specific time frames to remind person with dementia to do these everyday lifestyle tasks that they may have forgotten to do. If needed, these reminders can be given a second or third time with increasing, but always friendly, urgency. If the person performs the tasks within the designated timeframes, no verbal reminders are given. Caregivers can thus both gain an insight in the daily life pattern of a person with dementia and reduce the burden of care. Communication between both can be enhanced. In addition to improving care for the patient, such a technology can reduce caregiver's distress [29] and thereby extend the period that the informal caregiver can sustain the care needs for people with dementia [30].

EuroAge (2017–2020), an Iberian POCTEP (Programa de Cooperación Interreg VA España-Portugal) project focused on the development of innovative initiatives for the promotion of active aging in the EuroACE region (Alentejo and Centro (Portugal) and Extremadura (Spain)). Its objective was to promote active aging in the areas of physical, cognitive, and socio-emotional activity, with the primary objective of improving the quality of life and increasing healthy life expectancy through the integration of Portugal-Spain cross-border technical-scientific knowledge. One of the lines of work of this project was in the area of robotics, highlighting the great potential that exists in the EuroACE region, concerning Social and Assistive Robotics for the elderly or otherwise dependent individuals. In this project, the previous results from SocialRobot and GrowMeUp were extended with further integration with the home Internet of Things (IoT) infrastructure (e.g., camera network) and a virtual agent (e.g., human-like avatar) that can "coexist as an integrated solution."

My robot friend (2017–2019) is a project concerned with how older adults are often not included in the design processes and feedback loops of social robots and how this user participation can be improved – the project aimed to include older adults through elderly municipality councils as advisors and knowledge brokers. Here, we wanted to meet the elderly with an open mind and hear their impressions. We used different social robots, like the robot Pepper – developed by Softbank – and eWare's Tessa, as venture points for discussions and gained significant insight from the elderly on how robots could be used for being more social (Figure 16.2). One key insight was that it is not the robots in themselves that become the

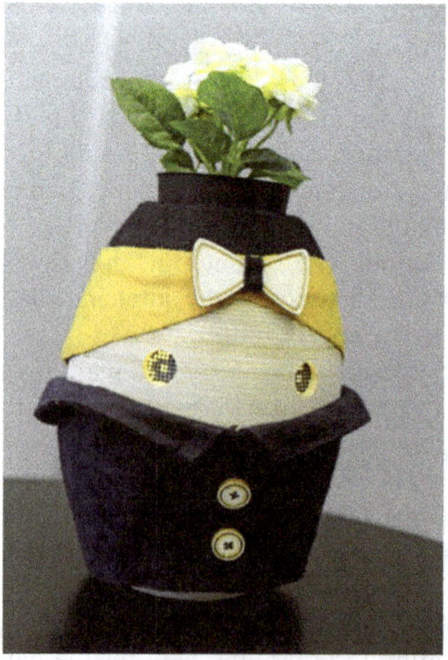

Figure 16.2 The Tessa robot from Tinybots used in the eWare project. Source: Picture provided by Kim Sørenssen/NTNU

important change agents in people's lives, but rather the intricate socio-networks of care that they make possible and strengthen.

LIFEBOTS Exchange (2019–2023): Lifebots is a project which seeks to increase cross-sectoral, international, and interdisciplinary collaboration in the area of social robotics technology, particularly within the care and health sector. This is facilitated by the exchange of personnel between multiple European countries and South Korea. While on the exchange, the personnel works on advancing the current maturity of social robotics and investigate how human users and social robotics can cohabitate. Having user organizations, Small and medium-sized enterprises (SMEs), and academic institutions as partners allows for a multifocal approach. The project is financed by the Research and Innovation Staff Exchange (RISE) program, which is part of the Marie Skłodowska-Curie Actions (MSCA) under the European Union's research and innovation framework programme, Horizon 2020. The project ties together knowledge from a lot of different projects on social robots, in order to learn from past interdisciplinary, international, and intersectoral collaborations.

16.4.2 Critical features of social robots

Based on the projects and robots described above, we here list certain essential elements to social robots that can be critical items to reflect upon when designing and implementing social robots that mitigate loneliness:

Table 16.1 Essential elements of social robots

Social features	The ability to provide emotional support, emotional care, and even love is an essential feature of social robots. In addition to the actions of the robot, this can include the possibility of enabling external communication and interaction with the outer world.
Natural interaction features	The capability of allowing interaction by means that feel "natural" to the user (e.g., gestures, speech, etc.) and adaptation to the user's general profile, specific needs, and intentions were identified as high priority requirements. In the AAL domain, these features must address the needs of users with cognitive or physical skills degradation (e.g., elderly or impaired people) and should aim to compensate for these limitations, hence enriching user experience and accessibility.
Robustness	Robots should not break down in the course of operation. Robots also need to be robust so that they do not break while interacting with humans. For instance, when robots tend to look more humanoid, there are often tendencies for spectators to want to shake the robots' hand, which often are not created for multiple humans squeezing their hands repeatedly. Depending on the context where the robot is, roboticists will have to take into account environmental aspects; for example, most robots are not that well fitted to deal with natural environments such as forests, mud, or rain.

(Continues)

Table 16.1 Essential elements of social robots (Continued)

Technical reliability	How humans use technology can depend on whether humans trust the robot to do what it is supposed to at the right time. When technical bugs and hardware or software malfunction makes robots behave in unexpected, or even dangerous ways, human acceptance rate can drop drastically. As Salem *et al.* [30] highlight, the reliability also refers to the level of trust that the designer's intentions are aligned to the needs of the user.
Privacy & security concerns	Who is listening on the other side of the robot's sensors is essential to protecting the privacy rights of the users. Robots inserted into the homes of users represent an interface with the most intimate place a person has. Behavioral and health data are highly sensitive and have special consideration under the European data protection legal framework and deserve the utmost protection.
Inter-operability	Social robots' ability to learn from different technological systems (e.g., integration with IoT devices for home) is critical to creating better user experiences. If one robot learns something crucial about human behavior, it is beneficial if other robots of the same type can inherit the knowledge and implement it in future interactions while still adhering to individual considerations of human users. The use of cloud robotics and standard interoperable systems may speed learning processes and ease mass implementation.
Usability	If robots are not easy to use; their usage does not last long. Intuitive plug-and-play technology could replace challenging, long tutorials. For different users, different thresholds of using robots exist; by making the user process as intuitive and straightforward as possible, robots can integrate into the life of everyday users more easily.
People-centered design	Taking into account users' needs and interests from the first stage of development increases the effectiveness of the future robot implementation process as well as the quality and usability of the final product. It also improves the accessibility of interactive systems by integrating theoretical models with practical user performance feedback. As the WHO notes, "integrated people-centred health services means putting the comprehensive needs of people and communities, not only diseases, at the centre of health systems, and empowering people to have a more active role in their own health." [31]
High cost	The pursuit of the most appropriate technological platform with the most advanced features usually leads to a price tag that is not compatible with the existing budgets both from individual buyers (the user at home and/or their families) and the national healthcare services. Thus, making cost reasonable is essential for the largescale adoption of technology.

16.5 Reflections on robots, the elderly, and loneliness

Implementing technology into the life of users is not a linear process. How social robots can become part of the daily life of older adults in their own homes is a significant challenge for welfare technology/AAL. In order to become a social resource for the elderly and act as an intermediary between people living at home, their relatives, and the municipal health and care services, social robots need either a certain level of intelligence or perception of intelligence. The potential of robots as assistive technology to supplement human contact in care may primarily address the goal of increasing individual autonomy, thus bridging the loneliness that public service users may experience due to functional reductions. However, whether such a technology is also used to replace human contact is currently being critically discussed within social science research on technology in care [32,33]. Europe is aware of this challenge and has reiterated that human contact is an essential aspect of social care, and that robot technologies should not replace [22,24]. Norwegian health and care authorities emphasize the same standpoint [34]. Transitions of welfare technology from having a supplementing role to replacing care personnel can be anticipated to take place at street-level in the services, where discrete conflicts about the distribution of resources within and between services take place.

Robot technology could be an interface that connects older adults in remote places to social networks, putting them in contact with relatives, friends, and doctors. However, the continuous use of companion robots could also intensify and exacerbate the loneliness these people feel. Although they would be "in contact" with other people, they may also experience this as a deprivation of the warmth of human-human encounters. In this sense, some European institutions try to understand to what extent the respect for family life should also include a possible "right to meaningful human contact" [35], although we wait for more guidance on the realization of such a right in specific situations.

Turkle [36] captures the long-term consequences of such technologies and warns that technologies, even if meant to combat loneliness, might make us be "alone together" staring blankly into our screen-worlds, forgetting the "real world" and being lonelier than we were before we had the technology. As robots are emissaries of the digital, good design is crucial to keep humans rooted in the offline world as well, in particular when it comes to healthcare, where illness exists not as digital representations but in real patients even if, on the other hand, virtual escape might lead to the forgetting of physical pains. Responsible technological development with a deep and interdisciplinary understanding of human affection is strongly needed.

The introduction of social robots in societies is a complex matter and requires including many different perspectives, including the gendered aspect of aging and technology. Women, in general, live longer than men. This demographic trend increases the older the sample population is. Designing robots with gender in mind is essential [37], as there might be physical or cultural differences between users based on gender [38]. Gender can be used both as an inclusive and an exclusion parameter, and it is, in our experience, essential to include a representative part of the population in planning, making, using, and analyzing technology.

16.6 Concluding remarks

This book chapter has explored how social robotic emotional care could mitigate isolation and loneliness. We first discussed the concept of being "social" and how that notion is changing with rapid digitalization. We paid particular attention to remote regions and explored the Scandinavian term "welfare technology," while also situating how loneliness can be a geo-cultural feeling both in the northern regions and southern locations – such as the Portuguese case. As a solution to these issues, we illustrated our case with different collaborative projects on human–robot interaction.

As Scandinavia is a wealthy region, but deficient in population numbers, situational understanding of robotic development and implementation in the region could provide highly fruitful for other regions doing similar tests. With increased globalization, new trade ways, technology brokering, and advancement, it becomes essential to ensure that society includes ways to connect individuals in remote places to the outer if they want. Having the choice of connecting to other individuals not only could reduce the negative aspects of loneliness but also improve their self-esteem and positivity. Social robots could be one component in achieving this goal as part of a seamless web of care practices.

Acknowledgments

This chapter has been partially funded by the LIFEBOTS Exchange project funded by the European Union's Horizon 2020 research and innovation programme under the Grant Agreement No. 824047; and by the LEaDing Fellows Marie Curie COFUND fellowship, a project that received funding from the European Union's Horizon 2020 research and innovation programme under the Marie Skłodowska-Curie Grant Agreement No. 707404.

References

[1] Lexico. *Definition of 'social'* [online]. n.d. Available from https://www.lexico.com/en/definition/social [Accessed 14 September 2019].
[2] Haraway D. Staying with the Trouble: Making Kin in the Chthulucene. Durham: Duke University Press; 2016.
[3] Haraway D. 'A manifesto for cyborgs: Science, technology, and socialist feminism in the 1980s' in Seidman S. (ed.). The Postmodern Turn: New Perspectives on Social Theory. Cambridge: Cambridge University Press; 1994 pp. 82–115.
[4] Hagerup, I. Mitt Kkip Seiler. Oslo: Aschehoug; 1951 (translated by authors).
[5] Cohen GD. 'Loneliness in later life'. American Journal of Geriatric Psychiatry. 2000; 8: 273–75.
[6] Sorkin D, Rook KS, and Lu JL. (2002). 'Loneliness, lack of emotional support, lack of companionship, and the likelihood of having a heart

condition in an elderly sample'. Annals of Behavioral Medicine. 2002; 24: 290–98.

[7] United Nations Development Programme. *Human Development Reports: Norway* [online] n.d. Available at [Accessed 14 September 2019].

[8] The World Bank. *GDP Per Capita (Current US$)* [online] n.d. Available at [Accessed 14 September 2019].

[9] Helliwell JF, Layard R, and Sachs JD. *World Happiness Report 2019.* Available at [Accessed 14 September 2019].

[10] *Ageing@Coimbra* [online] Available at [Accessed 14 September 2019].

[11] Moser I. (ed.) (2019) Velferdsteknologi – en ressursbok. Oslo: Cappelen Damm AS.

[12] Nakrem S and Sigurjónsson, JB. Velferdsteknologi i praksis. Oslo: Cappelen Damm AS; 2017.

[13] Broadbent, E. MacDonald, B., and Robinson, H. (2015) 'Group sessions with Paro in a nursing home: Structure, observations and interviews'. Australasian Journal on Ageing. 2016; 35(2): 106–12.

[14] Butter M, Rensma A, Van Boxsel J, *et al. Robotics for Healthcare: Final Report.* Brussels: DG Information Society, European Commission; 2008.

[15] Gorgey AS. 'Robotic exoskeletons: The current pros and cons'. World Journal of Orthopedics. 2018; 9(9): 112–19.

[16] World Health Organization. *Ageing and Health* [online]. 5 February 2018. Available from [Accessed 14 September 2019].

[17] Johnson S. 'Virtual visits: how Finland is coping with an ageing population'. *The Guardian* [online]. 26 June 2019 Available at [Accessed 14 September 2019].

[18] Kauranen A and Rosendahl J. *Record-low birth rate threatens Finland's welfare system: Finance Minister* [online]. 28 November 2018. Available at [Accessed 14 September 2019].

[19] Finnish Ministry of Social Affairs and Health. *Well-Being and Health.* AiRo programme; 2018. Available at https://stm.fi/en/artikkeli/-/asset_publisher/tekoaly-ja-robotiikka-parantavat-ihmisten-hyvinvointia-hyteairo-ohjelma-vauhdittaa-toteutuksia [Accessed 14 September 2019].

[20] Future of Life Institute. *Global AI policy: How countries and organizations around the world are approaching the benefits and risks of AI* [online]. n.d. Available at [Accessed 14 September 2019].

[21] European Parliament. Civil Law Rules on Robotics European Parliament resolution of 16 February 2017 with recommendations to the Commission on Civil Law Rules on Robotics (2015/2103(INL)). Available at [Accessed 14 September 2019].

[22] Fosch-Villaronga E. Artificial Intelligence, Healthcare, and the Law: Regulating Automation in Personal Care. Routledge; 2019.

[23] European Parliament. Report on a comprehensive European industrial policy on artificial intelligence and robotics (2018/2088(INI)). Available at [Accessed 14 September 2019].

[24] Quintas JM (2018). Context-based Human-Machine Interaction Framework for Artificial Social Companions. Doctoral dissertation, 00500: Universidade de Coimbra; 2018.

[25] International Federation of Robotics (2019). *Service Robots*. Retrieved from [Accessed 15 September 2019].

[26] Fong T, Nourbakhsh I, and Dautenhahn K. 'A survey of socially interactive robots'. Robotics and Autonomous Systems. 2003; 42(3–4): 143–66.

[27] Feil-Seifer D and Mataric MJ. 'Defining socially assistive robotics'. *IEEE 9th International Conference on Rehabilitation Robotics*, Chicago, IL, 2005. ICORR; 2005, 465–68.

[28] Duffy BR. 'Anthropomorphism and the social robot'. Robotics and Autonomous Systems. 2003; 42(3–4): 177–90.

[29] AAL Programme. *VictoryaHome* [online] n.d. Available at [Accessed on 14 September 2019].

[30] Salem M, Lakatos G, Amirabdollahian F, and Dautenhahn K. 'Towards safe and trustworthy social robots: ethical challenges and practical issues'. In *International Conference on Social Robotics*, 26 October 2015. Springer, pp. 584–593.

[31] World Health Organization. *WHO Framework on Integrated People-Centered Health Services* [online] n.d. Available at [accessed on 14 September 2019].

[32] Pols J and Moser I. (2009). 'Cold technologies versus warm care? On affective and social relations with and through care technologies'. ALTER, European Journal of Disability. 2009; 3(2): 159–78.

[33] Tøndel G. (2018). 'Omsorgens materialitet: trygghet, teknologi og alderdom [The Materiality of Care: Safety, Technology and Old Age]'. Tidsskrift for omsorgsforskning [Journal of Care Research]. 2018; 4(3): 287–297.

[34] Norwegian Ministry of Health and Care Services (2011). Innovation in the Care Services. White paper, 2011: 11.

[35] Parliamentary Assembly of the Council of Europe (PACE). Human Rights in the Robot Age: Challenges Arising from the Use of Robotics, Artificial Intelligence, and Virtual and Augmented Reality. The Hague: Rathenau Instituut; 2017. Available at https://www.rathenau.nl/sites/default/files/2018–02/Human%20Rights%20in%20the%20Robot%20Age-Rathenau%20Instituut-2017.pdf [Accessed 14 September 2019].

[36] Turkle S. Alone Together: Why We Expect More from Technology and Less from Each Other. Hachette UK; 2011.

[37] Søraa RA. 'Mechanical genders: how do humans gender robots?'. Gender, Technology and Development. 2017; 21(1–2): 99–115.

[38] Gendered Innovation. *Exploring Markets for Assistive Technologies for the Elderly* [online] n.d. Available at http://genderedinnovations.stanford.edu/case-studies/robots.html#tabs-2 [Accessed 14 September 2019].

Chapter 17

Healthcare robots for elderly people: A review of the robotic solutions, use cases, and barriers

Md. Rakibul Hoque[1,3], Sabin Huda,[1] and Md Rashadul Hasan[2]

17.1 Introduction

The elderly population, aged 60 and above, is increasing worldwide quicker than all other groups of people of younger age. As is anticipated in the World Population Ageing Report, the population of elderly people (age 60 years or more) is likely to be more than doubled by 2050, with a global increase from 962 million in 2017 to 2.1 billion in 2050 [1]. In the US context, it is estimated that the elderly population will increase by 26% by 2050 [2]. By 2050, the population of people over 80 is predicted to be more than 11% of their total population on average in many countries (e.g. Japan 17%, Spain 15%, and Germany 14.5%) [3].

Elderly people suffer from various health complications affected by various chronic diseases, such as diabetes, cardiovascular diseases, chronic respiratory diseases, Alzheimer's disease (causing dementia), depression, and cancer [4]. Fortunately, modernization of medical science has been always helping them to survive from such diseases and increase their longevity and total population ratio.

In general, a person who is aged 65 years or more is considered as elderly [5]. Though, when we talk about elderly people, we generally refer to those people who are more than 75 years old [6]. As the longevity of people increases, it creates an enormous demand of care needs for the elderly. In most developed countries, this issue of high aging population with a low number of caregivers is very prominent, with a shortage in both formal and informal caregivers of older people. In most of the industrial nations (e.g. Germany, Japan, and Korea), such a demographic change would cause overload for nursing care system [7]. For instance, in the Asian country Japan, a shortage of about 1 million caregivers by 2025 is projected in this regard [8]. Also, a shortage of native-born nurses is very common in developed countries like Germany. In Canada, the United Kingdom, and the United States,

[1]Department of Management Information Systems, University of Dhaka, Dhaka, Bangladesh
[2]Bhalo Achi Healthcare and Research Ltd., Dhaka, Bangladesh
[3]School of Business, Emporia State University, Emporia, KS, USA

foreign-born elderly caregivers consist up to 19–25%, responsible for costly care service [9]. In the context of African countries, the nursing care system is much unstructured and underdeveloped [10] that can properly provide nursing care for the elderly. Hence, the healthcare researchers from all around the world are avidly pursuing for developing and providing robot-assisted services as the alternatives of caregivers to make the elderly people capable of performing their daily tasks as much as is possible.

Yet again, the elderly people have less income and their income lessens even more as they get older. As a result, they rely heavily on health insurance and social security packages for their treatment and healthcare that can cause economic burden on a government [11]. The rise of elderly population in any country can cause the concerns of an overburden on healthcare service provision and healthcare expenditure. Then again, the elderly people's frailty depends on various factors like chronic disease and fitness conditions. As the longevity increases, the elderly people suffer from various forms of disabilities or physical limitations, which relate to sensory, cognitive, mobility, and self-care [12]; thus, they need support for their chronic disease management, basic self-care, and emotional motivation [13]. On top, two of the most common reasons that are associated with health-deterioration of elderly people are social isolation and loneliness. Often, elderly people live alone or pass their time at home alone, as their family members (e.g. their children) are mostly busy at workplace. More often, due to today's nontraditional family relationships and busy life, elderly people suffer from the lack of availability of later-life support more than ever before [14]. On the other hand, elderly people cannot do their daily tasks without the help of others or special equipment and the availability of caregivers as per the world's aging population is decreasing day by day. Therefore, researchers recommend for continuous study for elderly care to improve their age-specific activity limitations, poor functional capacity, and quality of living at home [12].

By developing elderly care robots for helping elderly people to overcome their functional limitations, keep them independent, and provide companionship, today's health researchers are keen to address the unmet demand of professional caregivers [15]. Therefore, the aim of the study is to review the scope of the application of robot-assisted services, their use cases and barriers in adopting the robot-assisted services or care robots. In this process, the study starts with an overview of the healthcare robots (Section 17.2) that exist in the market for elderly care. Then, Section 17.3 contains the methodology and Section 17.4 contains a review of the situations and scope relating to when and why assistive robots can be used and their use cases, while Section 17.5 provides an analysis of the barriers in adopting healthcare robots based on the existing literature. Finally, the study ends with a comprehensive discussion (Section 17.6) on the findings and future direction for the researches. This study provides a significant overview of the contemporary studies on healthcare robots developed and tested for serving elderly people. Such a study would not only contribute in improving the quality of lives of the elderly people but also contribute in development and adoption of robot-assisted healthcare services in various contexts and countries.

17.2 Existing robotic solutions for elderly care

Today's healthcare industry has been pursuing for a massive shift in the way that they provide care to the elderly people by introducing robot-assisted care increasingly. With the advancement of robotic industry, many believe that robots could be used as an alternative of medical staff and caregivers in many cases. According to Kachouie's review, assistive robots used for elderly care not only bring well-being but also reduce workload on caregivers [16]. In this regard, Japan, as a pioneer country in the healthcare robotic industry, is heavily investing in artificial intelligence to cope with the critical shortage of caregivers in the local market [17]. Research shows evidence that assistive robots are helpful in elderly care [18]. Currently, robots are used for assisting the elderly people in the occasions of providing companionship to reduce the feeling of loneliness and isolation [19], nursing [20], rehabilitation [21], assistance for elders with cognitive impairment and disability [22], telemedicine [23], and tele-presence [24]. Overall, the three main types of areas where assistive robots can be used are when there is a need for: (1) monitoring elderly people's behavior and health, (2) supporting elderly people in their daily tasks, and (3) providing companionship [25].

Robots in the healthcare context can be classified by their appearance, such as humanoid (human like), animoid (animal like), machine like, and pet like. They are used for providing mental, emotional, and psychosocial support. While the rehabilitation robots accomplish a physical task or make a job easier for elderly people, social robots are featured with interactive and likable interface for elderly people to provide companionship. Social robots can be classified into two groups as service robots and companionship robots [26]. When social robots are used for assisting elderly people to complete daily basic tasks, move, and live independently, they are usually known as service robots. Elderly people can interact with service robots with interactive interface. On the other hand, when the social robots are used for improving the quality of life of elderly people by becoming a companion to them, they are known as companion robots. In these ways, the robots can assist the elderly people to maintain and move on with their life independently and improve the quality of their lives by providing functional, psychological and certain medical assistance. The following sections will cover the methodology followed to select the articles for this review.

17.3 Methodology

The authors conducted an integrative literature review [27] that entails integrative synthesis of secondary data of any research topic of interest to find various perspectives on any topic. In this process, the authors searched for articles published since 2010 on the journal database namely: PubMed, Google Scholar, MEDLINE, Scopus, and EBCSO host. The keywords used were "elderly," "older people," "assistive technology," "robot," and "robotics." Additionally, hand searching was conducted following the references in the selected articles to find more relevant articles; even older articles published before 2010 when deemed significant. The inclusion criteria chosen were: (1) articles published in English only, (2) primary studies, (3) review studies, and (4) articles that were published between 2010 and 2019. On the other hand, articles were excluded when: (1) the articles were not methodologically studied, (2) not relevant to elderly care, (3) articles related to surgical robots, (4) articles related to non-robotic assistive technologies, (5) redundant articles, (6) articles did not focus on any robotic intervention, and (7) the articles on same intervention by some older authors.

After screening through inclusion and exclusion criteria, a total of 24 articles (Tables 17.1 and 17.2) were finally selected for review. The EndNote reference management software, used for screening the articles, was based on abstracts of the articles. Wherever an abstract of an article was found irrelevant, the article was excluded from selection for review. Finally, an integrative review approach was followed to evaluate the selected articles to synthesize information to build various insights on the scope of the application of robot-assisted services, their use cases, and barriers in adopting the robot-assisted services or care robots from the existing literature. The following sections will cover the discussions on the scope of using robots for elderly care, their user cases, advantages and disadvantages, and barriers to adopt robots for elderly care.

17.4 The use cases of healthcare robots

Various health issues that the elderly people have in their daily life create ample scope for introducing the use of assistive robots for elderly care. As the elderly people prefer to stay at home to feel comfortable and confident instead of care centers, which incur high cost for them, the scope of using robotic assistance for their self-care activities has widened [28]. Health issues of the elderly people can be of various types, such as decline of physical and functional abilities, cognitive abilities, psychosocial abilities and health management, and medical regime monitoring abilities [26]. The existing use cases of robotic technologies to assist elderly people cope with their gradually declining abilities are discussed under the subsections below according to the types of health inabilities. Also, Table 17.1 summarizes the functional capabilities and areas of use of some well-known assistive robots developed for elderly people.

17.4.1 Physical and functional decline

Elderly people suffer from waning of their physical and functional abilities as they age, it becomes essential to encourage them to maintain their independence in accomplishing their daily basic activities. In such a situation, the application of innovative technology such as assistive technology and smart home environment can support them in passing an active life. Of late, unlike before, the assistive robots are developed to work in smart home environments, which allows various new applications for elderly care [28]. One of the advantages of integrating the robots with smart home environment is to distribute the computational and

Table 17.1 Functional capabilities of assistive robots developed for elderly people

Robot name	Country/origin	Functional capabilities	Application context
EMOX robot [6]	France	A companion robot for human–robot interaction to improve the socio-interactional ability of the lonely elderly people and help them to give vocal commands to the robot to control the smart home environment.	Socially assistive robots
RiSH [28]	China	RiSH works in collaboration with the smart home environment and can recognize human body activity, which lets the home service robot to observe the environment through audio sound. Specifically used to detect and respond to human fall.	Fall and distress situation detection
Robot-Era [29]	European Seventh Framework Programme	Able to move and operate autonomously to accomplish daily housekeeping tasks.	Domestic service robot
Kobuki [30]	Japan	Able to detect someone falling near the robot, and then send message of the incident to someone who can help.	Robots dedicated to a specific task
TurtleBot [34]	China	Allows the elderly to contact to their families and doctors quickly whenever they need. Also, able to detect the target and estimate its pose.	Tele-presence
iPhonoid Robot [44]	Japan	Helps elderly people to organize their daily routine plans by providing information on weather condition, wind speed, and temperature.	Assistance
Giraff [42]	Italy	Allows social interaction from home to the outside world.	Telepresence
Pearl [35]	The USA	Provides reminders for routine activities such as eating, drinking, taking medicine, and using the washroom.	Personal assistant
CompanionAble [39]	European Seventh Framework Programme	Allows communication with family caregivers present outside home, provides predefined reminders, and specific recommendations. Also helps in cognitive stimulation to improve cognitive impairments.	Socially assistive robot
Hobbit [43]	European Seventh Framework Programme	An autonomous, multifunctional service robot, which is capable of smart home integration, speech recognition, fall detection and prevention, remote communication, and multimodal interaction for improving cognitive impairment.	Socially assistive robot

(Continues)

Table 17.1 (Continued)

Robot name	Country/origin	Functional capabilities	Application context
Care-O-bot [40]	Germany	Able to accomplish tasks in human environments and can additionally evoke positive emotions.	Manipulation robots
ROREAS [50]	Germany	Assists as a coach for walking and orientation training of post-stroke rehabilitation patients.	Socially assistive robot
Soft manipulator [51]	Italy	Assists elderly people in the task of bathing.	Personal assistant
RmRs [7]	Italy	Supports Activities of Daily Living (ADLs)	Independent living assistant
iCAR [52]	Sweden	Provides walking-support to the elderly people.	Assistive robot
ASTRO-MOBILE [46]	Italy	Accomplishes activities such as medicine delivery, stand support, reminding, and info-entertainment.	Ambient-assisted living
Auton Robot [53]	Turkey	The robot can learn from the exercise scenario and provide verbal feedback.	Robotic exercise tutor
BENDER [47]	Spain	Allows tele-presence tasks and has surveillance capabilities.	Ambient-assisted living
Tangibot [54]	Spain	Allows intuitive and appealing interactions to train elderly persons with cognitive impairment.	Socially assistive robot
CIRDO [31]	France	It can detect falls and distress situations.	Fall and distress situation detection
Kabochan [55]	Japan	A communication robot that can interact with humans to improve their cognitive ability.	Smile-supplement robot
LEGO robot [56]	Spain	Allows cognitive rehabilitation for the elderly by engaging them with memory and mathematical problem solving.	Assistive robot
RATULS robot [36]	The UK	Aids elderly stroke patients with upper limb impairment to accomplish specific exercise repetitively and constantly.	Assistive robot
Brian 2.1 [57]	Canada	Provides social interactions and cognitive stimulation to elderly people.	Socially assistive robots

processing load more to the smart home environment system instead of to the robots. It makes the robots more responsive and the total system more effective. The concept of integrating robots with smart home environment system also lowers the cost of robots. The newly developed robot-integrated smart home (RiSH) system can help elderly people in appliance control, room temperature control, communicating with friends, and rescuing from falling. Currently, RiSH can also supports elderly people with declined physical and functional conditions in performing activities of daily living (ADLs) (i.e. eating, drinking, taking shower, and managing other washroom functions) and in instrumental activities of daily living (IADLs) (i.e. maintaining medication regimen and preparing meals of proper nutrition) with the help of integrated sensors [28]. Similar to RiSH, Robot-Era was also developed as ambient-assisted system to work for elderly users indoors and in residential spaces [29]. The findings showed satisfactory level of performance and acceptance of the Robot-Era as a domestic service robot.

Among the elderly people, falling on the floor or ground is a serious issue as a report shows that 62.5% of falls for elderly people cause them injury [30]. To address this issue, Kobuki [30] and Cirdo [31] robots were reported as useful. On the other hand, rehabilitation robots are used for different rehabilitations (e.g. waist rehabilitation, ankle rehabilitation, and limb rehabilitation) caused by injury [20]. As the rehabilitation process requires a patient's active participation, where a robot can support uninterruptedly; hence, a major usefulness of the rehabilitation robot is that the frequency and intensity of the rehabilitation process can be enhanced according to the ability of the patients rather than the rehabilitation personnel [32]. Also, to help the infirm elderly people with limited functional abilities, independent nursing robots are used for cleaning an elderly person after defecation. Such robots also independently hold, feed, and disinfect the elderly persons, as well as clean and dehumidify their room [20].

Elderly people often suffer from hearing loss and immobility, and thus face difficulty in contacting with others when needed. According to the study by Kubota, Sekiya, and Tsuji, robot-assisted continuous muscle training can be useful to improve the limited ability of mobility of elderly patients [33]. Yet, considering the immobility problem of elderly people, Zhou *et al.* [34] developed a robot that allows its users to contact their families and doctors quickly whenever they need. Similarly, the MELVIN Robot can assist elderly persons by handling of trousers during their washroom visits [32]. Also, urinary incontinence, which is one of the worst declining fitness issues for elderly people, is addressed by Pearl robotic assistant [35]. However, assistive robots are not useful in all intended purposes. For example, the Rodgers *et al.* trialed a robot-assisted training program on elderly stroke patients to improve their upper limb function but did not find any significant evidence on its intended purpose [36].

17.4.2 Cognitive and psychosocial issues

Elderly people often suffer from cognitive, sensory, and motor impairments; hence, rehabilitation and companion robots are developed. The concept of coexistence of

Table 17.2 Findings and barriers in using some specific robots used for elderly care

Robot/project	Study findings	Barriers in adoption
EMOX robot [6]	The robot can help the isolated person and make them more efficient in the human–human communication.	Requires ethical considerations
RiSH [28]	Able to manage human activity monitoring, fall detection, and rescue with the help of remote caregiver.	Requires more testing in real environment and evidence.
Robot-Era [29]	The usability and acceptability of Robot-Era was satisfactory, however, suggested for second large field test.	High cost
Kobuki [30]	The robot's performance was reported with 80% success rate in fall detection in comparison to other conventional techniques.	Still needs improvement for real-life use case.
TurtleBot [34]	As a remote healthcare robot, TurtleBot may be used for remote elderly care.	Not mentioned
iPhonoid Robot [44]	The initial findings show that iPhonoid robot is useful to make various recommendations for elderly people based on weather conditions that can prevent them from health damage.	Not mentioned
Giraff [42]	Useful for reinforcing social ties of the elderly people and increasing social inclusion.	Depends on social participation of other peoples
Pearl [35]	The ultimate success of the project will depend on how the robot will be further developed according to proper and adequate knowledge of human behavior, aging, and disability.	Not mentioned
CompanionAble [39]	Able to provide useful service and enjoyable experience to elderly people who have cognitive impairment.	Longer field trials are required
Hobbit [43]	The robot helps the aged at home and thus postpones the need to move to a care center.	Needs more reliability tests.
Care-O-bot [40]	Able to assist the infirm person, and shows positive emotion in visceral, behavioral, and reflective levels.	Still requires real-world test and validation in interacting in particular emotional situations.

(Continues)

ROREAS [50]	Able to autonomously accompany the post-stroke patients in practicing their mobility exercise sessions.	Requires active participation and still needs trial in real clinical setting.
Soft manipulator [51]	Because of using soft robotic technologies, better compliance is achieved and safety is reported in human–robot interaction when used for intended purpose.	Not mentioned
RmRs [7]	The ultimate user acceptance of robotic micro-robot rooms (RmRs) is yet to be achieved.	Cost
iCAR [52]	Still in development phase.	Not mentioned
ASTROMOBILE [46]	The study concluded that robotic technology is promising and feasible for elderly care.	None; used user-centered design approach
Auton Robot [53]	The result shows that elderly people show willingness to do regular multiple sessions of exercise with the assistance of the robot.	Needs personally adaptable features to meet individual demands.
BENDER [47]	The robot-assisted service becomes cheaper and more effective when a service robot works on AAL system.	Still needs more technical improvement to make commercial version.
Tangibot [54]	Tangibot was found to be appealing to most users and showed promising performance to improve the cognitive abilities of the users with mild impairment through engaging the users with games.	Not mentioned
CIRDO [31]	The project is successful in establishing a link between needs, people, and technology.	Not mentioned
Kabochan [55]	The findings show that the elderly participants' anxiety decreased, and after interacting with Kabochan, their quality of improved due to improvement of their physical functioning.	Requires further studies
LEGO robot [56]	There is no significant advantage of using this robot over using mobile app for similar purpose.	Have alternative app for similar purpose
RATULS robot [36]	The result shows robot-assisted training cannot improve the upper limb function of stroke patients; thus, any clinical practice is not recommended for upper limb therapy.	Not useful
Brian 2.1 [57]	Most of the elderly users showed positive attitude toward Brian 2.1 robot for its intended uses.	Not mentioned

humans with robot partners is being vastly studied now to facilitate communication and companionship in lonely life [37]. For elderly people, often lack of motivation and emotional disorder is very common and is accompanied by depression and dementia [38]. By realizing the significance of active cognitive functions, robot like iPhonoid [37] was developed to engage elderly people in conversation and communication. At the same time, the game-based cognitive stimulation by companion robots can be potentially useful with these issues.

Both the positive and negative outcomes are reported in using robots for elderly people having mild cognitive impairment (MCI). While the study by Woo *et al.* reported that elderly participants showed negative attitude toward assistive robots [37], though the users also showed positive attitude toward the companion robot known as CompanionAble [39] that uses cognitive training application and games to improve the condition of mild cognitive impairment of elderly people. Similarly, Care-O-bot 4 [40], which is a more advanced companion robot and released as its fourth generation model, features as human-like behavior and it is reported to be as useful for increasing independence and quality of life of the elderly people through cognitive and empathetic interactions.

Social and emotional support is important for elderly people beside physical and functional support [23]. As elderly people stay for a longer time at home and spend their time alone, the socio-affective isolation is a common issue that affects their health [6]. Besides reducing the quality of life, such isolation has direct negative impact on their mental health and subsequent physical health. The socio-affective isolation leads to affective interactional degradation, especially in patients' conditions with Alzheimer's disease. For elderly people, a lack of social interaction often aggravates their psychological condition that can lead to dementia [41]. To address the psychological issue, the companion robot PARO was commercially successful in the early days of companion robot concept [25]. Another companion robot known as EMOX robot was found to be effective in improving the socio-interactional (e.g. communication) ability of elderly people [6].

Companion robots like tele-presence robots are mainly used to address psychological issues resulting from loneliness of the elderly people. The tele-presence robots allow interactions with remote environment and interpersonal communication [23]. One of the tele-presence robots from the early days of induction for assistive robots for elderly care is known as Giraff. The study reported that Giraff is useful for reinforcing social ties of elderly people and hence contributes in their social participation [42]. Similarly, study on tele-presence robot named ROBIN shows that tele-presence robot can foster the lonely elderly users' social participation [24]. However, unlike simpler robot like Giraff, the new generation robots are more intelligent. The improved version of Hobbit [43], for example, does not only accomplish the scheduled tasks and user's commands to support social functionalities but also autonomously adapts to different situations through machine learning-based users' behavioral pattern and adjacent environmental factors to provide elderly care. Such an adaptive ability is significant for sophisticated cognitive support offered through proactive interaction.

17.4.3 Mismanagement of medical regimes and health monitoring

Elderly people, as they age reasonably, face issues of mismanagement of their medical regimes and health conditions because of chronic illnesses and loss of abilities. This issue exacerbates furthermore when family members of an elderly person are unable to look after them because of their busy life. Now the nursing of the elderly is a social issue. Luckily, the innovation in technology has rendered the opportunity to use robots for nursing purpose. Till today, many nursing robots have been introduced. For instance, the Pearl robot, which is also known as Nursebot, was successfully used as a personal assistant that can help the elderly people in eating and taking medicine in due time by providing reminders [35]. On the other hand, considering the vulnerability and health damage of elderly people in adverse weather conditions, iPhonoid Robot can recommend to elderly people if they should wear warm or light clothes and the type of food they should take according to weather conditions [44]. In addition, a study by Łukasik, Tobis, Wieczorowska-Tobis, and Suwalska shows that elderly people have positive attitude for using assistive robots for nutritional support [45].

As technology advances, the newer generation assistive robot such as ASTROMOBILE [46] works in combination with Ambient Intelligent Infrastructure to identify users' needs and deliver medicine and reminders more efficiently. Also, in the BENDER robot development project by Pavón-Pulido *et al.*, it is shown that synergy between ambient-assisted living (AAL) system and assistive robot lowers the cost significantly, as well as makes real-time task planning by robots more feasible [47]. A comprehensive review on literature on AAL system by Al-Shaqi, Mourshed, and Rezgui reported that the application of the Internet of Things (IoT) concept might disrupt the current technologies used in developing geriatric care robots by enabling real-time health monitoring [48]. The integration of AAL with robots also provides opportunities to use environmental factors for analytics and decision-making in geriatric care. Similarly, in an attempt at integrating newer technology in geriatric care robots, Lera, Rodríguez, Rodríguez, and Matellán successfully integrated Augmented Reality technology (a technology of real-time identification of objects captured in camera and providing computer-generated information on those objects) in different tele-presence robots to assist elderly people with drug dose management and intake [49].

17.5 Barriers in adopting healthcare robots

The barriers in adopting healthcare robots are discussed below according to various related types of barriers that are commonly highlighted in the existing literature. Besides, Table 17.2 summarizes the findings and barriers in using some specific robots used for elderly care.

17.5.1 Users acceptance

Elderly people are unenthusiastic regarding robotic care in general. The adoption of healthcare robots can be negatively affected due to the possession of negative attitude by elderly people [25]. A study shows that gender, culture, context, prior experience, educational background, and type of application can negatively affect the attitude of the elderly people toward robots [25,58]. To increase the acceptability of the companion robots that interact with humans, researchers have recommended for in-depth understanding of the human behavioral nature first, especially of the elderly persons [32]. Such an understanding of human behavioral nature also differs because of different culture and demographic factors. Thus, in future artificial intelligence (AI) will be used to understand user behavior from long-term interaction with robots [59]. Even more excitingly, it is anticipated that in future the body of the robots will be composed of fluids, gels, and elastomers, so that the biological properties of the human skin are felt, which will ultimately increase the acceptance of the robots for elderly care [60]. Furthermore, user-centered development is emphasized in development of the elderly care robots for better acceptance [50].

According to the study by Pino, Boulay, Jouen, and Rigaud, a robot's appearance, features, and social interactive capabilities are important factors for their acceptance [61]. In the same way, compliance also plays an important role in adopting robotic care. As a result, researchers are giving importance on the emerging soft robotic technologies to maintain better compliance [51]. Also, Woo *et al.* [37] find that social influence is a significant factor in robot adoption for elderly care. Likewise, technology anxiety because of perceived complexity of technology in elderly people can be an important reason of impediment in adopting robot-assisted elderly care [62].

17.5.2 Usefulness and complexity

Usefulness is an important factor in the adoption of robots for elderly care. A study shows that elderly people's perception of usability of robot-assisted service is formed based on four main factors, namely safety, controllability, efficiency, and satisfaction [63]. In this regard, rehabilitation robots are often are not so effective in accomplishing their purpose, and hence still have low adoption rate. Most of the times, rehabilitation treatment requires specialized and human interaction intervention. Thus, often rehabilitation robot–assisted therapy is less useful in comparison to conventional therapy, especially in the case of post-stroke rehabilitation [32]. On the other hand, although studies show that elderly people have the capacity to use new technologies, the complexity in using assistive robots can arise when an elderly person has trembling hands, mobility problems, low vision capacity, and acoustic impairments, mostly because of various disease like arthritis and Alzheimer's disease [54]. Therefore, the use of a convenient and bigger tangible user interface for elderly users is suggested. However, it is also found in a survey that people's negative attitude regarding elderly people's association with technology might prevent elderly people from adopting new assistive technology [64].

17.5.3 Cost and inefficiency

Cost is always a big factor in adopting the robots for elderly care since the elderly people have low income. In a review on nursing robots by Jiang *et al.* [20], the cost and reliability were highlighted as the main barriers in nursing robot adoption. Similarly, Robot-Era, for example, was reported as much less likely to be adopted by the elderly because of high price despite satisfactory performance [29]. Besides cost, inefficiency is also a barrier in adopting robots for elderly care. For instance, while using robots, the inefficiency such as constant consumption of power is reported as an important barrier when the sensors of the robot have to track human movement always [30].

To address the cost issue, Koceska *et al.* [23] developed a low-cost assistive tele-presence robot and reported positive attitude and willingness to adopt their designed robot. Similarly, Zhou *et al.* [34] also developed a tele-presence robot known as TurtleBot that they claimed to be low-cost and reported positive outcome while testing the robot for its intended purpose. Additionally, the sensors used in the robots are becoming more affordable day by day, which can reduce the cost of robots in future.

17.5.4 Enjoyment, social attractiveness, and human dignity

Enjoyment is an important factor that can influence the engagement of the elderly people with robots. The study shows that human-like robot increases enjoyment level when used as a companion to assist in the ADL and other social activities [65]. Similarly, Hamada *et al.* [66] shows that the integration of recreational program in robot-assisted therapy for elderly users with dementia can make the use of assistive robots more enjoyable. Also, while evaluating the use of socially assistive robots for elderly care, Torta *et al.* found that users feel less enjoyment after a certain time; thus, they suggested for ensuring high level of users' enjoyment for long periods of time [67]. On the other hand, study on the Auton robot shows that the consideration of social attractiveness in the robot design process is important for acceptance of the robot as a fitness coach [39]. Additionally, consideration of human dignity is also important for the adoption of robots by the elderly people for their care [68]. Not understanding the dignity of vulnerable elderly people can have a negative impact on assistive robot adoption [69]. For instance, interaction with toy-like robots or the deprivation of human touch (e.g. robot-assisted cleaning) while using assistive technology can induce low self-esteem among elderly people, and can undermine their human dignity consequently.

17.5.5 Trust, safety, and evidence

Recent study shows that like cost issue, the lack of trust [70], and lack of evidence [32] on the usefulness of using robots for elderly care are other significant barriers for the adoption of assistive robots. As the newer generation of robots are being developed to work within AAL systems (e.g. smart home), the requirement of clinical evidence is identified as a significant factor for users' acceptance of robots for geriatric care [48]. On the other hand, when robotic assistance is used, there remain several safety concerns, such as the chance of collisions between elderly people and robots, which could lead to various injuries and loss because of mechanical and electrical failure. The reviews on the use of robots for geriatric care by Bodenhagen *et al.* [32] and Tanioka [73] specifically stressed on addressing the safety concern regarding potentially vulnerable elderly persons to increase adoption of elderly care robots.

17.5.6 Ethical consideration, privacy, and validation

There is always the involvement of ethical concern that robotic care should be a supplement to human care for elderly people, not a replacement [25,71]. It is reported that about 28 highly cited articles were published between 2002 and 2016 to address the ethical concern on using robots for elderly care [32]. Hersh [72], in his review on service robots for elderly people, has pointed out the necessity to use assistive robots sensitively and appropriately. The studies by Tanioka [73] and Coco, Kangasniemi, and Rantanen [74] also show that the ethical debate regarding the human-to-robot relationship is a significant consideration ignoring which can impede the adoption of nursing robots.

According to Körtner, ethical consideration in using assistive robots for the elderly encompass matters of dignity, privacy, safety, vulnerability, and consent of the users [75]. Beside the mere use intention, the ethical concern also expands into areas of the robot's functionality, shape, design, and conformation with cultural and religious background. Therefore, the ethical concerns are now addressed and evaluated during the design and development processes assistive robots. In this process, a scheme called Care-Centered Value-Sensitive Design (CCVSD) is devised that ensures that ethical concerns are addressed while designing robots for elderly care [76].

The privacy concern also leads to be a barrier in adoption [77], especially with the anticipation that robots used as personal assistants may involve with privacy breaching through the exchange of personal data with manufacturing or third party companies [32]. The assurance of privacy is also important for practicing autonomy or capacity to self-determination by the elderly users when they use assistive technology [78]. On the other hand, to ensure valid use of assistive robots for elderly people, researchers have recommended for having precise reasons in applying any robot intervention and taking validated measures to evaluate their usability [79].

17.6 Discussion and future direction

This study objectively reviews the non-technical aspects of the robotic solutions, use cases, and barriers in elderly care to provide a contemporary understanding of these. This review informs us that although since the last decade scientists and researchers are continuously integrating newer and innovative technologies (e.g. IoT, smart home, augmented reality, artificial intelligence, and machine learning) with the assistive robots used for elderly care, the results are mostly concluded with conspicuous barriers of various types in adoption and lack of clinical evidence. The review indicates that the assistive robot industry for elderly care will need a long time yet to meet user demand efficiently. Also, from the review, it is a significantly noticeable fact that hardly any assistive robot project was initiated in any developing country.

The review informs about different use cases for addressing different elderly related health management issues. The use cases and barriers in adoption were presented in groups under the above sections and subsections. The review shows that there is a significant lack of clinical evidence and comparative advantage other than the fact that assistive robots can be used as a mere partial supplement of an actual caregiver. Also, findings of most of the studies show that most of robot projects are in the initial stage (small-scale prototype), indicating low technical readiness level (TRL). Regarding barriers in adoption, lack of evidence and cost are still the bigger barriers. Besides, many studies have not evaluated users' acceptance methodologically, not to mention that Table 17.2 shows that one-third of the studies (8 out of 24 robots mentioned in the table) have not discussed any barriers in robot adoption by elderly people.

According to the studies reviewed, induction of robot-assisted elderly care is deemed as welfare in the society and the governments in the developed countries are keen to promote such use to address the overload on caregivers. However, the review shows that while the assistive robots are deemed as social entity, the relationship with humans is entangled with various ethical concerns (e.g. dignity, privacy, and consent). Thus, ethical evaluation is highly suggested in every trial for ensuring practical use sensitively and appropriately. Multiple studies discussed above highlighted the fact that assistive robots should not replace the actual caregivers but should be used as supplementary support. Besides, for more awareness and adoption, the necessity of learning on robot literature by the elderly people is rightly identified.

While considering the non-tangible aspects of the assistive robots for elderly care, the enhancement of the robots' social skills, adaptability, non-verbal communication, and apt behavior is significant for efficient human-to-robot relationship and coexistence [80]. On the other hand, while considering the tangible aspects, it is found that unlike previously the researchers are now more enthusiastically aiming for developing second or third-generation assistive robots by integrating newer technologies (e.g. ambient-assisted living). Such an integration of separate technologies with assistive robots not only supports developing multipurpose robots to enhance and prolong the independent living capacity of elderly people, but also lowers the cost significantly. Moreover, reviews show that researchers are increasingly focusing on soft robotic technologies instead of rigid robots for enhancing the interaction between humans and robots.

From this study and certain other observations, it has been noticed that in the developed western countries, expectations of older people regarding the appearance of the healthcare robot resembles pet animals and apart from medical support, they mainly seek companionship from their robots. Whereas in the developing Asian countries, the scenario is a bit different; here, the older people would prefer humanoid healthcare robots and like to get help from them in their daily activities.

The appearance of the healthcare robots should not resemble any light plaything, as older people prefer robots with serious aspects and should exhibit personality traits such as curiosity and humor, which is very important for their acceptance. The robot should be pleasing to touch or feel and it should be customizable. Devices that have a "presence" have the scope to provide companionship and improved social abilities as robots can promote positive effect on perceived enjoyment and fulfillment by users. The robot may provide visual stimuli, changing colors or sounds to provide a pleasing background. Also, unpredictability to some extent, i.e. not knowing what the robot is going to do next, is found to be desired by the users.

Some general characteristics, addressed for a healthcare robot by elderly people, which can be a great guideline while designing and producing the devices are as follows:

(i) Should be user friendly
(ii) Should be cost effective
(iii) Should possess more battery capacity
(iv) Should be easy to charge and maintain
(v) Should be capable of improving communication practices
(vi) Should be able to detect any unnatural occurrences, e.g. any fall, heart problems, severe breathing difficulties, etc.
(vii) Should be able to signal for help
(viii) Should be easy to install and repair
(ix) Spare parts should be easily available
(x) Should be networked with certain health service providers, e.g. doctors, nurses, hospitals, ambulances, etc.
(xi) Should be able to remind some regular daily activities, e.g. taking medicines, meals, bath, and exercises on time
(xii) Should be able to perform some regular health check-ups, e.g. measuring body temperature, blood pressure, glucose level, etc.
(xiii) Should be able to accompany older people when outside

Lastly, the authors argue that it will still be a long time before assistive robots are adopted for elderly care even by a large number of people [81], let alone mainstream adoption. However, it is obvious that despite being in the nascent stage of adoption, the researchers are eagerly working with the most advanced technologies to make the intervention of elderly care robots significantly useful and evidently imperative. Moreover, the authors conclude that continuous study and development process are essential for developing the next generation of affordable and effective assistive robots [82]. In this process, as the application of assistive robots for elderly care and its related studies are getting diverse day by day, the authors also suggest for the continuation of periodical scoping review [83] in the future, to identify the available evidence from the new literature, to make awareness of the evidence, and to inform about the knowledge gaps and new knowledge to aggregate newer perception of understanding to facilitate more adoption.

References

[1] UN. (2019). *Ageing*. Retrieved from https://www.un.org/en/sections/issues-depth/ageing/

[2] Parke, K., and Horow, J. M. (2015). Family support in graying societies. Pew Research Centre. https://www.pewresearch.org/wp-content/uploads/sites/3/2015/05/2015-05-21_family-support-relations_FINAL.pdf

[3] Deusdad, B. A., Pace, C., and Anttonen, A. (2016). Facing the challenges in the development of long-term care for older people in Europe in the context of an economic crisis. *Journal of Social Service Research*, *42*(2), 144–150. https://doi.org/10.1080/01488376.2015.1133147

[4] Nowson, C. A., Appleton, J., and Grieger, J. A. (2018). The impact of dietary factors on indices of chronic disease in older people: A systematic review. *The Journal of Nutrition, Health & Aging*, *22*(2), 282–296.

[5] Singh, S., and Bajorek, B. (2014). Defining “elderly” in clinical practice guidelines for pharmacotherapy. *Pharmacy Practice*, *12*(4), 489.

[6] Aubergé, V., Sasa, Y., Bonnefond, N., et al. (2014). The eee corpus: Socio-affective “glue” cues in elderly-robot interactions in a smart home with the emoz platform. In 5th International Workshop on Emotion, Social Signals, Sentiment & Linked Open Data (p. LREC. 2014).

[7] Linner, T., Güttler, J., Bock, T., and Georgoulas, C. (2015). Assistive robotic micro-rooms for independent living. *Automation in Construction*, *51*, 8–22.

[8] Muoio, D. (2015). Japan is running out of people to take care of the elderly, so it’s making robots instead. https://www.businessinsider.com/japan-developing-carebots-for-elderly-care-2015-11?IR=T

[9] Sloan, K. S. (2018). Filling the Care Gap – Foreign-born workers in aged care. Retrieved from https://globalageing.org/filling-the-care-gap-migrant-workers-in-aged-care/

[10] Bvumbwe, T., and Mtshali, N. (2018). Nursing education challenges and solutions in Sub Saharan Africa: An integrative review. *BMC Nursing*, *17*, 3. https://doi.org/10.1186/s12912-01–4

[11] Keehan, S. P., Stone, D. A., Poisal, J. A., *et al.* (2017). National health expenditure projections, 2016–25: Price increases, aging push sector to 20 percent of economy. *Health Affairs*, *36*(3), 553–563.

[12] National Academies of Sciences and Medicine, E., & Population, C. on. (2018). *Future Directions for the Demography of Aging*. Proceedings of a Workshop. National Academies Press.

[13] Uhlenberg, P. (2009). *International handbook of population aging* (*Vol. 1*). Springer Science & Business Media.

[14] Chen, Y., Ngo, V., and Park, S. Y. (2013). Caring for caregivers: Designing for integrality. In Proceedings of the 2013 conference on Computer supported cooperative work (pp. 91–102). ACM.

[15] Ferguson, W. Washington State University. (2019). Smart home tests first elder care robot. https://news.wsu.edu/2019/01/14/smart-home-robot/

[16] Kachouie, R., Sedighadeli, S., Khosla, R., and Chu, M.-T. (2014). Socially assistive robots in elderly care: A mixed-method systematic literature review. *International Journal of Human-Computer Interaction*, *30*(5), 369–393.

[17] Siripala, T. (2018). Japan's robot revolution in senior care. https://www.japantimes.co.jp/opinion/2018/06/09/commentary/japan-commentary/japans-robot-revolution-senior-care/#.XvH9-aa_PIU

[18] Khan, A., and Anwar, Y. (2019). Robots in healthcare: A survey. In Science and Information Conference (pp. 280–292). Springer International Publishing. https://doi.org/10.1007/978-3-030-17798-0

[19] Milner, M., and Rice, S. (2019). Robots are coming to a hospital near you.

[20] Jiang, J., Huang, Z., Huo, B., Zhang, Y., and Song, S. (2018). Research progress and prospect of nursing robot. *Recent Patents on Mechanical Engineering*, *11*(1), 41–57.

[21] Kim, J. (2018). Use of robots as a creative approach in healthcare ICT. *Healthcare Informatics Research*, *24*(3), 155–156.

[22] Tsun, M. T. K., Theng, L. B., Jo, H. S., and Lau, S. L. (2018). Potential of human tracking in assistive technologies for children with cognitive disabilities. In Wearable Technologies: Concepts, Methodologies, Tools, and Applications (pp. 972–993). IGI Global.

[23] Koceska, N., Koceski, S., Zobel, P. B., Trajkovik, V., and Garcia, N. (2019). A telemedicine robot system for assisted and independent living. *Sensors*, *19*, 834.

[24] Cortellessa, G., Fracasso, F., Sorrentino, A., *et al.* (2018). ROBIN, a telepresence robot to support older users monitoring and social inclusion: Development and evaluation. *Telemedicine and E-Health*, *24*(2), 145–154.

[25] Hudson, J., Orviska, M., and Hunady, J. (2017). People's attitudes to robots in caring for the elderly. *International Journal of Social Robotics*, *9*(2), 199–210.

[26] Robinson, H., MacDonald, B., and Broadbent, E. (2014). The role of healthcare robots for older people at home: A review. *International Journal of Social Robotics*, *6*(4), 575–591.

[27] Tan, C. C. L., Cheng, K. K. F., and Wang, W. (2015). Self-care management programme for older adults with diabetes: An integrative literature review. *International Journal of Nursing Practice*, *21*, 115–124.

[28] Do, H. M., Pham, M., Sheng, W., Yang, D., and Liu, M. (2018). RiSH: A robot-integrated smart home for elderly care. *Robotics and Autonomous Systems*, *101*, 74–92.

[29] Hendrich, N., Bistry, H., and Zhang, J. (2015). Architecture and software design for a service robot in an elderly-care scenario. *Engineering*, *1*(1), 27–35

[30] Sumiya, T., Matsubara, Y., Nakano, M., and Sugaya, M. (2015). A mobile robot for fall detection for elderly-care. *Procedia Computer Science*, *60*, 870–880.

[31] Bouakaz, S., Vacher, M., Chaumon, M.-E. B., *et al.* (2014). CIRDO: Smart companion for helping elderly to live at home for longer. *Irbm*, *35*(2), 100–108.

[32] Bodenhagen, L., Suvei, S.-D., Juel, W. K., Brander, E., and Krüger, N. (2019). Robot technology for future welfare: Meeting upcoming societal challenges–an outlook with offset in the development in Scandinavia. *Health and Technology*, *9*(3), 197–218.

[33] Kubota, K., Sekiya, M., and Tsuji, T. (2019). Robot-assisted eccentric contraction training of the tibialis anterior muscle based on position and force sensing. *Sensors*, *19*(6), 1288.

[34] Zhou, B., Wu, K., Lv, P., *et al.* (2018). A new remote health-care system based on moving robot intended for the elderly at home. *Journal of Healthcare Engineering*, 2018, 11 pp. Article ID 4949863. https://doi.org/10.1155/2018/4949863

[35] Pollack, M. E., Brown, L., Colbry, D., *et al.* (2002). Pearl: A mobile robotic assistant for the elderly. In AAAI workshop on automation as eldercare (Vol. 2002, pp. 85–91).

[36] Rodgers, H., Bosomworth, H., Krebs, H. I., *et al.* (2019). Robot assisted training for the upper limb after stroke (RATULS): A multicentre randomised controlled trial. *The Lancet*, 6;394(10192):51–62.

[37] Woo, J., Botzheim, J., and Kubota, N. (2014). Conversation system for natural communication with robot partner. In 2014 10th France-Japan/8th Europe-Asia Congress on Mecatronics (MECATRONICS2014-Tokyo) (pp. 349–354). IEEE.

[38] Perugia, G., Díaz Boladeras, M., Barakova, E., Català Mallofré, A., and Rauterberg, M. (2017). Social hri for people with dementia: one size fits all? In Proceedings of the Companion of the 2017 ACM/IEEE International Conference on Human-Robot Interaction (pp. 257–258). ACM.

[39] Schroeter, C., Mueller, S., Volkhardt, M., *et al.* (2013). Realization and user evaluation of a companion robot for people with mild cognitive impairments. In 2013 IEEE International Conference on Robotics and Automation (pp. 1153–1159). IEEE.

[40] Kittmann, R., Fröhlich, T., Schäfer, J., Reiser, U., Weißhardt, F., and Haug, A. (2015). Let me introduce myself: I am Care-O-bot 4, a gentleman robot. Mensch Und Computer 2015–*proceedings*.

[41] Saczynski, J. S., Pfeifer, L. A., Masaki, K., *et al.* (2006). The effect of social engagement on incident dementia: The Honolulu-Asia Aging Study. *American Journal of Epidemiology*, *163*(5), 433–440.

[42] Cesta, A., Coradeschi, S., Cortellessa, G., Gonzalez, J., Tiberio, L., and Von Rump, S. (2010). Enabling social interaction through embodiment in ExCITE. In ForItAAL: Second Italian Forum on Ambient Assisted Living (pp. 1–7).

[43] Bajones, M., Fischinger, D., Weiss, A., *et al.* (2018). Hobbit: Providing fall detection and prevention for the elderly in the real world. *Journal of Robotics*, 2018, 20 pp. https://doi.org/10.1155/2018/1754657

[44] Szeles, J., Kubota, N., and Woo, J. (2017). Weather forecast support system implemented into robot partner for supporting elderly people using fuzzy logic. In 2017 Joint 17th World Congress of International Fuzzy Systems Association and 9th International Conference on Soft Computing and Intelligent Systems (IFSA-SCIS) (pp. 1–5). IEEE.

[45] Łukasik, S., Tobis, S., Wieczorowska-Tobis, K., and Suwalska, A. (2018). Could robots help older people with age-related nutritional problems? Opinions of potential users. *International Journal of Environmental Research and Public Health*, *15*(11), 2535.

[46] Cavallo, F., Aquilano, M., Bonaccorsi, M., *et al.* (2014). Improving domiciliary robotic services by integrating the ASTRO robot in an AmI infrastructure. In Gearing up and accelerating cross-fertilization between academic and industrial robotics research in Europe: (pp. 267–282). Springer.

[47] Pavón-Pulido, N., López-Riquelme, J. A., Ferruz-Melero, J., Vega-Rodríguez, M. Á., and Barrios-León, A. J. (2014). A service robot for monitoring elderly people in the context of ambient assisted living. *Journal of Ambient Intelligence and Smart Environments*, *6*(6), 595–621.

[48] Al-Shaqi, R., Mourshed, M., and Rezgui, Y. (2016). Progress in ambient assisted systems for independent living by the elderly. *SpringerPlus*, *5*(1), 624.

[49] Lera, F. J., Rodríguez, V., Rodríguez, C., and Matellán, V. (2014). Augmented reality in robotic assistance for the elderly. In International Technology Robotics Applications (pp. 3–11). Springer

[50] Gross, H.-M., Scheidig, A., Debes, K., *et al.* (2017). ROREAS: Robot coach for walking and orientation training in clinical post-stroke rehabilitation—prototype implementation and evaluation in field trials. *Autonomous Robots*, *41*(3), 679–698.

[51] Ansari, Y., Manti, M., Falotico, E., Mollard, Y., Cianchetti, M., and Laschi, C. (2017). Towards the development of a soft manipulator as an assistive robot for personal care of elderly people. *International Journal of Advanced Robotic Systems*, *14*(2), 1729881416687132.

[52] Solis, J., Teshome, T. D., and De la Rosa, J. P. (2015). Towards developing a multipurpose assistive vehicle robot capable of providing assistance to caregivers and support to elderly people. In 2015 IEEE International Conference on Automation Science and Engineering (CASE) (pp. 1145–1150). IEEE.

[53] Görer, B., Salah, A. A., and Akın, H. L. (2017). An autonomous robotic exercise tutor for elderly people. *Autonomous Robots*, *41*(3), 657–678.

[54] Garcia-Sanjuan, F., Jaen, J., and Nacher, V. (2017). Tangibot: A tangible-mediated robot to support cognitive games for ageing people—a usability study. *Pervasive and Mobile Computing*, *34*, 91–105.

[55] Tanigaki, S., Kishida, K., and Fujita, A. (2018). A preliminary study of the effects of a smile-supplement robot on behavioral and psychological

symptoms of elderly people with mild impairment. *Journal of Humanities and Social Sciences*, *45*, 19–26.

[56] Lopez-Samaniego, L., Garcia-Zapirain, B., and Mendez-Zorrilla, A. (2014). Memory and accurate processing brain rehabilitation for the elderly: LEGO robot and iPad case study. *Bio-Medical Materials and Engineering*, *24*(6), 3549–3556.

[57] Louie, W.-Y. G., McColl, D., and Nejat, G. (2014). Acceptance and attitudes toward a human-like socially assistive robot by older adults. *Assistive Technology*, *26*(3), 140–150.

[58] Nomura, T., Kanda, T., Suzuki, T., and Kato, K. (2009). Age differences and images of robots: Social survey in Japan. *Interaction Studies*, *10*(3), 374–391.

[59] Kiesler, S., and Goodrich, M. A. (2018). The science of human-robot Interaction. *ACM Transactions on Human-Robot Interaction (THRI)*, *7*(1), 9.

[60] Rossiter, J., and Hauser, H. (2016). Soft robotics—the next industrial revolution. *IEEE Robot. Autom. Mag. 23*(3), 17–20.

[61] Pino, M., Boulay, M., Jouen, F., and Rigaud, A. S. (2015). "Are we ready for robots that care for us?" Attitudes and opinions of older adults toward socially assistive robots. *Frontiers in Aging Neuroscience*, *7*, 141.

[62] Iancu, I., and Iancu, B. (2017). Elderly in the digital era. Theoretical perspectives on assistive technologies. *Technologies*, *5*(3), 60.

[63] Moon, M. K., and Kim, S.-C. (2017). Usability evaluation of movement support service robot for elderly. In Advances in Ergonomics Modeling, Usability & Special Populations (pp. 517–526). Springer.

[64] Yusif, S., Soar, J., and Hafeez-Baig, A. (2016). Older people, assistive technologies, and the barriers to adoption: A systematic review. *International Journal of Medical Informatics*, *94*, 112–116.

[65] Moro, C. (2018). Learning socially assistive robot behaviors for personalized human-robot interaction. http://hdl.handle.net/1807/82909

[66] Hamada, T., Kagawa, Y., Onari, H., Naganuma, M., Hashimoto, T., and Yoneoka, T. (2016). Study on transition of elderly people's reactions in robot therapy. In *The Eleventh ACM/IEEE International Conference on Human Robot Interaction* (pp. 431–432). IEEE Press.

[67] Torta, E., Werner, F., Johnson, D. O., *et al.* (2014). Evaluation of a small socially-assistive humanoid robot in intelligent homes for the care of the elderly. *Journal of Intelligent & Robotic Systems*, *76*(1), 57–71.

[68] Can, W. S. R., and Seibt, S. D. J. (2016). Social robotics, elderly care, and human dignity: A recognition-theoretical approach. *What Social Robots Can and Should Do: Proceedings of Robophilosophy 2016/TRANSOR* 2016, 290, 155.

[69] Sharkey, A. (2014). Robots and human dignity: A consideration of the effects of robot care on the dignity of older people. *Ethics and Information Technology*, *16*(1), 63–75.

[70] McMurray, J., Strudwick, G., Forchuk, C., *et al.* (2017). The importance of trust in the adoption and use of intelligent assistive technology by older

adults to support aging in place: Scoping review protocol. *JMIR Research Protocols*, *6*(11), e218.

[71] Parviainen, J., and Pirhonen, J. (2017). Vulnerable bodies in human–robot interactions: Embodiment as ethical issue in robot care for the elderly. https://www.researchgate.net/publication/313717892_Vulnerable_Bodies_in_Human-Robot_Interactions_Embodiment_as_Ethical_Issue_in_Robot_Care_for_the_Elderly

[72] Hersh, M. (2015). Overcoming barriers and increasing independence–service robots for elderly and disabled people. *International Journal of Advanced Robotic Systems*, *12*(8), 114.

[73] Tanioka, T. (2019). Nursing and rehabilitative care of the elderly using humanoid robots. *The Journal of Medical Investigation* (*Vol. 66*). https://doi.org/10.2152/jmi.66.19

[74] Coco, K., Kangasniemi, M., and Rantanen, T. (2018). Care personnel's attitudes and fears toward care robots in elderly care: A comparison of data from the care personnel in Finland and Japan. *Journal of Nursing Scholarship*, *50*(6), 634–644.

[75] Körtner, T. (2016). Ethical challenges in the use of social service robots for elderly people. *Zeitschrift Für Gerontologie Und Geriatrie*, *49*(4), 303–307.

[76] Van Wynsberghe, A. (2016). Healthcare robots: Ethics, design and implementation. Routledge.

[77] Pal, D., Triyason, T., and Funikul, S. (2017). Smart homes and quality of life for the elderly: A systematic review. In *2017 IEEE International Symposium on Multimedia (ISM)* (pp. 413–419). IEEE.

[78] Sorell, T., and Draper, H. (2014). Robot carers, ethics, and older people. *Ethics and Information Technology*, *16*(3), 183–195.

[79] Abdi, J., Al-Hindawi, A., Ng, T., and Vizcaychipi, M. P. (2018). Scoping review on the use of socially assistive robot technology in elderly care. *BMJ Open*, *8*(2), e018815.

[80] Bedaf, S., Draper, H., Gelderblom, G.-J., Sorell, T., and de Witte, L. (2016). Can a service robot which supports independent living of older people disobey a command? The views of older people, informal carers and professional caregivers on the acceptability of robots. *International Journal of Social Robotics*, *8*(3), 409–420.

[81] Korchut, A., Szklener, S., Abdelnour, C., *et al.* (2017). Challenges for service robots—requirements of elderly adults with cognitive impairments. *Frontiers in Neurology*, *8*, 228.

[82] Song, W.-K. (2016). Trends in rehabilitation robots and their translational research in National Rehabilitation Center, Korea. *Biomedical Engineering Letters*, *6*(1), 1–9.

[83] Munn, Z., Peters, M. D. J., Stern, C., Tufanaru, C., McArthur, A., and Aromataris, E. (2018). Systematic review or scoping review? Guidance for authors when choosing between a systematic or scoping review approach. *BMC Medical Research Methodology*, *18*(1), 143. https://doi.org/10.1186/s12874-018-0611-x

Chapter 18

The integration of robots and wearables

Mingzhong Wang[1] and Don Kerr[1]

18.1 Introduction

The ageing population has become a global challenge to the society. He, Goodkind, and Kowal [1] forecasted that the percentage of people aged 65 and over will jump from 617 million (8.5% of the world population) to about 1.6 billion (17%) by 2050. The rapid rising proportion of the aged population has a fundamental impact on economy. As the proportion of people in working age shrinks, the labour supply and cost will inevitably rise, resulting in insufficient supply towards the increasing demand of age care.

Ageing population is a more prominent problem in developing countries. Many developing countries will experience faster ageing process than developed countries due to their faster fertility transitions [2], which means they will have abrupt change in the supply and demand of aged care. Moreover, they will become 'older' before being 'rich' [3], which indicates that they will have fewer resources available for caring their aged population. For example, World Health Organization [4] forecasted that the proportion of the population aged 60 and over in China will increase from 12.4% in 2010 to 28% in 2040; and, for every younger couple, there will be four or more older family members who will require daily care and assistance. Moreover, its populations in rural areas will have higher proportions of older people.

To ensure the well-being of the elderly, we are in urgent demand of high-quality but low-cost care services for the ageing population. In addition to traditional health and aged care solutions, innovative assistive technologies become promising to improve the quality of life along with reducing costs [5]. Vichitvanichphong, Talaei-Khoei, and Kerr [6] define assistive technologies as a product, equipment or device, usually electronic or mechanical in nature, which facilitates seniors to maintain their independence or improve their quality of life. They [6] found that smart home and remote care, robots and supportive devices are among the top innovative solutions.

[1]USC Business School, University of the Sunshine Coast, Queensland, Australia

The authors of Refs. [7–9] found that robot-based technologies can enhance well-being of the elderly while decreasing the workload for carers. Moreover, Kachouie *et al.* [7] summarise six categories of benefits after reviewing related work, including improvement in feeling and mood, increase in physical activities, increase in social interactions and activities, decrease in depression, sense of achievement and positive psychological effect.

Broadbent *et al.* [10] discovered that the elderly care more about the functionalities of robots than the appearance, and the top wish list includes fall detection, calling for help, lifting and location reporting. However, most of these requirements constrain that one robot can only serve one user each time. Moreover, switching from one user context to another requires manual reconfiguration by experts or technicians. Consequently, the cost of robot-based aged care will remain high due to its single-user mode.

In comparison with robots, the wearable devices can achieve many tasks, such as fall detection and location reporting, more conveniently at much lower costs. Moreover, as wearable devices are attached to specific users, they can be used as the key to unlock the multi-user mode in robots. Therefore, this chapter proposes the integration of robots and low-cost wearable devices to achieve the following benefits:

- Robots become scalable regarding to its functionalities. Wearable devices can be considered as plugins of robots to extend the capabilities according to the actual needs.
- Robots become accessible and affordable, especially in developing countries, due to much lower cost per capita when multiple users can share the same robot. The integration of wearable devices helps to automate the context switching between multiple users.
- Robots become wireless regarding health and activity monitoring. The data collection is accomplished by wearables, which can be synchronised to the robots remotely.

The chapter is organised as follows. A literature review on the application of robot and wearable technologies for the elderly is provided first. Then, a cost-effective and scalable mHealth platform, which integrate robots and wearables, for the elderly is introduced. Two key measurements, multi-user maturity model and personalised information maturity model, are proposed to guide the integration progress of robots and wearables in the context of aged care.

18.2 Robots for the elderly

Various types of assistive robots have been deployed and studied in the context of aged care. It is generally agreed that robots could improve the quality of life for the elderly with reduced dependency and increased social interactions [11]. For example, Sung *et al.* [12] trialled Paro, a seal-type robot pet, in East Asian culture and confirmed that interacting with companion robots helps to improve the activity participation and communication skills of the elderly. Khosla, Nguyen, and Chu [13] trialled Matilda, a social robot, from 2010 until 2013 with 115 participants in Australian residential aged care facilities and found that there is a statistically significant improvement in emotional, visual and behavioural engagement of older people with social robots over the years.

Bedaf, Gelderblom, and de Witte [14] identified 107 robots for the elderly, which claim to support different types of tasks, including:

- Physical activities of users, including standing, carrying, fetching, dressing, washing, walking and cooking. For example, Paro, ALIAS Robot, Cafero Robot and Carebot.
- Non-physical applications, including agenda and medication reminding, health and environment monitoring, information acquisition, social interaction and entertaining. For example, Mealtime Partner, Walk Assist Robot, Sanyo Bath Robot and Winsford Feeder.
- Non-specified tasks, including housework, self-care, medication and daily chores. For example, Flo Robot, Hector and Jarow.

Vandemeulebroucke, de Casterlé, and Gastmans [15] studied the same topic from an end-user perspective, which focuses on the experience and perceive of the elderly towards the robots. It showed that users commonly use vocal or physical (involving part of their body) approach to interact with the robots. Moreover, users, in general, assign five different roles to robots for their services.

- Servant. Robots are capable of doing servant-like tasks and helping with physically demanding chores, including carrying heavy objects and getting objects on high shelves.
- Safety system. Robots should be capable of detecting fall and sending alerts in case of emergencies. Moreover, they can be virtual doctors or nurses supporting continuous health monitoring.
- Cognitive assistant. Robots should behave as a reminder for events and activities, such as appointments and medications. Moreover, robots can recommend exercise plans to improve the health.
- Entertainer. Robots should support playing radio, music and games on demand. In addition, robots can help with presenting the news and weather forecast.
- Companion. The interaction with robots may help to alleviate the feeling of loneliness or isolation.

Shishehgar, Kerr, and Blake [16] identified nine types of robots in aged care, which are, in the order of usage frequency, (1) companion, (2) telepresence, (3) rehabilitation, (4) manipulator service, (5) reminder, (6) health monitoring, (7) entertainment, (8) domestic and (9) fall detection/prevention robots. They are applied to address eight key categories of tasks in aged care, which are, in the order of research interest, (1) social isolation, (2) dependent living, (3) physical or cognitive impairment, (4) mobility problems, (5) poor health monitoring, (6) lack of recreation, (7) memory problems and (8) fall problems.

Although robots are promising for assisting the elderly, Johnson *et al.* [17] highlighted that just robots are insufficient because they lack the capacity to collect information and interact with the home environment. Therefore, the KSERA (Knowledgeable SErvice Robots for Aging) project was proposed to integrate smart home technology with robots to enhance independent living for the elderly. In its design, the robot becomes the communication interface between the elderly, the smart home and the external world.

Although assistive robots demonstrate great potential to support the elderly, the cost factor has been largely ignored. Almost all designs, trials and research assume:

- either there is a one-on-one setting between the robot and user or the robot does not provide personalised services, and
- the robot is the final product, which has predefined and fixed set of capabilities.

The first assumption suffers from high deployment and usage cost, making robots infeasible to the public and developing countries. We argue that, in aged care facilities or villages, a single robot should be capable of serving multi-users with personalised services. In this way, the average cost per capita can be reduced to an acceptable level, making robots an economic choice.

The second assumption hinders the scalability of robots. As users have different demands of functionalities, it is impossible to create one robot to fit all with affordable cost. Moreover, with new requirements from the users, it would be costly to update or even replace existing robots. Therefore, we argue that, as in PC industry, modularised design should be adopted, which transforms a robot to a hub for plugins/gadgets of various functionalities. Users can customise the components of a robot to meet their needs and update easily in the future by adding or removing the plugins. For example, if the health monitoring, such as heart rate and activity level, is required, a fitness tracker can be worn. Moreover, depending on the accuracy requirement of heart rate measurement, users can choose a tracker at different price range. Therefore, the next section will provide an overview about the usage of wearable devices in the context of supporting the elderly.

18.3 Wearables for the elderly

Wearable devices are enablers for low-cost, continuous and non-invasive monitoring of health and activity of users. Godfrey *et al.* [18] attributed its promising future to its low-cost ability to gather habitual data in a discrete manner for longitudinal periods in any environment.

Wearable sensors or devices appear in various shapes, sizes and capacities, such as bracelet, wristband, watch, necklace, shoes, belt, cloths, gloves, glasses and even implants. In addition to a common usage of activity tracking, wearable devices can monitor a wide range of vital signs [19–21], including:

- Electrocardiogram (ECG), which captures the cardiac electrical cycle to help with the diagnose of cardiovascular diseases.
- Heart rate, which is a simple health indicator of the cardiovascular and psychophysiological status.
- Blood pressure, which is one of the most important cardiopulmonary parameters.
- Oxygen saturation, which measures the fraction of oxygen-saturated haemoglobin in the blood. It is helpful to diagnose hypoxia.
- Blood glucose, which is essential for people with diabetes.
- Skin perspiration, which helps to detect mental stress.

Kekade *et al.* and Alharbi *et al.* [22,23] demonstrated current available wearable devices are reliable and feasible to monitor physical activity and energy expenditure of the elderly. Moreover, the use of wearables in monitoring vital signs would aid in the early detection and prevention of emergencies, particularly in cardiac patients.

Malwade *et al.* [24] argued that one of the major challenges for caring the older population is to provide continuous and personalised care, and wearable technologies are the right tools for this purpose because they support efficient information exchange and communication with care staff on a regular and continuing basis, allowing identification of elderly in need of healthcare assistance. Unfortunately, wearable solutions are underutilised in daily medical care and elderly care [25].

As wearable devices have limited storage, processing and battery capacity due to the size, they commonly utilise a two-tier processing architecture, as shown in Figure 18.1. Most commercial wearable devices are paired with a more powerful intermediate system, such as smart phones or computers, and they behave like data

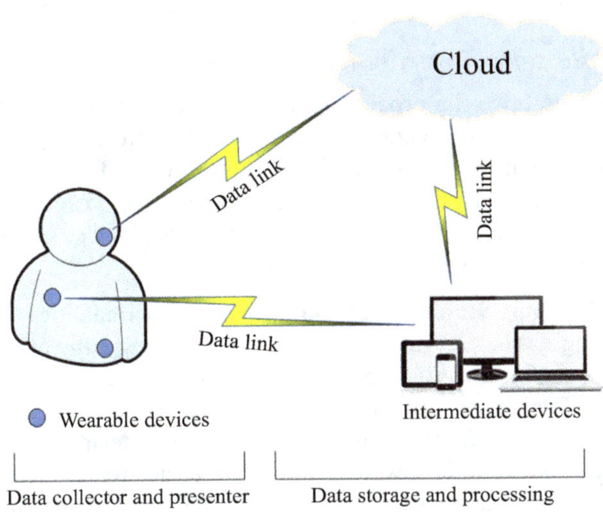

Figure 18.1 Application platform for wearable devices

Table 18.1 Features of wireless protocols in wearable devices [21]

Wireless protocol	Max range	Max data rate	Power consumption
Bluetooth (<v4.0)	100 m	1–3 Mbps	2.5–100 mW
Bluetooth Low-Energy	100 m	1 Mbps	10 mW
NFC	10 cm	400 Kbps	0
Wi-Fi	>150 m	54 Mbps	1 W
ZigBee	100 m	250 Kbps	35 mW

collectors with little local processing and synchronise with the intermediate system. They usually utilise cloud services as the long-term storage or intelligent processing platforms, thus benefiting from the features of scalability, economy and availability in cloud computing [26]. The communication between wearables and intermediate systems is in general wireless based, as summarised in Table 18.1. Bluetooth is a popular choice because of its balanced configurations and wide availability on smartphones and computers.

It is evident that there is frequent overlap between the functionalities of robots and wearable devices, such as fall detection and remote health monitoring. In fact, wearable devices can usually achieve these tasks more accurately and cost-effectively. Therefore, we argue that robots, instead of providing these capabilities directly to users, can find a better fit to act as an open and mobile intermediate station to manage the wearable devices. The next section provides a detailed explanation to this design.

18.4 Cost-effective and scalable mHealth platform for the elderly

18.4.1 Mobile servicing robot with wearable plugins

Following the general two-tier processing architecture in wearable applications, we propose a cost-effective and scalable mobile health platform for the elderly care which employs a mobile robot as the intermediate station (Figure 18.2) to benefit from both robots and wearables. The key idea is to deploy a robot as the mobile hub, which allows connections from various wearable devices of multiple users. The platform has the following features in its design.

- **Customisable and scalable capability**: New functionalities can be added without changing the design of robots. Instead of integrating all functionalities into a robot itself, wearable devices are used as plugins to enable relevant capabilities. Each user can customise the set of wearables he/she needs. Wearables are better at distributed and continuous health and activity monitoring than robots due to lower cost and higher accuracy. Outsourcing these functionalities to wearables, a robot can focus on its strength of mobility and become a primary data processing and integration centre due to its abundant

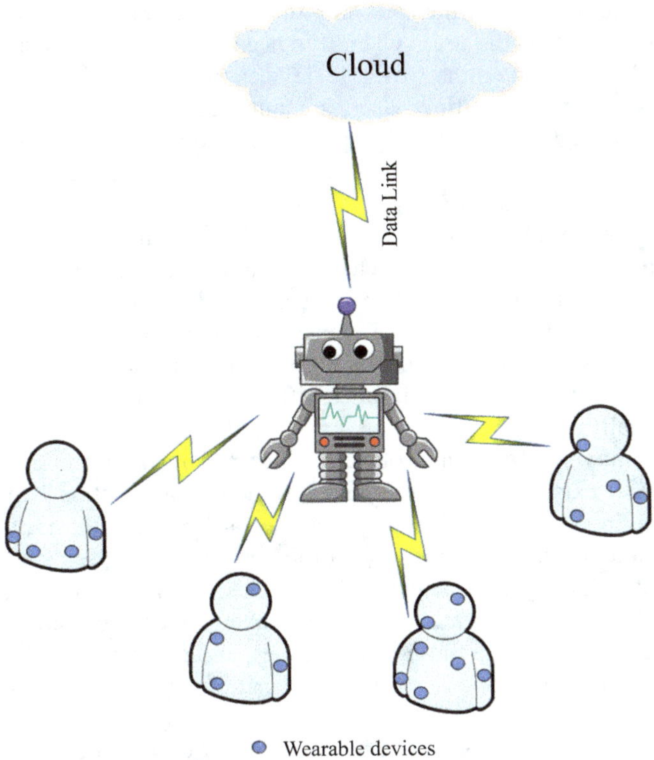

Figure 18.2 Scalable multi-user robot platform with wearable devices

computation, storage, power and communication resources. Moreover, with the hub design, a robot becomes the bridge for data exchange and communication between end-users and cloud centres.

- **High reliability and maintainability**: The system collects accurate data about the users and it is easy to repair or upgrade relevant components. The data accuracy and timeliness are critical in the aged care context. Therefore, multiple wearable devices with redundant capabilities can be deployed to improve the reliability and availability of the health and activity monitoring process. Moreover, the robot, which is an integration hub of wearables, can analyse the data from multiple wearable plugins to detect any malfunction. As these functionalities are provided by external components, they can be easily replaced for repair or upgrade.
- **Mobility**: Robots can patrol around to serve wearables and users. In traditional wearable applications, users need to visit the intermediate devices if they need to synchronise the data or update the configurations of their wearables. However, this setting is not practical or convenient for the elderly people because moving around may not be easy for them. In comparison, with a

mobile robot as the intermediate hub, the hub becomes always on and it can manoeuvre towards the users when it is needed. In addition, a summon function can be installed on the wearable devices to call up the robot.

- **Non-contact authentication**: Users are automatically authenticated to a robot by their wearable devices. To get personalise services, users need to authenticate themselves to the robot first. For the elderly people, traditional methods, such as passwords and fingerprints, are not practical or convenient because they require the robot is next to a user before providing any services. In ideal situation, the robot, which services multiple users, should be capable of authenticating a user even when they are in different places. As wearable devices are attached to individuals, they are sound tools to support automatic and remote authentication and authorisation. For example, with Bluetooth installed, elderly people within up to 100 m can be recognised by the robot automatically.
- **One-to-many support**: One robot provides personalised services to multiple users. Most existing research assumes a one-on-one relation between robots and users in deployment due to the lack of automatic authorisation solution. With wearable-based authorisation, a robot can remotely 'see' and identify all nearby users based on the signals of wearables. At the initial stage, a profile is created for each user with all his/her wearable devices registered. At the run-time, the robot can loop through all profiles, and tailor personalised decisions on when and how to push or pull information for each user and wearable device.
- **Low usage cost per capita**: The average deploy cost per user is affordable to the public, especially in developing countries. Although a single robot may cost hundreds or thousands of dollars, it can be shared by multiple users to lower the average cost per user to a favourable level. In general, the major cost of a robot can be attributed to its mechanical parts, especially for the advanced services, such as lifting and carrying. However, these services, which are generally not urgent, are only occasionally requested by a single user. Therefore, sharing a robot does not degrade its service level. Moreover, with the shift of focus onto integration, the standalone robots become less specialised regarding functionalities and capabilities. Consequently, open standards and off-the-shelf components can be adopted to the design and manufacturing to lower the cost. Finally, in comparison with purchasing a robot with many capabilities unused, our design allows users to customise types and models of wearables to suit their actual needs, leading to less waste of resources.

18.4.2 Architecture

The abstract architecture of the integrated platform for robots and wearables is illustrated in Figure 18.3. To enable the proposed design, five key components should be provided.

- Device manager provides controls on wearable devices, which help to add/remove/update a device, and pull/push the data from/to a device.

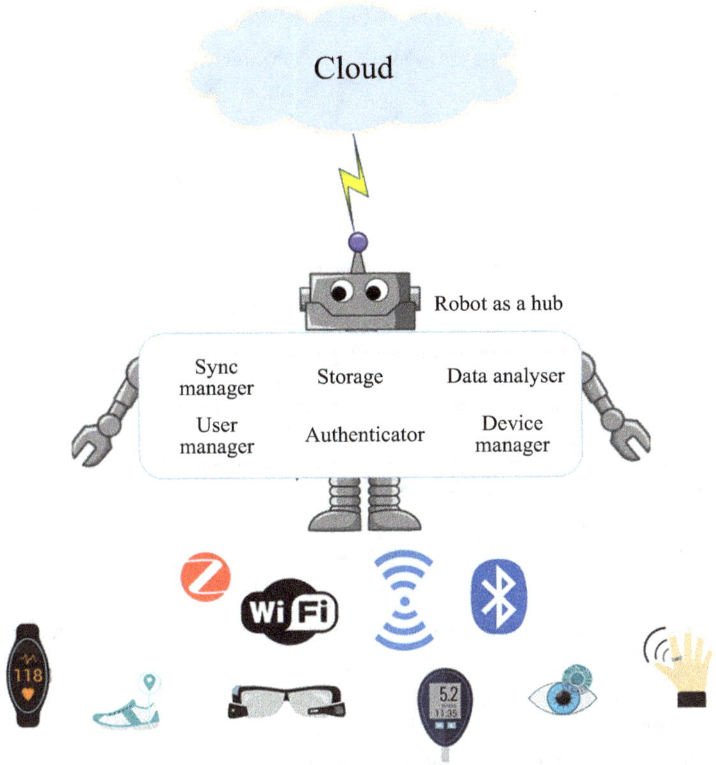

Figure 18.3 Architecture of integrated platform for robots and wearables

- User manager provides the management of users, which can add/remove/update a user, and load/delete/save the profile of each user. A profile is the virtual space for a user, which contains not only the user registration details but also the data collected from his/her wearable devices and analysing results.
- Authenticator is in charge of linking/unlinking each wearable device to/from a specific user, and verify the connection request from wearable devices.
- Storage manager supports the local storage for the records of users, devices, data from the devices and analysis results.
- Data analyser integrates and analyses the data collected from wearables locally.
- Sync manager controls the communication between the robots and back-end clouds.

Storage manager, data analyser and clouds share many overlapped functionalities regarding to data management and processing. The decision on the distribution of data storage and processing workload being either local or cloud depends on many different factors, such as local processing capacity, network availability, speed and latency.

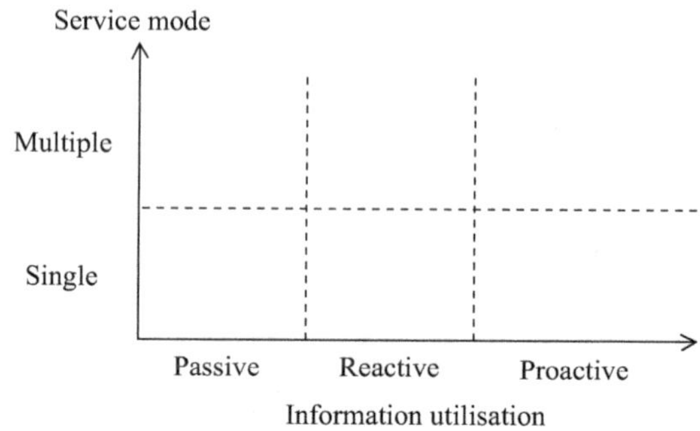

Figure 18.4 Maturity model for robots in aged care

18.4.3 Maturity model for multi-user robots in mHealth

This section discusses potential levels of applying robots for the elderly regarding the information utilisation. Following Godinez *et al.* [27], Figure 18.4 illustrates three levels of information usage, including:

- Passive which relies on analysing the data collected in the past for decision-making. However, the decision is not optimised and even outdated due to the lack of latest information.
- Reactive which relies on analysing the data collected both in the past and runtime for better decision-making. Reactivity is essential in a changing and dynamic environment for sound and appropriate executions.
- Proactive which tries to predict and evaluate future events and their effects based on data collected both in the past and runtime for decision-making. This is the best solution as it may find out the best available solution by evaluating the results of possible solutions to future events.

Most existing research on applying robots onto the aged care falls in the category of single user mode in passive or limited reactive level due to the lack of real-time monitoring mechanisms, or multiple user mode in passive level due to the lack of automatic user authentication. In the solution proposed in this chapter, with the inclusion of wearable devices, which continuously collect health and activity data of users, the use of robots can be promoted to the full reactive level. In addition, with the artificial intelligence support by the backend clouds, it can be further improved to the proactive level to benefit the elderly.

Moreover, with the automatic authentication supported by wearable devices, our solution can achieve, with low cost for individual users, full reactive and proactive usage levels in multiple user mode.

18.4.4 Illustrative user scenarios

In this section, we describe two example user scenarios in a fictitious aged care village in China to illustrate the proposed solution.

18.4.4.1 Personal assistant

The village tenants demand some help with their daily activities, such as reminders for medicine and agendas, guidance on physical training and assistance to video-chatting with other family members. To satisfy the demand, the village needs to hire at least two staff for shifting, which is very costly in the long-term. Another solution is to introduce mobile robots, but one robot per tenant has high purchasing, maintenance and management cost. Therefore, a robot that can be shared becomes a feasible solution.

After consulting with the tenants, the village finds that most tenants are unlikely to use the robot at the same time. Moreover, not almost all requests are urgent, which means it is acceptable for a user to wait for a while until he/she gets serviced. With some analysis, the village decides to have one robot servicing seven tenants, which is the optimal trade-off between the cost and user experience.

The IT team distributes a wrist tracker to each tenant, and then remotely creates a user profile by linking the tracker with a robot. Thereafter, the robot polls through all registered users to provide personalised services to each user.

18.4.4.2 Emergency plans

The government introduces a new policy that all aged care facilities should have plans for life-threatening emergencies. To satisfy this policy and improve the service quality, the village decides to introduce 24/7 monitoring and detection of potential fall and heart attack.

As the robots are modularly designed, the support of new functionalities can be easily and economically achieved by equipping a new wearable device for each resident. In comparison with purchasing specialised devices or hiring new staff, the cost is reduced by at least an order of magnitude.

18.5 Conclusion

Assistive robots and wearable devices are two promising solutions to provide high-quality but low-cost care for the elderly people. However, each technology alone is not appropriate due to either the cost factor or poor usability. Therefore, in this chapter, we propose to transform a robot to a hub, which openly hosts multiple wearable devices as plugins for various specialised health and activity monitoring functionalities.

With the inclusion of wearable devices into a robot, the data collection or monitoring becomes distributed and wireless. Moreover, wearable devices can serve as keys to automatic and remote user authentication as they are personal belongs. Therefore, one-to-many servicing mode between the robot and users can be simply achieved. With this design, the average cost per capita can be dramatically reduced because (1) multiple users share the robot to reduce the usage cost, and (2) robots themselves become standard and open units to reduce the design and build cost. Moreover, information-centric services, such as health and activity monitoring, become more customisable, convenient and reliable due to the distributed and wireless deployment of wearables.

The abstract architecture to implement the proposal is introduced and discussed, which has the key components of user, device, authentication, storage and cloud synchronisation management.

In the future, the collaboration between multiple robots should also be considered. For example, it is a common scenario that a retirement village has several robots deployed, and each has a confined servicing area. The users may move from one corner to another and need to switch the hub robots accordingly. In this case, the mesh network of multiple robots becomes a practical requirement.

References

[1] He W., Goodkind D., and Kowal P. 'An Aging World: 2015'. (U.S. Government Publishing Office, 2016)

[2] Bongaarts J. 'Fertility transitions in developing countries: Progress or stagnation?'. *Studies in family planning*, 2008, **39**, (2), pp. 105–110.

[3] Butler R.N. 'Guest editorial: Report and commentary from Madrid: The United Nations World Assembly on Ageing'. *The Journals of Gerontology Series A: Biological Sciences and Medical Sciences*, 2002, **57**, (12), pp. M770–M771.

[4] World Health Organization. 'China country assessment report on ageing and health'. (World Health Organization, 2015)

[5] World Health Organization. 'World report on ageing and health'. (2015)

[6] Vichitvanichphong S., Talaei-Khoei A., Kerr D., and Ghapanchi A.H. 'Assistive technologies for aged care: Supportive or empowering?'. *Australasian Journal of Information Systems*, 2014, **18**, (3), pp. 75–96.

[7] Kachouie R., Sedighadeli S., Khosla R., and Chu M.-T. 'Socially assistive robots in elderly care: A mixed-method systematic literature review'. *International Journal of Human-Computer Interaction*, 2014, **30**, (5), pp. 369–393.

[8] Robinson H., MacDonald B., and Broadbent E. 'Physiological effects of a companion robot on blood pressure of older people in residential care facility: A pilot study'. *Australasian Journal on Ageing*, 2015, **34**, (1), pp. 27–32.

[9] Broadbent E., Kerse N., Peri K., *et al.* 'Benefits and problems of health-care robots in aged care settings: A comparison trial'. *Australasian Journal on Ageing*, 2016, **35**, (1), pp. 23–29.

[10] Broadbent E., Tamagawa R., Patience A., *et al.* 'Attitudes towards health-care robots in a retirement village'. *Australasian Journal on Ageing*, 2012, **31**, (2), pp. 115–120.

[11] Sharkey A., and Sharkey N. 'Granny and the robots: Ethical issues in robot care for the elderly'. *Ethics and Information Technology*, 2012, **14**, (1), pp. 27–40.

[12] Sung H.-C., Chang S.-M., Chin M.-Y., and Lee W.-L. 'Robot-assisted therapy for improving social interactions and activity participation among institutionalized older adults: A pilot study'. *Asia-Pacific Psychiatry*, 2015, **7**, (1), pp. 1–6.

[13] Khosla R., Nguyen K., and Chu M.-T. 'Human robot engagement and acceptability in residential aged care'. *International Journal of Human–Computer Interaction*, 2017, **33**, (6), pp. 510–522.

[14] Bedaf S., Gelderblom G.J., and de Witte L. 'Overview and categorization of robots supporting independent living of elderly people: What activities do they support and how far have they developed'. *Assistive Technology*, 2015, **27**, (2), pp. 88–100.

[15] Vandemeulebroucke T., de Casterlé B.D., and Gastmans C. 'How do older adults experience and perceive socially assistive robots in aged care: A systematic review of qualitative evidence'. *Aging & Mental Health*, 2018, **22**, (2), pp. 149–167.

[16] Shishehgar M., Kerr D., and Blake J. 'A systematic review of research into how robotic technology can help older people'. *Smart Health*, 2018, **7–8**, pp. 1–18.

[17] Johnson D.O., Cuijpers R.H., Juola J.F., *et al.* 'Socially assistive robots: A comprehensive approach to extending independent living'. *International Journal of Social Robotics*, 2014, **6**, (2), pp. 195–211.

[18] Godfrey A., Hetherington V., Shum H., Bonato P., Lovell N.H., and Stuart S. 'From A to Z: Wearable technology explained'. *Maturitas*, 2018, **113**, pp. 40–47.

[19] Chan M., Estève D., Fourniols J.-Y., Escriba C., and Campo E. 'Smart wearable systems: Current status and future challenges'. *Artificial Intelligence in Medicine*, 2012, **56**, (3), pp. 137–156.

[20] Fontecha J.F., Gónzalez I.G., Villarreal V.V., and Bravo J.B. 'Ambient intelligence for health: Advances in vital signs and gait monitoring systems within mHealth environments'. In 'Human Monitoring, Smart Health and Assisted Living: Techniques and technologies' (Institution of Engineering and Technology, 2017), pp. 183–202

[21] Dias D., and Paulo Silva Cunha J. 'Wearable health devices—Vital sign monitoring, systems and technologies'. *Sensors (Basel)*, 2018, **18**, (8).

[22] Kekade S., Hseieh C.H., Islam M.M., *et al.* 'The usefulness and actual use of wearable devices among the elderly population'. *Computer Methods and Programs in Biomedicine*, 2018, **153**, pp. 137–159.

[23] Alharbi M., Straiton N., Smith S., Neubeck L., and Gallagher R. 'Data management and wearables in older adults: A systematic review'. *Maturitas*, 2019, **124**, pp. 100–110.

[24] Malwade S., Abdul S.S., Uddin M., *et al.* 'Mobile and wearable technologies in healthcare for the ageing population'. *Computer Methods and Programs in Biomedicine*, 2018, **161**, pp. 233–237.

[25] Hentschel M.A., Haaksma M.L., and van de Belt T.H. 'Wearable technology for the elderly: Underutilized solutions'. *European Geriatric Medicine*, 2016, **7**, (5), pp. 399–401.

[26] Wang M., and Kerr D. 'Confidential data storage systems for wearable platforms'. *Managing Security Issues and the Hidden Dangers of Wearable Technologies*, 2017, pp. 74–97.

[27] Godinez M., Hechler E., Koenig K., Lockwood S., Oberhofer M., and Schroeck M. 'The Art of Enterprise Information Architecture: A Systems-Based Approach for Unlocking Business Insight'. (IBM Press, 2010, 1st edn.)

Chapter 19
The usability of smart speakers for seniors

Jacqueline Blake[1]

19.1 Introduction

Smart homes and smart devices are becoming more common with Marikyan et al. [1] describing the transforming of devices into smart devices as a 'wave of transformation'. Smart devices are connected to the Internet and are part of the Internet of things (IoT) paradigm. IoT devices are often wearable such as watches or sensors; however, this study investigates smart speakers. Smart speakers are Internet-enabled speakers containing microphones to pick up instructions for a digital assistant, usually Google assistant, Amazon Alexa or Apple's Siri, giving the device the ability to be voice-controlled. They have become a common, relatively low-cost item for people to add to their home network. The ambient natural language processing given by the digital assistant means the speaker has the capacity to answer questions, play music and provide a low-cost entry to home automation.

Digital assistants are available in other devices such as mobile phones and computers; however, usage of the assistants on smart speakers was shown to be much higher [2]. Abramovich [3] reports that in August 2018 in the United States, 32% of people surveyed already owned a smart speaker; however, in the 65 years and older age group this drops to 23%. The same study showed that people who were comfortable with using digital assistants on a smart speaker were also comfortable using digital assistants on other devices such as their phones. Smart speaker owners also reported using the assistants more often than on other devices, 71% at least once a day. Smart speakers can form part of a smart home infrastructure; however, Shuhaiber and Mashal [4] in their Jordanian study state that a smart home is often seen as a sign of wealth and luxury. This may also be true in many of the belt and road regions, but a single smart speaker can create a smart space or room, with many manufacturers offering small low-cost versions of the speakers.

Digital assistants are available on other devices; however, the ambient, always listening nature of smart speakers may suit individuals who are resistant to using smartphone technology/apps. Berenguer et al. [5] detail how seniors who are users

[1]Business School, University of the Sunshine Coast, Australia

of smartphones tend to restrict the use of the device to the standard applications of making and receiving voice calls and texting. Therefore, while the facilities that a smart speaker offers are available on other devices, seniors tend not to use the functions. In some regions making up the belt and road region such as India, Pakistan, Russia and Romania had low smartphone penetration rates in the age group 55 and older in 2015. Russia had the highest rate of 10.5% while China had 19.8% [5]. These characteristics demonstrate that while it is an attractive proposition to use a smartphone and existing apps to provide services for seniors, other types of interactions and devices should be explored to improve adoption.

19.2 Methodology

In this study, 10 seniors over 65 years old who had Internet available in their homes and a willingness to interact with a smart speaker were recruited. They were each given a Google Home for a 4-week period. The seniors had been participants in previous technology research projects and therefore, in general, had a positive approach to new technology. The smart speakers used were the standard Google Home devices, which were chosen based on their relatively low cost and the wide range of mobile phones incorporating Google Assistant. A researcher went to a participant's home, installed the smart speaker, linked a music service (Google Play Music) and offered some assistance with how to use the smart speaker. The participant was also given a handout giving some instructions for the devices gesture controls and a list of possible commands such as 'OK Google set a timer for 15 minutes' or 'OK Google tell me a fun fact'. They were then asked to use the smart speaker how they wished for 4 weeks.

A pre- and post-questionnaire was administered to the participants by the researcher. The questionnaires were a pen and paper form which could be completed within 10 minutes. Questionnaires contained qualitative questions to assist with gauging initial perceptions and knowledge of the device. How useful the device was for the individual during the user period and the likelihood of them adopting this technology in the future.

Social risks were mitigated by not using any Google accounts the users might already have, instead using university research Google accounts created and used for each Google Home device with corporate telemetry switched off for the duration of the test. Only the active researchers had access to these Google accounts. Query information was collected by accessing on https://myactivity.google.com and selecting Assistant from the filters. All information gathered was aggregated into groups within a document to preserve privacy for the user and to allow for aggregation of the collected data. The query information includes the audio of unsuccessful requests. The recording was used to discern what underlying issue caused a failed query. Any private information recorded by the device was generalised and aggregated. Users were notified and shown how the information was collected prior to the installation with any questions answered during installation.

19.3 Results

19.3.1 Pre-questionnaire

Table 19.1 shows that six participants had either heard of IoT devices or had researched IoT devices on the Internet before starting the study. Eight participants had heard of smart speakers and Google Home either through friends and family or through the Internet research on IoT devices. Only two participants had already had experience with smart speakers through their family. When asked about what they thought their experience would be using the Google Home, three participants replied with statements that they wanted to gain knowledge about new technology, test how the technology works and share that knowledge with others. Another three participants wanted to use and explore the limits of a new device, two more wanted to be able to use voice requests. One person had no preconceived idea. When asked how easy they expected the Google Home to be to use, six people thought that they would find the device easy to use, one person moderate difficult, one person moderate and two who thought it would be difficult. All participants access the Internet through tablets, mobile phones and a laptop/desktop computer. Eight participants were unconcerned about the always listening nature of smart speakers and two who indicated some concern.

19.3.2 Post-questionnaire

At the end of trial, the participants were asked questions about their experience. The first question was how was their experience with the Google Home? All participants considered that their experience was positive. There was an obvious learning curve when first using the Google Home but all persevered with using the device and learned how to ask a Google assistant understandable query. Comments collected are shown in Table 19.2.

When asked if they found the Google Home easy to use, every participant answered yes; however, six people added that learning to phrase the question in the required format took some trial and error. Nine participants from the ten replied that they would consider buying a Google Home or hoped to be gifted a device. All participants stated that they would recommend the Google Home to friends and family; however, this was tempered for two participants as they thought their friends would not be interested. For the question, what they liked least about the Google Home, five people made statements about Google Home failed to understand their query. Two people had trouble with connections to music or radio stations; however, both participants still said they were happy with their experience. While the participants gave a range of answers for what they liked most. Five participants mentioned quick or correct response to questions, four people mentioned the availability of music and news, and one person also mentioned the quality of the sound. Three people commented that they enjoyed not having to use a keyboard and two participants stated they liked something to talk to or a voice in the background. The comments in Tables 19.2 and 19.3 show that listening to music is the most popular smart speaker activity.

Table 19.1 Pre-questionnaire

Question	No. of no responses	No. of yes responses	Comments
Have you heard anything about the Internet of things (IoT) before?	4	6	• Home gadgets connected to the Internet can be controlled by a (a) smartphone; (b) computer; (c) Google Home and (d) hackers (!!) – no idea how to make them secure: 'Big Brother is Watching'!! • Everything that is connected to the Internet, for example, Google Home • Through the Computer Club • Siri (speaker technology) and through the Computer Club
Have you heard of Smart Speakers before?	2	8	• Done some research • Through my son • I've done some research • My son-in-law has one • Ditto (PLUS my son who has a Google Mini) • Through a friend who's got it (a niece who is an excellent cook – she uses it a lot of recipes) • Through the Computer Club
Have you heard of the Google Home before?	2	8	• I'd heard about it and looked it up on the Internet. • The Computer Club and my son • Through my research.
Have you had any experiences with a similar device before? If so what were those experiences?	8	2	• Through my son. Many advantages but maybe time-wasting? Because you end up playing with it all day!
What do you think you will experience in this study?			• Wanted to gain knowledge about new technology, test how the technology works and share that knowledge with others • Knowledge – to know more about it. Social meetings at the Clubhouse – I could demonstrate the GH and bring subjects to talk about • Learning about a new device so I can help people at the Club

(Continues)

Table 19.1 (*Continued*)

Question	No. of no responses	No. of yes responses	Comments
			• I like experimenting with new things; broadening my knowledge of the new world and embracing new technology • Use and explore the limits of a new device • I like experimenting with new things; broadening my knowledge of the new world and embracing new technology • Wanted to use voice control for requests • To ask questions instead of having to type into my computer • To communicate on our behalf – to express our needs/instructions verbally instead of typing on a keyboard • Confusion • Confusion! I would like to be able to turn on the lights (remotely) • I don't know • I don't know – no idea really
How easy do you think the Google Home will be to use?	4	6	• Easy: • No problem • Not too hard, I'd expect • Fairly easy/shouldn't be too hard • I think it will be easy because I only have to talk to it • Quite easy, we'd expect • I don't think it will be difficult • More difficult • I don't think it will be easy • Frustrating – when she doesn't answer me • Not easy to easy – let's say moderate
What kind of technology do you currently have to access the Internet?			• iPad, tablet, laptop and smartphone • Tablet × 2, laptop, desktop and smartphone × 2

(Continues)

Table 19.1 (Continued)

Question	No. of no responses	No. of yes responses	Comments
			• Tablet, smartphone, desktop, smart TV (YouTube, iView, SBS on Demand) • PC, Apple iPhone, tablet plus (indirectly) an Internet-enabled TV + security system • PC, laptop, android tablet, iPad, smartphone and iPhone • iPad, laptop and desktop • iPad, iPhone and PC (I have Siri on my phone) • Smartphone, Smart TV, laptop × 2, desktop × 2 and tablet × 2 • Laptops × 3, smartphone and tablet • Android tablet, smartphone, desktop and laptops × 2
How do you feel about speaking into a room and having a computer answer your questions for you?			• Doesn't worry me. I talk to the cat! • Google does this for you anyway – I'm not afraid of this technology • Doesn't worry me but more concerned about what I will do (I expect to feel frustrated) • Not an issue for me • Elma: If it was spouting all the time, I'd tell it to 'shut up'! Peter: doesn't bother me • I think I'd feel strange! • Terrifying (at least to begin with). I think it would take you out of your comfort zone! • Doesn't worry me! • No problem with that! • Maybe a bit awkward, off-putting. But I am enthusiastic about trying new technology

Table 19.2 Post-questionnaire

Question	No. of no responses	No. of yes responses	Comments
How was your experience with the Google Home?		10 Positive responses	• Fine – I talked to it every day that I was home . . . If I had a problem, I got it sorted and once I got Google Assistant on my phone I could do more • GH would always respond to me – great potential for using more senses and connections (e.g. smart lights). I would like to have it synch with my contacts and my diary – and maybe have U3A run a course on this • Thought it was just a gadget to start with, then found it good and convenient • Useful particularly with playing music. It frees up the need to go to the keyboard and type something. Very positive overall! • Positive. We probably didn't make such a lot of use out of it because of our lifestyle. We see it being good for people who have a lot of 'smart devices' in their home • I kept trying to persevere, asking for recipes and for it to play music but I really started to appreciate it when my son visited, and he asked it lots of different questions • I enjoyed the quality of the music sound but had some difficulties giving her the right terminology. Overall, when asking other questions, I find that googling directions from the iPad achieves more details results • Surprisingly good – far better than I expected! • It was quite pleasant for the most part. She understood most of my questions
	1	9	• Solved my own problems • Needed some improvements

(Continues)

Table 19.2 (Continued)

Question	No. of no responses	No. of yes responses	Comments
Did you find the Google Home easy to use?			• Not proficient yet but had adequate skills to get through • Once you understood the limitations and how she worked • Yes. Although GH didn't always understand us – maybe the Aussie vernacular? • I wasn't comfortable with it. I felt I always had to walk over close to speak to it • Not really – it took a little while to learn how to phrase questions to get the best answers
Would you consider buying a Google Home or similar device in the future?	03 – Maybe	7	• Yes – definitely! I have already been looking online at prices plus Amazon Alexa • Yes – He may get one for Christmas • Yes – definitely! • Yes – At the beginning, I would have said 'probably not' but after using it for a while, I would now say 'definitely YES'! • Maybe – very doubtful but we enjoyed the experience
Would you recommend the Google Home to friends and family?	0	10	• She talks to everyone! And people everywhere are interested • We recognise that GH has generation-specific benefits – for the younger generation: using it for 'fun things' (our grandkids) – and if it could be taught to the older generation, it would be more beneficial – our generation really doesn't know about this sort of technology • Could imagine that people who would appreciate how voice control makes it easier • Why? Because it's nice to have but not essential. It's a simpler way to do things, for example Play ABC News

(Continues)

Table 19.2 (*Continued*)

Question	No. of no responses	No. of yes responses	Comments
			• I would but I really can't think of any of my friends as a lot of them aren't into technology that much • Yes to family definitely. Our friends (old people) probably wouldn't appreciate the technology
What did you like most of the Google Home?			• The instantaneousness of it • You can ask questions and get answers. You didn't need to go to your smartphone or computer • Music, news in the morning, thinks it would be perfect for elderly and give them something to talk to • To request music and not have to go to a keyboard. And the quality of the sound was good • The music • The convenience • The fact that you could ask her any question . . . . .The response time is what impressed me • The fact that you can use it for so many different things. Music is fine and she has played everything I've asked • The fact that at any time, I can be doing work around the place and she provides a bit of a background
Was there anything that you did not like about the Google Home? (if so, what?)			• Yes – it's nor fully functional yet. I learnt to use it within its limitations. For example, I learn to rephrase, not be too long-winded. I learnt you've got to speak clear and use shorter sentences • You had to be careful of your words – how you say them and spell it out to her. And I thought it didn't give me all the things that I knew it could! It would be good if you could customise your requests • Yes – when GH didn't understand instruction

(*Continues*)

Table 19.2 (*Continued*)

Question	No. of no responses	No. of yes responses	Comments
			• Not knowing its limitations and having to rephrase requests until she understood • I found it a little difficult adjusting volumes using my hand. But I could use my voice, for example '70% level' • Overall, nothing specific that we did not like – very positive overall
What functionality do you think was most useful to you?			• Number 1: Drive time; Number 2: telephone numbers – not so much used for a request for knowledge or facts; Number 3: instant day-to-day stuff especially reminders (I used it a lot for reminders) • We used it a lot for music, weather, Google maps – and for languages (German) and translation, plus alarms (for cooking recipes) • Music playing • Mainly used for music (e.g. 'soft jazz' in the mornings) and the news, plus distances between one location and another and what are the times to travel between them • I was amazed at some of the things it knew and that it could interpret some of the names I gave it, for example, Queensland place names • The music • Radio and music • Music – the quality of the sound is better than I thought it would be. I have played a lot of music and the radio. Plus, setting reminders and alarms • At night-time, I would disconnect her and move her to my bedroom – so I liked the fact that she was so portable. Plus, the music. Plus, the immediacy of information that you may want

Table 19.3 Reported frequency of functions used the most in Google Home

Functions used the most	Frequency
Play music	7
Setting alarms	3
Drive time/distance between places	2
Listening to news	2
Asking general knowledge questions	2
Listening to the radio	2
Asking questions for entertainment	2
Portability	1
Language translation	1
Google maps	1
Weather	1
Business phone numbers	1

Recorded requests illustrate the problem with beginning users using natural language to request information from the Google Home such as 'OK Google talk to me' or to having a long pause after 'OK Google'. However, as can be seen in Table 19.4, the rate of unsuccessful queries does decrease as the participants use the Google Home. Table 19.4 also shows that eight of the ten participants' usage decreased over the 4 weeks.

However, still most participants had multiple interactions per day. Some participants discussed friends and family enjoying playing with and asking queries of the smart speaker which may have skewed the number of interactions. One of the benefits for the participants seemed to be having something new to demonstrate to their visitors, shown in the comment 'Everyone, of my friends and family have visited and used my GH. The children (grand-children) used her for a Trivia Quiz'.

19.4 Discussion

The participants in this study all reported enjoying the experience of trialling Google Home and all planned to either purchase a Google Home or hoped to be given one. All the participants were comfortable with technology and used a range of devices (laptop/desktop, tablet and mobile phone). Although the Google Home removes the need to interact with the device using a keyboard request, queries still needed to be made using a set syntax. Familiarity and comfort interacting with their other devices may have increased the participants' willingness to adopt the new technology of a smart speaker [3].

The results from this study have shown that the seniors (over 65 years old) in this study did engage with and enjoy using a smart speaker with the most common use was listening to music. Can the familiarity with the smart speaker built up through the request for music be leveraged into using the digital assistant for practical outcomes of a smart home such as operating lights, setting medication timers and making calls using a voice command? Making or answering calls using

Table 19.4 Frequency of successful/unsuccessful queries by participant

	Query	Week 1	Week 2	Week 3	Week 4
One	Successful	75	0	0	3
	Unsuccessful	35	0	0	2
	Total	110	0	0	5
Two	Successful	94	17	18	45
	Unsuccessful	61	12	10	34
	Total	155	29	28	79
Three	Successful	58	42	21	11
	Unsuccessful	18	10	4	4
	Total	76	52	25	15
Four	Successful	55	8	18	Away
	Unsuccessful	24	5	11	
	Total	79	13	29	
Five	Successful	39	85	98	118
	Unsuccessful	20	11	15	23
	Total	59	96	113	141
Six	Successful	49	19	61	122
	Unsuccessful	12	2	20	9
	Total	61	21	81	131
Seven	Successful	79	39	29	17
	Unsuccessful	46	19	8	10
	Total	125	58	37	27
Eight	Successful	85	55	35	42
	Unsuccessful	41	20	15	16
	Total	126	75	50	58
Nine	Successful	177	102	150	39
	Unsuccessful	51	16	34	11
	Total	228	118	184	50
Ten	Successful	207	57	94	96
	Unsuccessful	42	8	16	16
	Total	249	65	110	112

voice command is useful for those people who might miss calls because they have limited or no movement or have difficulty hearing phone calls due to hearing aid function. Currently, Google restricts making hands free calls using Google Home in the United States, Canada and United Kingdom. However, we can assume that availability of this feature will spread globally soon. A smart speaker can be considered like a smartphone to be a general-purpose technology, with the capabilities of the smart speaker tailored using Google Actions or in the Echo's case Amazon Alexa Skills. One consideration when choosing a smart speaker might be that the purchase locks you into a digital assistant for interoperability with other smart home devices.

As of January 2019, only 4.26% of available Actions on Google Home fall into the health and fitness category, 4.03% social and communication with a further 6.91% in the home control category [6]. Therefore, there is unlikely to be a suitable package for users in the belt and road region focused on seniors needs for health and communication. However, it is possible for packages of Google Home Actions to be constructed tailored around the needs of the population of the regions along the belt and road trail. The Google Home actions can be generated using a provided workflow and do not require a high level of technical ability. The 'Activities' packages could be made up from components to individualise the smart home speaker capabilities for instance, for those people with mobility problems the ability to turn a light off and on, change a station on a radio or television or call for help. Again, while these activities could be recreated using a smartphone as Berenguer et al.'s [5] research showed adoption of activities beyond calling and texting are unlikely to be adopted by seniors.

Tran et al. [7] detail some of the issue in installing a multi-resident sensor system in smart homes such as having to use wearable sensors or identification of users using visual images. Lower cost versions of the smart speakers such as the Amazon Echo Dot and Google Home mini have become available decreasing the financial barrier to ownership. These speakers have the potential to be deployed in developing countries as low-cost voice-activated sensors and communication devices. For instance, in telemedicine, smart speakers could be used to communicate the well-being of a patient by voice responses to questions without the patient being required to physically manipulate a device. If a space is Internet-enabled, the simple installation of plugging in and connecting to a Wi-Fi network would enable the ad hoc installation of a support system that could be removed when no longer required. For example, if an aged person was recovering from a fall and required some monitoring, a smart speaker could be installed and the patients contacted multiple times a day with well-being and medication reminders, the system could then be removed and deployed elsewhere on recovery. Robinson et al. [8] ran a study investigating smart speaker use in public places testing the applicability of natural language interaction with computers in resource-constrained regions. One of the aims of this research was to expose people to and promote spoken language-driven technology. The research did show that the devices were more inclined to be used in public spaces by younger people.

19.5 Implications for the Belt-and-Road region

A smart speaker can be viewed as a luxury item in a connected lifestyle; however, there is also potential that a smart speaker could be used as a portable relatively low-cost medium for transmitting and receiving audio information. This audio information might be used for purposes such as telehealth, keeping in touch with friends and family and to facilitate an independent lifestyle. A smart speaker can form part of a short-term support solution for a person, as it is a lightweight piece of equipment which might be moved from room to room, automatically reconnecting as required. Interaction with the smart speaker is by voice negating any need to have computer knowledge. The vocal interactions can be very structured which means that a person can be given a small set of easily learned instructions which are not context-dependent unlike a lot of computer instructions.

Lelkes [9] asks the question if Internet-assisted contact in seniors will ask as a substitute for in-person contact? The belt and road region on the whole is one that emphasizes strong family connections and collectivism [10]. Hui and Triandis [11] viewed collectivism as having seven characteristics: consideration of ones actions on the wider society, sharing of material resources, sharing of nonmaterial resources, conforming to social group mores, a focus on gaining social group approval, sharing of outcomes and a feeling of involvement in the lives of other members of the social group. However, in this region, China has in recent decades has increasing rural-urban migration and aging [12], with an increasing median age [13]. Some of the seniors follow the family into urban areas to help with childcare and maintain the family unit. Bianji [14] writes how away from their old home with different dialects and customs the seniors feel cut-off and invisible with high levels of mental health issues such as depression. Lelkes [9] research showed a relationship between Internet use and well-being, the smart speaker provides a computer-person interaction mode that removes the need for keyboard skills and provides a conversational means of instruction.

19.6 Conclusion

This research demonstrated that seniors found the smart speaker as a standalone device usable and were interested in extending how they were using the device. The next stage of this research would be if the seniors would be prepared to use the smart speakers as a controller for home automation such as smart lighting systems and as a voice-activated communication device to send and receive voice calls and text messages. This research had the limitation of a small group of users who had an interest in new technology and in most cases were proficient users. The use of smart speakers by seniors in the belt and road region will depend on the development of smart speaker skills or activities that provide a compelling reason for learning how to interact with the device. Another limitation is the availability of Internet connectivity and the cost of that connection for the user. However, a smart speaker does provide another way of interacting with seniors beyond a smartphone or tablet for functions such as telehealth or to reduce feelings of social isolation.

References

[1] Marikyan D., Papagiannidis S., and Alamanos E. 'A systematic review of the smart home literature: A user perspective'. *Technological Forecasting and Social Change*. 2019;138:139–154.

[2] Kinsella B. Smart speaker owners use voice assistants nearly three times a day. 2018. Available from https://voicebot.ai/2018/04/02/smart-speaker-owners-use-voice-assistants-nearly-3-times-per-day/ [Accessed 12 Mar 2019].

[3] Abramovich G. Study finds consumers are embracing voice services. Here's how. 2018. Available from https://www.cmo.com/features/articles/2018/9/7/adobe-2018-consumer-voice-survey.html#gs.7u1812. [Accessed 28 Apr 2019].

[4] Shuhaiber A., and Mashal I. 'Understanding users' acceptance of smart homes'. Technology in Society, 2019;58:101110. Available from https://www.sciencedirect.com/science/article/abs/pii/S0160791X18300484.

[5] Berenguer A., Goncalves J., Hosio S., Ferreira D., Anagnostopoulos T., and Kostakos V. 'Are smartphones ubiquitous?: An in-depth survey of smartphone adoption by seniors'. *IEEE Consumer Electronics Magazine*. 2016;6(1):104–110. Available from https://www.researchgate.net/publication/311740678_Are_Smartphones_Ubiquitous_An_in-depth_survey_of_smartphone_adoption_ by_seniors

[6] Sterling G. Google Actions vs. Alexa Skills is the next big App Store battle. 2019. Available from https://searchengineland.com/google-actions-vs-alexa-skills-is-the-next-big-app-store-battle-312497 [Accessed 29 Jun 2019].

[7] Tran S., Zhang Q., Smallbon V., and Karunanithi M. Multi-resident activity monitoring in smart homes: A case study. 2017. Available from https://searchengineland.com/google-actions-vs-alexa-skills-is-the-next-big-app-store-battle-312497

[8] Robinson S., Pearson J, Ahire S, *et al*. 'Revisiting "hole in the wall"; Computing: private smart speakers and public slum settings'. *Proceedings of the 2018 CHI Conference on Human Factors in Computing Systems*; Montreal QC, Canada. 3174072: ACM; 2018. pp. 1–11.

[9] Lelkes O. 'Happier and less isolated: internet use in old age'. *The Journal of Poverty and Social Justice*. 2013;21(1):33–46.

[10] Yang F., Zhang J., and Wang J. 'Correlates of loneliness in older adults in Shanghai, China: Does age matter?'. *BMC Geriatrics*. 2018;18(1);300–300.

[11] Hui C. H., and Triandis H. C. 'Individualism-collectivism: A study of cross-cultural researchers'. *Journal of Cross-Cultural Psychology*. 1986;17(2):225–248.

[12] World Population Review. 'China population 2019'. 2019.

[13] Han S. 'Median age of the population in China from 1950 to 2100 (in years)'. 2019.

[14] Bianji L. J. 'Migrating elderly people feel invisible in China's cities'. People's Daily Online, 2018.

Section V

mHealth for chronic illnesses

Chapter 20

The status of healthcare service delivery systems: comparison, mobile health, and healthcare service design

Saradhi Motamarri[1], Shahriar Akter[1] and Pradeep K. Ray[2,3]

20.1 Introduction

Services industry, including healthcare services are transforming with the new powerful, anytime and anywhere accessible delivery channels: Internet and wireless mobile communications. These are a direct consequence of advances in information and communications technologies (ICT). The Internet had played a dominant role in the resource-rich countries resulting in the *digital divide* between developed and developing nations. However, this situation is drastically altering due to the exponential growth of mobile wireless communications in developing nations [1]. It is a startling fact that populations of these nations have in possession of mobile devices, while they still struggle for access to basic healthcare, as is apparent from the selected healthcare system indicators shown in Table 20.1 [2,3].

Along with the advances in Internet technologies, there is a corresponding impetus in various industries to leverage the Internet as an additional or in some instances as the sole delivery channel to offer products/services which have led to the emergence of *electronic commerce*. Healthcare is still in the catching-up race with the other sectors even in the developed world in transforming itself to leverage the flexible and accessible Internet and wireless communications channels [4,5]. Interestingly the widespread adoption of mobile phones in the developing world is offering a viable, cost-effective and ubiquitous channel to deliver healthcare services. The authors believe that progressively mobile technologies will play a vital complementary role in not only raising the bar of healthcare in these counties but may also help in achieving the millennium development goals set by the World Health Organisation (WHO) [2,6–8]. In order to achieve this goal, mobile

[1]School of Management, Operations and Marketing, University of Wollongong
[2]School of Public Health and Community Medicine, University of New South Wales Sydney, Australia
[3]Centre for Entrepreneurship, University of Michigan-Shanghai Jiao Tong University Joint Institute, China

Table 20.1 Sample health system indictors for selected countries. Adapted from [2]

Country	Births attended by skilled health personnel (%)	Hospital beds per 10,000 population	Total health workers per 10,000 population
Bangladesh	20 (2006)	3 (2001)	5 (2001)
India	47 (2006)	9 (2003)	14 (2003)
Mexico	83 (2005)	11 (2002)	28 (2001)
Pakistan	54 (2006)	12 (2005)	12 (2003)
Russia	100 (2006)	97 (2006)	128 (2003)
United Kingdom	99 (1998)	39 (2004)	75 (2001)
United States	100 (2004)	32 (2005)	125 (1999)

healthcare services (mHealth) need to adopt a rational approach across the services life cycle in fulfilling the market opportunity.

Services marketing literature is abound with discussion on *service quality*, its characteristics and measurement [9,10]. There have been efforts to characterise the perceived service quality of mHealth services [11,12]. Service quality is an antecedent to service delivery, design and opportunity. While marketing literature is abound on product life cycle [13], there has been little focus on the services life cycle [14,15]. It is possible that services term has been used extensively by marketing, operations and computer science with different connotations [16]. Given this opportunity to fill a research gap on both services life cycle and antecedents to healthcare service quality, the authors propose a services life cycle model and then proceed with a discussion on utilising this model to understand the phases of services life cycle and how it can be applied in the design of healthcare services.

The healthcare imperatives of the developing nations, the potential of mHealth as a powerful delivery alternative, the factors that influence and position mHealth services on par with incumbent services, prompted us to investigate healthcare service design with specific reference to mHealth. The ensuing sections will detail the lessons learnt from the extant literature and chart an approach for mHealth service design. The chapter concludes with specific research questions to address in future research endeavours in order to achieve robust mHealth services offering that would benefit the developing nations.

20.2 Services life cycle

An unfulfilled need is a trigger point for the emergence of a new service opportunity in the marketplace. The need of a buyer becomes an opportunity for a service provider. The requirements of the need may not be concrete whereby

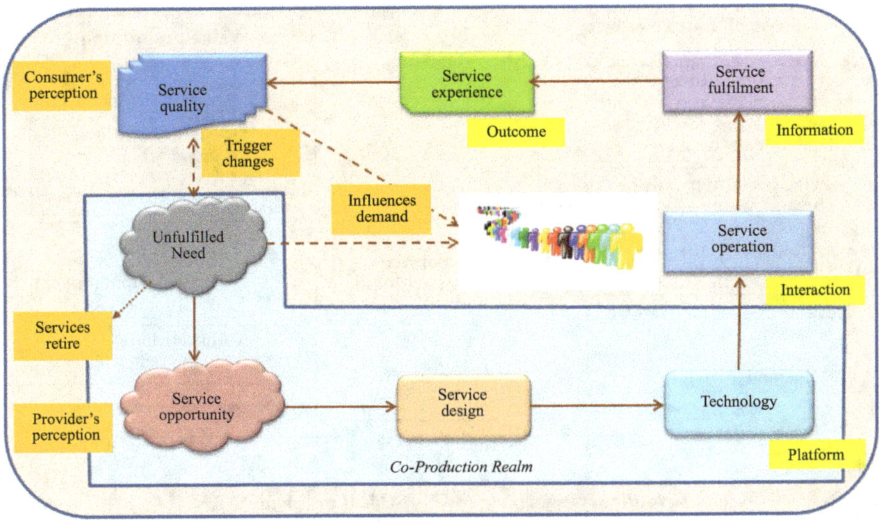

Figure 20.1 Services life cycle. Adapted from [60]

service providers perceive it depending on their core strengths and structure their assets in transforming the opportunity into a service offering. Technology plays a vital role in designing the service or it can also mean that for the same opportunity different technologies give rise to as service alternatives. The next stage to design is operation where the buyer interacts with the provider. This leads to the fulfilment of the need for the buyer and generates an experience with the service vis-à-vis his original need. One can imagine the service quality in the perception of the buyer as the extent to which the experience matches to his original need. This is one of the reasons that service quality may be perceived differently by different people. Figure 20.1 is a portrayal of these phases as services life cycle. Thus, the important antecedents to service quality are *service operation* and *service design*.

With respect to healthcare services, a doctor uses his/her clinic as the technology to deliver a face-to-face consultation to a patient, which has been in existence for a long time. In this instance, the doctor uses mobile wireless communications as the technology and this leads to mHealth as an alternative for the face-to-face consultation service. mHealth has to provide a better overall value to the patients so that they can switch to this alternative over the incumbent services in a healthcare market. Keaveney's Customer Switching Model [17] proposes the factors that may induce consumers to switch from one service provider to another. As shown in Figure 20.2, the model underscores on factors: service quality, interaction, handling of feedback, price, inconvenience and other behavioural factors. Healthcare service providers can utilise these insights during their services strategy, design and operation phases in order to successfully deliver as well as sustain their services offering.

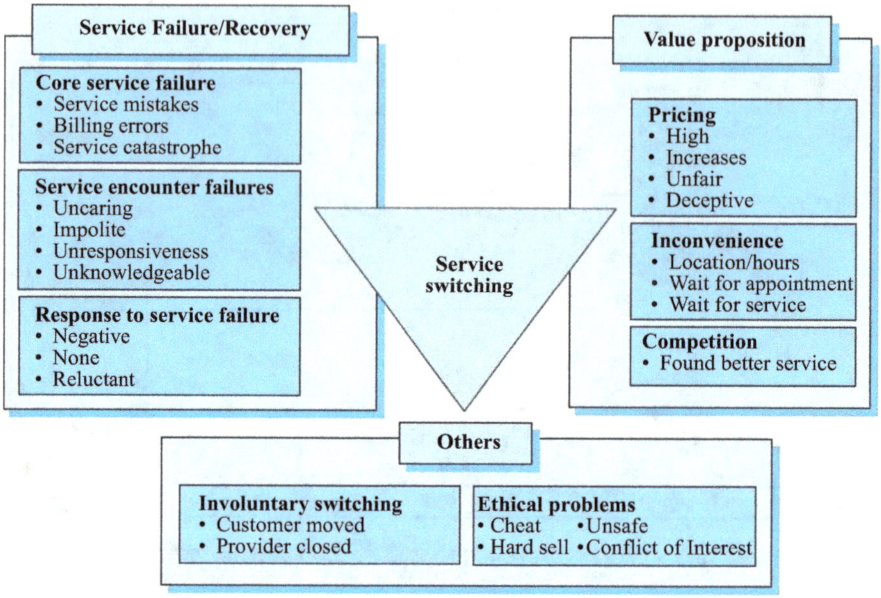

Figure 20.2 Customer service switching behaviour model. Adapted from [17]

20.3 Methods

The primary objective of this research is to understand the requirements of healthcare services design. However, the search in various sources like PubMed, Google Scholar and SciVerse databases has not yielded any specific study that was devoted to healthcare services design itself keeping aside mHealth. Table 20.2 presents the results of some of these search terms. A reconnaissance of the results has not pointed to any artefacts that focused on the design of healthcare services. Considering the complexity and inter-disciplinary nature of this endeavour, the research calls for assimilation of knowledge from several disciplines as shown in Figure 20.3.

An assimilation of inter-related areas connected to mHealth like, ICT, IT infrastructure library (ITIL), quality of service and house of quality (HoQ) yielded interesting insights on healthcare services in developing countries. These insights have significant impact and benefit healthcare service providers, governments and public, and is highlighted alongside the discussion on healthcare services design framework.

20.4 Healthcare services scenario

20.4.1 Patients' evaluation of general practice

Service delivery is challenging. Services marketing and management pose special challenges because services deal with 'processes rather than things, with

Table 20.2 Literature search for healthcare service design artefacts

No	Search terms	PubMed	Googlescholar
1	Healthcare health care service	400,170	1,550,000
2	Healthcare health care service design	39,059	828,000
3	Healthcare health care service design mobile mHealth	1,004	2,210
4	Mobile health m-health health care healthcare service design	0	173
5	Mobile mHealth m-Health health care healthcare service design	11	174
6	Health care service system design	14,596	2,260,000
7	Health care service system design mobile	208	341,000
8	Health care service delivery system design mobile	24	92,400
9	Health care service delivery system comparison	554	542,000
10	Health care service delivery system comparison mobile	6	63,600
11	Health care service delivery system comparison mobile mHealth	0	1,280

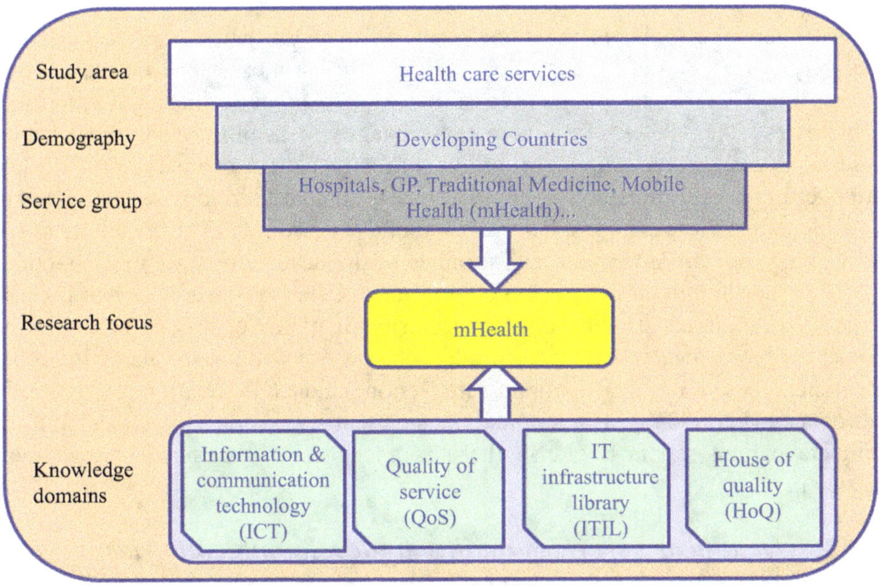

Figure 20.3 Healthcare services design – knowledge domains. Adapted from [61]

performances more than physical objects' [14]. Three management functions – marketing, operations and human resources – are intimately joined in what Lovelock has dubbed the '*service trinity*,' to create and deliver services. Ascertaining and promotion of quality in general practice and primary care is not only a necessity but also essential in retaining the service portfolio and continual assessment helps to alter and tailor the services to suit the consumers [18]. Similar motivations have driven Thorsen et al. [19] to study the purpose of general practice consultation from the patients' perspective. Other researchers like van den Brink-Muinen et al. [20] have explored the basic question of whether doctors' talks with patients meet the patients' expectations. They observe that patients want an attentive, friendly, frank and empathetic doctor who listens well of their bio-medical concerns and advises and tries to alleviate their issues. They also recommend the GPs that they can gather patients' feedback after their consultation.

Petek et al. [21] have performed a longitudinal survey ($n = 7{,}472$) in which they have collected patients' evaluations of European General Practice (GP). As there is a dearth of internationally standardised longitudinal data on the patient evaluation of healthcare, they are motivated to carry on a longitudinal assessment. The respondents are chronic care illness patients. The research objective is to compare patients' evaluation of the current study of 2009 with a previous similar study done in 1998. They have used EUROPEP questionnaire consisting of 23-items. Petek et al. have not found any major changes between 1998 and 2009 for all the countries combined. However, they noticed that English patients are more positive towards general practice in 2009, whereas German patients have become slightly less positive.

An interesting point is that more than 80% of the patients rated GP most positively (4 or 5 on the Likert scale), but they are not most happy on the factors: waiting time (72.1%), telephone accessibility (82.7%) and dealing with emotional problems (83.2%). Petek et al. note that changes in healthcare systems, health professions and patient population might influence patient evaluations of healthcare over time. Unfortunately, no internationally standardised longitudinal data are available to test these changes. Petek et al. found accessibility over the phone to GP and waiting time are important determinants of the healthcare system satisfaction.

The other important conclusion comes out of Petek et al. study is that there is no good correlation between patients' assessments of the quality of care and the respective biomedical outcomes. Similar observations are also made by other researchers based on their patient satisfaction studies in relation to total hip arthroplasty [22]. Finally, Petek et al. conclude that service providers must aim for complete patient satisfaction else there is a chance that patients change their physician.

20.4.2 Healthcare services quality in developing countries

Andaleeb [23] in his work on healthcare delivered to children in Bangladesh summarises the previous studies on the status overall health sector as performing in a dismal state, due to lack of medicines, separate consultation rooms, water, electricity, poor quality of medicines and apathy of healthcare workers and extra payments for supposedly free services. Based on the user satisfaction survey he suggests that nurses must provide service that is good, prompt, caring, helpful, assures confidence and finally demonstrates expertise in order to alter the patients' image of them. When coming to doctors he suggests that they need to demonstrate expertise, respond to queries, foster confidence and be available to the patients. He

Table 20.3 Healthcare service delivery indicators for Bangladesh. Adapted from [25]

Sl. no.	Service delivery indicator	Public	Private	Traditional
1	Treatment service users used (%)	13	27	60
2	Median waiting time (min)	30	20	5
3	Mean cost paid to provider (in Taka)	188	451	100
4	User satisfaction with service provider behaviour (%)	56	91	90

concludes that by making customers' voice publicly available will exert some social pressure on healthcare workers and influence behavioural changes else children will be neglected of basic care. Assessing the overall situation in terms of healthcare services in developing countries, the World Bank did an elaborate analysis and was very dissatisfied with state-of-affairs. They summarised that

> *Services are falling because... they are inaccessible and prohibitively expensive. But even when accessible, they are often dysfunctional, extremely low in technical quality, and extremely unresponsive to the needs of a diverse clientele* [24].

20.4.3 Healthcare service delivery indicators for Bangladesh

The Canadian Institute for Energy Training (CIET) under the project *Bangladesh Health and Population Sector Programme 1998–2003* compiled an interesting assessment report *The Third Service Delivery Survey 2003* [25] in which they have provided detailed information on the healthcare delivery systems in Bangladesh. Table 20.3 provides a snapshot of some of the delivery system indicators. Unqualified practitioners are the major providers of curative healthcare. Traditional medicine practice is highly prevalent in Bangladesh at that time as 60% of the population subscribing to it. Based on the reviews presented earlier on Bangladesh healthcare status, it is no surprise that the public hospitals cost twice that of traditional medicine and private practice costs four times of the traditional practice.

The public service is highly inaccessible and supposed to be free of cost, but to the ill social practice of baksheesh, it costs twice that of a visiting a traditional practitioner to the average Bangladeshi patient. The mean waiting times are again worse with public services in comparison to traditional and private providers. It is also interesting to note from these indicators that the average patient satisfaction with traditional or private is twice that of public service.

20.5 The advent of ICT and mobile communications

Information and communication technology (ICT) has had a very transforming role in several industrial segments like banking/finance, manufacturing, commerce, logistics, services, etc., and it has improved the general productivity of these sectors of the economy. However, there is enormous potential for its transformative role in the health sector [4]. Ever since the invention of telecommunication, there has been a certain degree of its application in the medical sector. The advent of the Internet in the mid-nineties has given impetus to many researchers to apply these innovations in improving healthcare delivery. These efforts have culminated into the development of '*Telemedicine*,' '*Telehealth*' and '*Electronic Health or eHealth*' [26–28].

Global mobile subscriptions have topped 6 billion, a nine fold increase from 0.7 billion in 2000 [1]. In developing countries, wireless communications are the fastest growing sector [29–31], and it overtook fixed-line communications. The developing world has a surprising share of over 75% of these subscriptions or close to 4.5 billion. International Telecommunication Union (ITU) also observes that the growth in mobile phones outweighs a slow increase in the adoption of computers in this part of the world.

Thanks to the phenomenal innovation in mobile communications technologies in the last decade, the developing world has leap-frogged fixed-line communications that facilitated in narrowing down of the global digital divide [31]. Furthermore, continual technological innovation is fuelling a rapid increase in mobile device capabilities and functionalities, coupled with a decrease in device costs. Despite this amazing penetration of wireless mobile technology in the developing world, the state-of-affairs concerning education and health remain very unsatisfactory as noted in Table 20.1. Poor people are yet to travel several kilometres to avail of basic medical services [24].

National Intelligence Council prepared a typology map depicting the healthcare system status across the world [32]. It has classified the healthcare system into five categories: excellent, good, fair, poor and unstable. A greater number of countries are rated fair or below. It is also clear that to a greater part of the world healthcare is not even a priority of their respective governments. The World Health Organisation's (WHO) health indicators show a large divide in healthcare between developed and developing nations [2,33] which the authors term as '*health care divide.*'

20.5.1 The emergence of eHealth/mHealth

Mobile health is transforming healthcare in developing countries by serving the unserved [34]. This transformation is driven by the dramatic growth in mobile phones. The affordability, ubiquity and ever-increasing capabilities of mobile phones positioning are an alternate delivery medium for healthcare services. This leads to the emergence of *Mobile health* or *mHealth*. Mobile phones offer easy accessibility, personalised solutions and location-based services [34]. Globally the mobile phone wireless networks expanded massively, they were able to provide widespread coverage to the remotest corners and at times, to geographically inaccessible locations. In some parts of the world where the wired phone was never heard of, today the populations have adopted mobile phones with ease. The ready availability of low-cost mobile phones makes it a formidable platform for healthcare delivery. The mobile technology can scale well to handle the healthcare challenges with its low cost and simplicity to use [34].

Electronic health (eHealth) encompasses any form of health service rendered electronically. Mobile Health (mHealth) is a specific case of eHealth where the delivery of service depends on wireless cellular technology. With the ongoing innovations in communications technologies and the availability of a wide variety of devices at affordable prices to the individual users, the mHealth frontiers are ever-expanding. What was viable technically but not operationally in the past now is becoming a possibility. In view of this, mHealth is defined to encompass the spectrum of services possible by Global Observatory for eHealth (GOe) as [6]:

mHealth or mobile health as medical and public health practice supported by mobile devices, such as mobile phones, patient monitoring devices, personal digital assistants (PDAs), and other wireless devices. mHealth involves the use and capitalization on a mobile phone's core utility of voice and short messaging service (SMS) as well as more complex functionalities and applications including general packet radio service (GPRS), third and fourth generation mobile telecommunications (3G and 4G systems), global positioning system (GPS), and Bluetooth technology.

The UN Foundation and Vodafone Foundation report in 2009 has presented six categories of applications based on mobile technology for the healthcare sector, namely: education and awareness, helpline, diagnostic and treatment support, communication and training for healthcare workers, disease and epidemic outbreak tracking, remote monitoring and remote data collection [35]. Mobile phones are anticipated to serve as the universal patient terminal in telemedicine scenarios as well as data collection and monitoring device in the self-management of diabetic patients [36].

Free et al. conducted a systematic review protocol of mHealth technologies exploring the effectiveness of mobile phones for health and health services [31]. By reviewing various publications since 1990, they have collated useful evidence of mHealth interventions. The review comprehensively looked at publications that incorporated mobile communications technology or computing to enhance health, health service or quality. They have grouped the publications into three broad categories:

- Interventions designed to improve diagnosis, investigation, treatment, monitoring and management of the disease;
- Interventions to deliver treatment or disease management programs to patients and health promotion and
- Interventions to improve healthcare processes, for example, appointment attendance, result notification and vaccination reminders.

20.5.2 mHealth: the next generation of telemedicine?

Waegemann [37] argues that within a short span Internet evolved and transformed into Internet 2.0 and Internet 3.0 and became a trusted source of information. It has profoundly helped society to chart new paths. Similarly, he foresees that mobile phones will eventually transform healthcare due to the connectedness it enables between the patient and care provider. He terms this evolution as a connected health system. He foresees an evolution of *patient-centric* healthcare from the currently dominant practice of *doctor-centric* mode resulting in the care processes shift from the physician's office (or clinic, hospital or another provider setting) toward the patient. This will bring different specialties of the medicine to be connected and are orchestrated by the physician in delivering care to the patient. Yet again, he terms this as *participatory medicine* or *participatory health*.

Waegermann [37] further argues that this vision comes to reality when the telemedicine is conceived more than just connected healthcare system. Telemedicine 1.0 that is based on the premises of dedicated wired internet connection are to be abandoned and needs to embrace mHealth that is ubiquitous (wireless). The mHealth revolution can enable communication-based care in which the patient is at the centre of care circumscribed by wellness and healthcare providers. He foresees the worldwide movement of mHealth might materialise and countries like Brazil and India may leapfrog to advanced mHealth systems. Finally, Waegemann stresses that mHealth may also need to discern the concerns of security and privacy, and hopefully newer generations of smartphones may overcome this hurdle and help in realising the mHealth revolution.

In contrast to Waegemann's assertions, the mHealth literature is filled with anecdotes that eHealth is not cost-effective. In a recent systematic reviews on eHealth, Black et al. [38] have studied the impact of eHealth on the quality and safety of healthcare. They conclude that there is a large gap between postulated and empirically demonstrated benefits of eHealth technologies. They also argue that the technologies have not yet demonstrated their cost-effectiveness. They also quote paucity of evidence in relation to improvements accrued due to eHealth. Average researcher will be bewildered by these conflicting assessments. But it appeals that these reviews have ignored potential mHealth applications that are practically working and enhancing the lives of people in developing countries. Black's review does not include a comprehensive assessment of working mHealth solutions done by Ivatury et al. [2].

Turning mobile technologies into solutions that become routine operational processes among various healthcare providers and stakeholders is not necessarily a simple process. It requires organisational changes and progressive resolution of non-technological hurdles [39,40]. Yu et al. [41] also argue that one of the critical success factors for the mobile health application is its compliance to regulatory requirements apart from benefiting in operations and offering cost advantages. Several years ago commenting on American healthcare systems, Shortell [42] observed that hospital systems did not achieve their stated objectives due to lack of their systemness. Shortell ponders that in the evolving space of consumer demands and uncertainties, the biggest question is whether organisational arrangements are evolving horizontally and vertically. Hopefully, mHealth with its ingrained promise for connected health can fulfil those decades' long gaps in healthcare systems.

20.6 The need for healthcare services design framework

In manufacturing, finance and other services industries, continual innovation has brought new forms of delivery, giving rise to new forms of services [43]. Competition in healthcare delivery has led to newer forms of services such as outpatient surgery centres, executive wellness programs, independent nursing group practices, hospices, nursing homes, intermediate care facilities and home healthcare programs [44]. To these range of alternatives to healthcare services, mHealth is one of the emerging alternatives.

Considering the broad agenda of better healthcare for all, the dire situation of healthcare status in the developing countries and the vast potential and promise of mHealth, there is a significant opportunity for the research community to direct attention towards service design and service operation. While ITIL [45] comes in handy with its systematic framework to address the service operation phase, there are hardly any studies on how to bring the patients' perspective to the service providers and guide them in devising healthcare services. Our multi-disciplinary search pointed us to review *House of Quality* (HoQ) as a potential framework to rely on for services design. HoQ is a basic design tool and part of the management approach *Quality Function Deployment* (QFD). Hauser and Clausing's [46] classic paper on HoQ has brought its significance to the worldwide community. With its widespread success in bringing together various functional divisions of manufacturing, HoQ has been applied in various forms and to various degrees of sophistication in manufacturing, engineering and subsequently in the design of services [47]. HoQ inter-links customer requirements, their rankings, engineering characteristics, performance measures, competitive products/services and thereby elicits in a single diagram the areas of improvements required to win in the market.

Deming's famous PDCA Cycle is the underlying foundation for QFD and ITIL. While ITIL focuses on the operational aspect of Services Management, HoQ essentially deals with the design of products and services. Figure 20.4 presents a typical portrayal of HoQ Matrix consisting of eight rooms, each room exemplifying a stage of service design [47]. As shown in the figure, HoQ not only helps in the design of products/services but also in drawing conclusions about their competitive position in the market. This comparative evaluation of market helps in examining the strengths and weaknesses and thereby provides input for product positioning and creating an action plan to bridge the identified deficiencies. In the event, a service provider ignores these competitive insights; Keaveney's model suggests that the customers may switch providers thereby either leading to the eventual decline/disappearance of a product/service from the market. In either case, both HoQ and Keaveney's models point to the importance of understanding the comparative analysis of healthcare services. A good service design and consistent operation of the service are essential to raise the bar of user satisfaction [45].

Researchers have investigated patient perceptions of service quality in general [18,19,21,48–51] and mHealth in particular [12]. While there has been research on

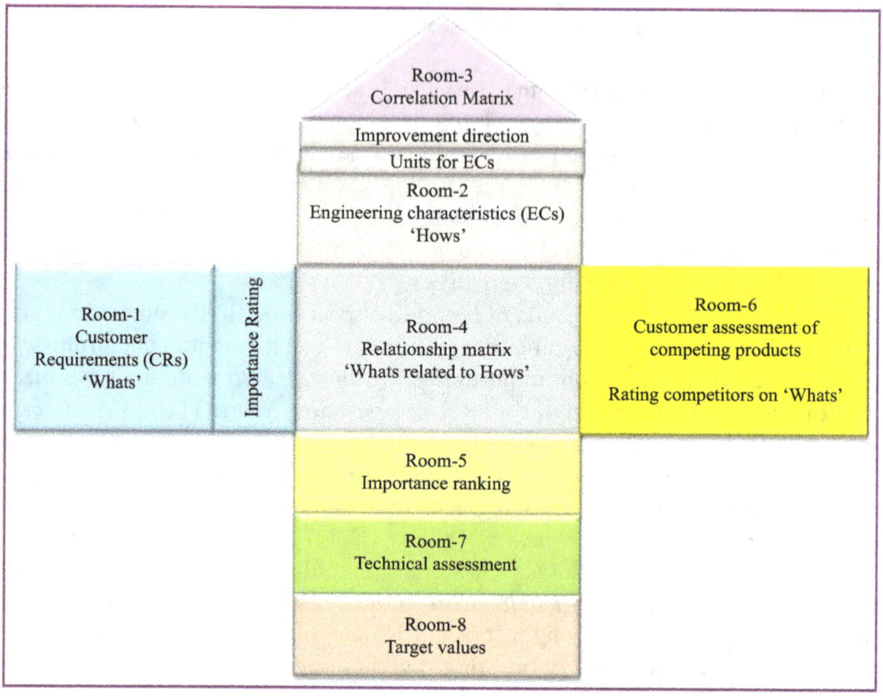

Figure 20.4 House of quality (HoQ) matrix. Adapted from [47]

the aspects of service quality of mHealth from patients' perspective [11,12,34,52], it has not addressed how mHealth is different from other healthcare delivery systems. These insights provided motivation to search the literature for comparative analysis of healthcare delivery systems. In the extant literature, there are very few studies devoted to the comparison of healthcare delivery systems. And there has not been any study that is devoted to a comparative analysis of mHealth with respect to other healthcare alternatives. Competition within healthcare sector can be understood in two basic forms: (1) intra-system (e.g. hospital vs. hospital) and (2) inter-system (e.g. GP vs. mHealth). Section 20.7 will briefly review these comparative studies.

20.7 Healthcare services quality, satisfaction and comparative studies

Physicians are used to acting as surrogate decision-makers for the patient. However, with drastic changes in healthcare, this model is replaced by consumer-centric model which recognises the patient's increasing role in both influence and selection stages of the healthcare decision process [44,53,54]. Lim and Zallocco, for the first time, studied inter-system competition by analysing the consumer attitudes towards divergent healthcare systems, namely, hospitals, home healthcare, nursing homes and outpatient clinics. Their research objectives are:

- to determine consumer attitudes toward the four healthcare delivery systems;
- to determine how consumers' perceptions of these systems vary on specific attributes and
- to identify dimensions that most clearly discriminate the four systems.

Lim and Zallocco conducted a survey in Toledo, Ohio, USA, through a self-administered, structured questionnaire and respondents were selected through a modified area sampling technique. Respondents were questioned about their attitudes towards four healthcare delivery systems along ten attributes: quality of medical care, safety, speed of recovery, quality of medical personnel, risk of complications, cleanliness, convenience, comfort, privacy provided and cost. A 6-point Likert scale ranging from strongly agree (6) to strongly disagree (1) was used for responses. After data clean-up, they got 102 usable questionnaires.

Overall mean scores put hospitals as more safe, clean and of better quality. However, hospitals are perceived as more expensive. Nursing homes have the most negative image with respondents. In terms of the lowest cost, outpatient clinics are rated more positively. On the dimensions of convenience, comfort, privacy and likelihood of speedy recovery, home healthcare is most positively rated. They performed multiple discriminant analysis (MDA) to classify the delivery systems. Lim and Zallocco have found that the three dimensions: personalised care, quality of medical care and value distinguish the four healthcare delivery systems. MDA has provided insights into which dimensions a delivery system is positively viewed thereby providing useful inputs for service providers, healthcare researchers and policymakers. For example, home healthcare service providers can highlight their strengths as perceived by consumers in comfort, privacy, medical quality and the likelihood of speedy recovery as differentiating factors to offer better services.

20.7.1 Intra-system comparisons

Andaleeb [33] has studied the quality of services provided by public and private hospitals in Bangladesh. He notes that large segments of the population in developing countries are deprived of a fundamental right: access to basic healthcare. Quoting a World Bank 1987 study, he obverses that the situation is acute in Bangladesh as only 30% of the population have access to primary healthcare. Due to Bangladesh government's regulatory reforms, during 1982–1996, there is an increase of 346 private hospitals and 5,500 beds. Though there are signs of improvement in numbers in capacity, there is a dearth of information about the quality of the services offered by hospitals. Public hospitals being subsidised by the government have a marginal tendency to improve their services, while private hospitals which primarily run on patients' patronage are obligated to improve their services and be competitive among peers.

To gauge patients' assessments of the hospital services they have received in the past, Andaleeb has used a modified framework to that of SERVQUAL of Parasuraman et al. [9]. Through qualitative interviews, Andaleeb established that a prominent cultural concept, *baksheesh* (facilitation payments) was prevalent in Bangladesh and needs to be included in the modified framework. They collected data from 216 interviews of which the final valid cases were 207. He applied two group DA to determine whether service quality ratings (along with education and income) predicted the choice of hospitals; which factors accounted most for the differences in the scores and how reliably the patients could be grouped into public or private hospital users. Of the 207 cases, only 191 found to have valid data, consisting of 91 respondents of public hospitals and 100 used private hospitals or clinics.

The DA identified one significant discriminant function that produced a classification accuracy of 70.16%. The accuracy is 25% greater than that obtained by chance [55,56] confirming a satisfactory predictive power of the model. Private hospitals were evaluated better on responsiveness, communication and discipline. Thus, supporting Andaleeb's premise that market incentives would explain differences in perceived quality of services provided by public and private hospitals. Furthermore, he concludes that even in the private hospitals, level of service having not measured up to the satisfaction of some of the affordable patients, they are switching to services in foreign countries thus costing the economy on foreign exchange front. This is an important conclusion that there is a vast opportunity to improve healthcare services in Bangladesh. It can be noted that the emergence of mHealth service as one of the favourable alternative in Bangladesh is not a major surprise due to the prevailing structural failure of the healthcare delivery in Bangladesh. This conclusion is well supported by a detailed study undertaken by the World Bank on the status of services in developing countries [24].

Moving forward on the works of Andaleeb, Siddiqui and Khandaker [57] compared services of public and private hospitals of Bangladesh and then compared private hospitals with foreign counterparts from the perspective Bangladesh patients. They have quoted several prior studies that essentially concluded that public hospitals are used 30% or lower due to the facts of unavailability of doctors and nurses, their attitudes and behaviour, lack of drugs, waiting time, travel time, etc. They collected questionnaires from 400 randomly selected patients. Their analysis showed that private hospitals were doing better in terms of availability of drugs, tangibility, perceived costs, the empathy of nurses and responsiveness. It has also been derived that foreign hospitals are doing even better on these dimensions compared to private hospitals. Public hospitals also fared lower in the aspects of tangibility compounded by the factors of cleanliness, water supply and availability of equipment. The cost has been studied as patients' perception of costs that includes consultation, diagnostics, accommodation, etc. Based on their analysis they concluded that the overall quality of service was better in foreign hospitals than the private hospitals in Bangladesh in all the factors, including 'perceived cost' factor.

20.8 Conclusions

20.8.1 Research questions

The review of healthcare services, mHealth, healthcare systems' status in developing countries, services management framework and HoQ has brought to fore very important questions for healthcare in general and mHealth about the importance of services design. It is possible to draw a comparative analysis of existing healthcare services from a qualitative perspective. However, as the patients are the ultimate consumers of mHealth services, it is worthwhile to understand how patients perceive mHealth vis-à-vis other healthcare delivery systems. Such a research endeavour shall possibly answer [58,59] from the patients' perspective in developing countries:

- Are different healthcare services distinguishable from each other?
- Is mHealth distinct from other existing services? and
- If so, what factors contribute to service differentiation?

20.8.2 Research contribution

The exploding global population and the healthcare divide will pose far more challenges in the ensuing years unless a careful multi-disciplinary study is undertaken. Given its ubiquity, affordability and high penetration even among the poor population, mHealth can be a potential healthcare service delivery alternative, to compliment other forms of healthcare delivery, for the developing countries to reach the underserved and unserved population groups. Thus, this research on mHealth can help bridge the healthcare divide and assist the developing countries in achieving better healthcare for all.

20.8.3 Conclusions

The multi-disciplinary search on healthcare services has uncovered several interesting facts about healthcare services, provided a framework to understand the antecedents for a quality healthcare service and proposed that HoQ can be utilised in the process of healthcare services design. The discussion highlighted the lack of comparative evaluation of healthcare service alternatives and how such an evaluation can contribute to the design of efficient healthcare service alternatives to address the healthcare challenges of the developing nations.

References

[1] ITU. *World ICT Data and Statistics*. 2011. Available from http://www.itu.int/ITU-D/ict/statistics/ [Accessed 12 Mar 2012].

[2] Ivatury G., Moore J., and Bloch A. 'A doctor in your pocket: Health hotlines in developing countries'. *Innovations: Technology, Governance, Globalization*. 2009;4(1):119–153.

[3] Sharma C. State of the Global Mobile Industry, Annual Assessment-2012 [online]. Available from: https://www.slideshare.net/chetansharma/annual-state-ofglobalmobileindustry2012chetansharmaconsulting [Accessed 01-Jun-2020].

[4] Agarwal R., Gao G.G., DesRoches C., *et al.* The digital transformation of healthcare: Current status and the road ahead. *Information Systems Research*. 2010;21(4):796–809.

[5] PWCC. *Healthcare Unwired*. Health Research Institute, PWCC; 2010. p. 40.

[6] WHO. *mHealth: New Horizons for Health Through Mobile Technologies: Second Global Survey on eHealth*. Switzerland: WHO; 2011. p. 112.

[7] Mechael P.N. 'The case for mHealth in developing countries'. *Innovations: Technology, Governance, Globalization*. 2009;4(1):153–168.

[8] HIMSS. Advancing global health IT: A consultation with the World Bank at HIMSS12. In: *A HIMSS G7 Advisory Report*. 2012, HIMSS. p. 8.

[9] Parasuraman A., Zeithaml V.A., and Berry L.L. 'SERVQUAL: A multiple-item scale for measuring consumer perceptions'. *Journal of Retailing*. 1988; 64(1):12–40.

[10] Brady M.K., and Cronin J.J. 'Some new thoughts on conceptualizing perceived service quality: A hierarchical approach'. *Journal of Marketing*. 2001;65(3):34–49.

[11] Akter S., D'Ambra J., and Ray P. 'Service quality of mHealth platforms: development and validation of a hierarchical model using PLS.' *Electronic Markets*. 2010;20(3):209–227.

[12] Akter S., D'Ambra J., and Ray P. *User Perceived Service Quality of m-Health Services in Developing Countries*. In *18th European Conference on Information Systems*. 2010.

[13] Levitt T. 'Exploit product life cycle'. *Harvard Business Review*. 1965;43(6):14.

[14] Lovelock C., and Wirtz J. *Services Marketing: People, Technology, Strategy*. 7th edn. 2010.

[15] McGuire L.I. *Australian Services: Marketing and Management*. Macmillan Education Australia; 1999.

[16] Alter S. 'Service system fundamentals: Work system, value chain, and life cyle'. *IBM Systems Journal*. 2008;47(1):16.

[17] Keaveney S.M. 'Customer switching behavior in service industries: An exploratory study. *Journal of Marketing*. 1995;59(2):71–82.

[18] Ramsay J., Campbell J.L., Schroter S., *et al.* 'The General Practice Assessment Survey (GPAS): Tests of data quality and measurement properties'. *Journal of Family Practice*. 2000;17(5):372–379.

[19] Thorsen H., Witt K., Hollnagel H., *et al.* 'The purpose of the general practice consultation from the patient's perspective: Theoretical aspects'. *Journal of Family Practice*. 2001;18(6):638–643.

[20] van den Brink-Muinen A., van Dulmen A.M., Jung H.P., *et al.* 'Do our talks with patients meet their expectations?' *Journal of Family Practice*. 2007; 56(7):559–68.

[21] Petek D., Künzi B., Kersnik J., *et al.* 'Patients' evaluations of European general practice—revisited after 11 years.' *International Journal for Quality in Health Care*. 2011;23(6):621–628.

[22] Haverkamp D., Sierevelt I.N., van den Bekerom M.P., *et al.* 'The validity of patient satisfaction as single question in outcome measurement of total hip arthroplasty'. *Journal of Long-Term Effects of Medical Implants*. 2008;18(2): 145–50.

[23] Andaleeb S. 'Caring for children: a model of healthcare service quality in Bangladesh.' *International Journal for Quality in Health Care*, 2008; 20(5):7.

[24] Worldbank. *World Development Report: Making Services Work for Poor People*. New York: Worldbank; 2004.

[25] Cokroft A., and Milne D., and Anderson N. *Bangladesh Health and Population Sector Programme: Third Service Delivery Survey 2003: Final Report*. Ottawa: CIET, Canada; 2003. p. xxiii, 85.

[26] Bashshur R., Shannon G., Krupinski E., *et al.* 'The taxonomy of telemedicine'. *Telemedicine and e-Health*, 2011;17(6):484–494.

[27] Bashshur R.L., and Reardon T.G., and Shannon G.W. 'Telemedicine: A new health care delivery system'. *Annual Review of Public Health*. 2000;21(1): 613–637.

[28] Moore M. 'The evolution of telemedicine'. *Future Generation Computer Systems*. 1999;15:10.

[29] ITU. *Mobile Overtakes Fixed: Implications for Policy and Regulation*. International Telecommunications Union (ITU); 2003. p. 39.

[30] Banks K., and Burge R. *Mobile Phones: An Appropriate Tool for Conversation and Development?* Cambridge, UK: Fauna & Flora International; 2004. p. 72.

[31] Free C., Phillips G., Felix L., *et al.* 'The effectiveness of M-health technologies for improving health and health services: a systematic review protocol'. *BMC Research Notes*. 2010;3(1):250.

[32] National Intelligence Council (NIC). *Typology of Countries by Health-Care Status*. NIC: Washington, DC; 2003.

[33] Andaleeb S.S. 'Public and private hospitals in Bangladesh: service quality and predictors of hospital choice'. *Health Policy and Planning*. 2000; 15(1):95–102.

[34] Akter S., and Ray P. *mHealth – An Ultimate Platform to Serve the Unserved. IMIA Yearbook of Medical Informatics*. Germany: Schattauer; 2010. pp. 94–100.

[35] Vital Wave Consulting. *mHealth for Development: The Opportunity of Mobile Technology for Healthcare in the Developing World.* Washington: United Nations Foundation, Vodafone Foundation; 2009, p. 70.

[36] Giménez-Pérez G., Gallach M., Acera E., *et al.* 'Evaluation of accessibility and use of new communication technologies in patients with type 1 diabetes mellitus'. *Journal of Medical Internet Research*. 2002;4(3).

[37] Waegemann P. 'mHealth: The next generation of telemedicine?' *Telemedicine and e-Health*. 2010;16(1):3.

[38] Black A.D., Car J., Pagliari C., *et al.* 'The impact of eHealth on the quality and safety of health care: A systematic overview'. *PLoS Medicine*. 2011;8 (1):e1000387.

[39] Essén A., and Conrick M. 'New e-service development in the homecare sector: Beyond implementing a radical technology'. *International Journal of Medical Informatics*. 2008;77(10):679–688.

[40] Venkatesh V., Morris M.G., Davis G.B., *et al.* 'User acceptance of information technology: Toward a unified view'. *MIS Quarterly: Management Information Systems*. 2003;27(3):425–478.

[41] Ping Y., Wu M.X., Yu H., *et al.* The challenges for the adoption of M-Health. In: *IEEE International Conference on Service Operations and Logistics, and Informatics, 2006. SOLI '06*. 2006.

[42] Shortell S.M. 'The evolution of hospital systems: Unfulfilled promises and self-fulfilling prophesies'. *Medical Care Research Review*. 1988;45(177):39.

[43] Hwang J., and Christensen C.M. Disruptive innovation in health care delivery: A framework for business-model innovation. *Health Affairs*. 2008;27(5):1329–35.

[44] Lim J.S., and Zallocco R. Determinant attributes in formulation of attitudes toward four health care systems. *Journal of Health Care Marketing*. 1988; 8(2):25–30.

[45] OGC. *ITIL, Version 3*: London: Office of Government Commerce, The Stationery Office; 2007.

[46] Hauser J.R., and Clausing D. 'The house of quality'. *Harvard Business Review*. May-June, 1988.

[47] Ray P.K. *Integrated Management from E-Business Perspective: Concepts, Architectures and Methodologies*. New York: Kluwer; 2003.

[48] Heje H.N., and Olesen F. 'Patients' evaluations as quality measurements in general practice'. *Ugeskrift for Laeger*. 2002;164(46):5386–5389.

[49] Andaleeb S.S. 'Service quality perceptions and patient satisfaction: A study of hospitals in a developing country'. *Social Science & Medicine*. 2001; 52(9):1359–1370.

[50] Andaleeb S.S., Siddiqui N., and Khandakar S. 'Patient satisfaction with health services in Bangladesh'. *Health Policy and Planning*. 2007;22(4): 263–273.

[51] Ware J.E.J., Wright W.R., Snyder M.K., *et al.* 'Consumer perceptions of health care services: implications for academic medicine'. *Academic Medicine*. 1975;50(9):839–848.

[52] Akter S., D'Ambra J., and Ray P. 'Trustworthiness in mHealth information services: An assessment of a hierarchical model with mediating and moderating effects using partial least squares (PLS)'. *Journal of the American Society for Information Science and Technology*. 2011;62(1):100–116.

[53] Berkowitz E.N., and Hillestad S.G. 'Evolution of tripratite model of hospital selection'. *Proceedings from Advances in Health Care Research*. Association for Consumer Research; 1982.

[54] Wright N.D., and Parsons R.J. Consumers' Selection of Hospital Maternity Care. In: *Proceedings from Advances in Health Care Research*. Snowbird, UT: Association for Consumer Research; 1982.

[55] Malhotra N. *Marketing Research: An Applied Orientation*. 4th edn. Upper Saddle River, NJ: Pearson Education; 2004.

[56] Hair J.F.J., Black W.C., Babin B.J., *et al. Multivariate Data Analysis: A Global Perspective*. 7 edn. Upper Saddle River: Pearson Prentice Hall; 2010.

[57] Siddiqui N., and Khandaker S.A. 'Comparison of services of public, private and foreign hospitals from the perspective of Bangladeshi patients'. *Journal of Health, Population and Nutrition*. 2007;25(2):221–230.

[58] Motamarri S., Akter S., Ray P., *et al.* 'Distinguishing 'mHealth' from other healthcare services in a developing country: A study from the service quality perspective'. *Communications of the Association for Information Systems*. 2014;34(1):669–690.

[59] Motamarri S., Akter S., Ray P., *et al.* Mhealth: A better alternative for healthcare in developing countries. In: *PACIS-2012 Proceedings, Paper 29*. Ho Chi Minh City, Vietnam; 2012.

[60] Motamarri S. *The Convergence of SDL and STD Towards Co-creation*. Paper presented at the ANZMAC-2015, UNSW, Sydney, Australia, Nov-Dec, 2015.

[61] Motamarri S. Distinguishing mHealth from other health care alternatives in developing countries: A study on service characteristics'. MPhil Thesis, UNSW Business School, The University of New South Wales, Sydney, Australia, 2013; p. 1:191.

Chapter 21

What is going on in digital health communities? A typology of support exchanges for cancer patients

Babak Abedin[1], David Milne[2] and Shadi Erfani[2]

The use of online health communities (OHCs) for informational and emotional social support seeking is on the rise. However, still little is known about type of exchanges in these communities. In this chapter, we draw on and contribute to the digital health literature by critically studying online support exchanges in a major Australia OHC for cancer patients. We examine about 2,500 messages from 2009 to 2018 and develop a novel annotation scheme of support topics that comprise of five overarching themes: informational support provision, emotional support provision, request for help, self-reflection and disclosures, and conversational cues. Findings revealed that members of OHCs overwhelmingly disclose personal reflections to bond with the community and many members actively post to the community solely to provide informational and emotional support to others. We present implications of our finding to the practice as well as to the theory and discuss potentials for future studies.

21.1 Introduction

An online health community (OHC) is an Internet-based text forum in which people share health-related information, experiences and feelings and provide support and encouragement to other community members [1]. Online communities are fluid organisations with a dynamic environment for interactions between the community owner, individual participants and the technology [2]. The use of these platforms is on the rise [3] as interactions in these communities can supplement the traditional communications between doctors, patients and caregivers. Often the user-generated health contents in these communities provide information and support that is not available elsewhere [4].

Past studies have widely discussed users' motivations for joining OHCs such as on-going management of health conditions [5], exchanging support and learning

[1]Macquarie Business School, Macquarie University, Sydney, Australia
[2]Faculty of Engineering and IT, University of Technology Sydney, Sydney, Australia

from one another's experience [6], accessing informational and emotional help about rare and socially stigmatised health conditions [7,8], alleviating distress and improving the mood [9] and adopting information and forming close relationships with like-minded people [10]. Yet, the literature is still unsettled about how individuals use the community in terms of what support they exchange in these communities [11,12]. In this chapter, we draw on theory of attraction-selection-attrition (ASA) for online communities (OCASA). The theory is comprised of three stages, which explain user behaviours in online communities: attraction (expectations and goals that encourage people to join the community), selection (how they use the community and whether the community serves their purpose) and attrition (people leaving the community as their needs were not satisfied). The key focus of the theory is to help making decision for enhancing the user experience and assessing the impact of such decisions on how communities grow or diminish.

Thus, the objective of this chapter is to develop an annotation scheme of support topics exchanged between community users and discuss what topics are discussed in the initial conversations of new OHCs users. This chapter also makes an important contribution to the practice by informing policy making and advocacy in health, particularly for cancer health initiatives. We do this in light of recent call by Wainwright et al. [13] for taking an evidence-base practice for information systems (EBPIS) approach to place the focus of the academic research on practitioners' problem and to produce new knowledge to inform professional policy making. The remainder of this chapter is structured as follows. First, we present the background of the study with an overview of the OCASA theory as well as OHCs research for cancer patients. We then introduce the environment under study, which is a well-established online community for cancer patients in Australia. We then discuss our research design and present the procedure for collection of textual conversation as well as the process of developing an annotation scheme for data analysis and interpretations. We then present our findings and discuss theoretical and practical implications, and conclude the chapter with recommendations for future research.

21.2 Research background

21.2.1 Attraction-selection-attrition theory for online communities

Butler et al. [14] later extended ASA theory (Schneider, 1987) to the online community context and coined ASA theory for online communities (OCASA). They did so with an idea that attraction of members to an online community, their selection to stay and engage in that community, and the community attrition are central to the emergence of community characteristics. While some online communities can attract and maintain a large number of members, research shows that most communities fail do to so and struggle to grow and retain members [15], which in turn damages the dynamic of engagements within the community and limits its sustainability. Butler et al. [14] argue that the community's size and resilience are critical for its success as they create a self-reinforcing loop: a small community that cannot retain its members limits members' engagement and contributions, which consequently brings down the benefits and outcome for its members. They base the theory on three stages:

1. *Attraction*: People join a community such as online community with a hope to find a match between their personal interests and the community's dynamic, activities and topics. Thus, the critical issues are how much a community may meet such expectations, and how wide the gap is between the new member's expectation and the community's actual dynamic and content.
2. *Selection*: When new members expose themselves to activities and discussions after joining the community, their fit expectations change. These expectations evolve as members use the community resources and exchange interactions with others. Members may experience a variety of benefits from using online communities such as sense of community [16] and access to expert advice. Members' perceived value from their first-hand experience leads them to revise their expectations about the future availability of such benefits, and thus decide whether to stay in the community as well as how much they should stay active and engaged in the community.
3. *Attrition*: The third stage of the theory focuses on when individuals leave an online community due to their perception that the community's future activities diverge from their own interests.

Butler et al. [14] extended the ASA theory to a commercial online community, with an assumption that a particular cost–benefit logic explains members' participation decisions. However, they acknowledge that this transactional approach is not the only reason that underlies individuals' behaviours. While a transactional approach may explain members' attrition motive for commercial and for-profit communities, non-profit and bond-based communities such as OHCs pose different motives for members to stay or leave the community [6,14].

21.2.2 OHCs for cancer patients

Extant literature has shown that using OHCs can have both positive and negative impacts on the wellbeing of the community members [6,10], and thus adopting a careful structure for the community management, activities and content is crucial [1]. OHCs allow members to meet like-minded people, exchange emotional and social support, and even receive professional health advice, which can significantly improve psychological wellbeing of the members. In particular, these online communities enable isolated people and those with a rare or socially stigmatised condition to access informational and emotional support networks [7]. This is because earlier studies have shown that members of online communities have intrinsic motivation for social acceptance and desire to help others, which in turn can drive interactions in online communities and build close relationships between members despite them being personally unknown to one another [17]. On the other hand, using OHCs may have adverse health outcomes. For instance, unfiltered and unmoderated health content [18] or excessive use of online communities without a balance with offline activities and support can lead to adverse health outcomes for the members of the community.

Diagnosis of cancer is a life-changing event and takes a great toll on a person's psychological well-being and quality of life. Emotional support and informational support can reduce some of the distress experienced by cancer patients [19] and can benefit patients in terms of improving mood, handling potentially difficult situations and managing stress. Patients frequently cannot get adequate support because the disease itself often closes off communication with family and friends. Friends or relatives are uncertain about what they should or should not discuss with the patients. Patients themselves may be unwilling to share their distress with their family because they do not wish to put further burdens on them and may look for other support channels such as talking with other patients with similar diagnoses. Support resources should be convenient, timely, anonymous, under the user's control and flexible enough to adapt to differing coping styles. Online support groups open a platform for such exchanges [20].

21.3 Study context

We studied an OHC owned and moderated by Cancer Council NSW (CCNSW). This organisation is an independent charity that is 94% community funded. They host a set of active online communities for people with or who have had cancer as well as for their family members and friends, to exchange information and emotional support with other community members. Various cancer support topics are discussed in this community every day and they are increasingly attracting more users from across Australia and beyond.

Members' engagement in these communities is guided by a set of guidelines, one of which is in regards to the moderation of the content that encourages moderators to rarely intervene in the conversations of community members to encourage peer-led conversations. Given this moderation style, moderators' comments were rare and thus not examined in this study.

21.4 Research design

We applied an online ethnographical, or netnographical, approach. Netnography applies ethnographic approaches to online exchanges and refers to passively following individuals' online conversations, actively engaging with participants through direct questioning or becoming a member observer in online communities [21]. We took a passive observational perspective and conducted a thematic analysis of 2,463 community messages. We then used a systematic approach for conducting the literature review for developing the annotation scheme for practical research [22,23] as has been previously applied in other studies for comprehensively review extant literature [24].

The data collection process covered textual conversations about people with cancer from the 1st of April 2009 and the 1st of July 2018. This resulted in

859 collected users. For each user, we gathered the conversation stemming from their first post: namely their first message and all other messages posted within 7 days in the same thread. These messages included messages written by the identified user (i.e. the conversation starter), by affiliated community members (i.e. replying moderators) and other unaffiliated community members (i.e. replying peers). The 859 users/conversations yielded a total pool of 2,463 messages available to be annotated.

21.4.1 Development and validation of the annotation scheme

The meaning of exchanges between community members became explicit through multiple cycles of interpretations between the authors and the online community advisory team in three steps:

1. Understanding: (i) Literature searching: this first step refers to an analytic development of key concepts, theories and assumptions; and (ii) classifying and mapping: we then systematically listed all extracted topics from the previous step, and classified them into five themes based on their similarities. Each theme included two or more topics (Table 21.1).
2. Explanation: The objective here was a critical assessment and validation of Table 21.1. This step includes a broad analysis of what types of knowledge are produced, and how useful they are in explaining the problem of interest. We did this in two steps: first, we randomly selected ten threads (approximately 100 messages) from the forum and annotated them using the classifying scheme in the previous step. This ensured all sentences (and the corresponding meaning) could be captured by the classifying scheme. Authors separately and manually annotated the text and then met to discuss agreements and resolve disagreements. Second, we presented the annotation scheme to the community experts for feedback. This rectified issues related in the clarity of descriptions and in aggregating similar topics.
3. Interpretation. This phase includes building an argument from the earlier classification and leading to a construction of a problematisation for the

Table 21.1 Review of topics and support exchanges in online health communities

Source	ISP				ESP				RS		CC			SR&D	
	ID	IT	IR	CC	E	E&S	ES	S	RIS	RES	S&C	A&A	HQ	DI	DE
[23]											✓	✓	✓	✓	
[10]	✓	✓			✓	✓			✓	✓					
[25]	✓	✓	✓	✓	✓	✓	✓	✓	✓	✓				✓	
[26]	✓	✓	✓	✓		✓		✓		✓				✓	✓
[27]											✓	✓	✓	✓	✓
[28]	✓	✓	✓	✓	✓	✓	✓	✓	✓	✓				✓	✓
[11]	✓	✓		✓	✓		✓		✓						
[29]	✓	✓				✓			✓	✓		✓			

research. Thus, we critically assessed our classification in Table 21.1 and produced an annotation scheme that addresses a gap in the knowledge of cancer-related topics exchanges in OHCs. This resulted in a scheme comprised of fifteen discussion topics grouped in five themes (Table 21.2).

Informational support provision (ISP) reflects explicit informational support provided to the community members. In OHCs, this reflects exchanges about cancer-related diagnosis and treatment information or referrals. Emotional support

Table 21.2 The annotation scheme

Themes	Discussed topics	Descriptions
Informational support provision (ISP)	Illness (cancer) diagnosis (ID)	Information and symptoms about cancer diagnosis
	Illness (cancer) treatment (IT)	Information about treatment options and factors to consider when making treatment decisions
	Illness (cancer) recurrence (IR)	Information on procedures for regular self-monitoring, lifestyle changes such as dietary changes, to reduce the likelihood of recurrence of cancer
	Care and coping (CC)	Advice on how to cope with cancer
Emotional support provision (ESP)	Encouragement (E)	Support in persistence in facing challenges; hope/prayers that their situation improves
	Empathy and sympathy (E&S)	Expressing condolences or the ability to understand and share the feelings of another
	Esteem support (ES)	Appreciation for the value of an individual and his or her accomplishments
	Solidarity (S)	Expressions of team spirit so members would not feel alone in their treatment
Request for support (RS)	Request for informational support (RIS)	Explicit request for advice or help about cancer-related questions or matters
	Request for emotional support (RES)	Explicit request for advice or help about emotionally coping with cancer
Self-reflection and disclosure (SR & D)	Disclosure of information (DI)	Revealing details of the author's situation, problems faced, etc., or sharing news/events
	Disclosure of emotions (DE)	Revealing details of the author's thoughts and feelings
Conversational cues (CC)	Salutations and closings (S&C)	An expression of greeting or goodbye, usually at the opening or closing of the posting
	Acknowledgements and appreciations (A&A)	Recognising or acknowledging the helpfulness, ideas, comments, capabilities and experiences of other participants in the conversation
	Horizontal questions (HQ)	Questions which do not have a 'correct' answer, but for which discussion might produce consensus or deeper understanding of the problem

provision (ESP) reflects providing emotional support to peers in form of empathising, sympathising, solidarity, encouragement and esteem support. Request for support (RS) refers to explicit requests for emotional or informational help or questions about cancer care.

As per Table 21.1, extant literature has widely reported RSs, ISPs and ESPs as explicit support exchanges in OHCs. However, less has been done to capture implicit support topics. This group of exchanges is important as earlier research in the broader online communities' literature has reported the existence of off-task (e.g. posts not directly health-related) content in peer to peer exchanges [30,31]. Thus, we included self-reflection and disclosures, and conversational cues in our annotation scheme. The conversations were annotated using a web application that was developed specifically for this experiment. The system randomises the order in which conversations are given, using blocked random allocation with a block size of 10.

21.5 Results

Table 21.3 lists, for each type of forum member, the proportion of conversations that contain at least one example of each of the different annotation topics.

Almost all of these conversations contain self-disclosure from the new visitor. In almost all cases this includes informational disclosure, and in 43% of cases,

Table 21.3 Distribution of support exchanges in the online community

	New visitor	Replying peers
Self-reflection and disclosure	93.6%	49.3%
Disclosure of information	92.4%	48.9%
Disclosure of emotions	42.7%	20.2%
Request for support	41.1%	5.3%
Request for informational support	39.6%	5.3%
Request for emotional support	15.8%	0.9%
Support provision	36.2%	40.9%
Informational support provision	12.2%	21.1%
Cancer diagnosis	2.4%	4.4%
Cancer treatment	6.0%	10.2%
Cancer recurrence	1.3%	0.2%
Cancer care and coping	6.4%	14.0%
Emotional support provision	33.8%	38.9%
Encouragement	25.1%	29.1%
Empathy and sympathy	7.8%	15.6%
Esteem support	9.6%	13.8%
Solidarity	8.7%	13.1%
Conversational cues	67.6%	45.6%
Salutations and closings	62.2%	43.6%
Acknowledgements and appreciations	22.4%	12.0%
Horizontal questions	8.0%	5.8%

emotional disclosure. Thus, while new visitors almost invariably describe their diagnosis and other aspects of their situation, they are less likely to discuss their thoughts and feelings openly. Roughly 40% of new visitors make an explicit request for support, and in almost all cases, these requests focus on informational support. Explicit requests for emotional support are comparatively rare. Interestingly, many new visitors seem to join the forum with the intention of giving rather than receiving help and tend to provide encouragement ahead of other forms of support.

Peers are quick to share the facts of their own situation when welcoming new users, presumably with the intention of showing the visitor that they are not alone, but among people who share similar burdens. However, peers are less likely to discuss their thoughts and feelings about their situation, with only 20% of conversations including any form of emotional disclosure. When providing support to new users, peers tend to focus on providing emotional support—particularly encouragement—ahead of informational support.

21.6 Discussion

OHCs help people to share common health concerns and exchange support with like-minded people and health professionals [32]. The increasing prevalence of online communities for health support within and outside the information systems and technology management research has been the driving force behind their increasing use by health professionals, patients and carers.

From a theoretical point of view, we developed and tested a novel annotation scheme that revealed and systematically organised support topics in OHCs, particularly for cancer patients. It included five support topics: informational support provision, emotional support provision, request for help, self-reflection and disclosures, and conversational cues. The scheme relied on initial posts made by new members, and took into consideration the community reactions to these posts, to determine active or passive status of individuals in terms of actively posting to versus lurking the community. Following this, we applied the scheme to a well-known Australian OHCs to examine what topics were discussed in the initial conversations of new users. Initial posts are important in understanding new members' attraction to the community. Our results showed that almost all of these conversations contained self-disclosure from the new visitors, and in almost all cases this included informational disclosure and in almost half of cases emotional disclosure. Furthermore, we found that almost half of new visitors make an explicit request for support, and in almost all cases, these requests focus on informational support and rarely on emotional support. Emotional support and disclosure are important, as earlier research has stressed on the deeply remedial potential of emotional reciprocity [33]. Many new visitors seem to join the forum with the intention of giving rather than receiving help and tend to provide encouragement ahead of other forms of support. This is in line with Butler et al. [14] about characterising bond-based communities as a space where members act altruistically for the good of the community. Peers are quick to share the facts of their own situation when welcoming new users, presumably with the intention of showing the visitor that they are not alone. However, peers are less likely to discuss their thoughts and feelings about their situation, with only 20% of conversations including any form of emotional disclosure.

This study applied the OCASA theory and showed that how cancer patients often act altruistically and exchange support for the good of OHCs. In particular, this study highlighted that OHCs members engage in reciprocal exchanges of self-disclosure coupled with provision of information and emotional support as well as social niceties and solidarity. We found that these exchanges are often a way for members to express desire to connect with others and develop relationships. Smithson et al. [34] have pointed to a similar finding, as they found the same OHCs members who posted the conventional advice on healthcare often initiate new posts asking for advice in similar situations. These findings extend and contribute to earlier studies by Yan et al. [11] that reported personal benefits (i.e. reputation enhancement, perceived social support and a sense of self-worth) and avoidance of costs (i.e. executional and cognitive costs) are key drivers of memberships in OHCs.

From the practical approach, this study also offers support and sheds light on OHCs practical applications. We do this in light of recent call by Wainwright et al. [13] for taking an EBPIS approach to place the focus of the academic research on practitioners' problem and to produce new knowledge to inform professional policy making. We closely worked with online community managers and cancer health professionals in one of the major non-profit organisations in Australia, which led to a number of important implications for the practice. First, OHCs managers and owners should explicitly highlight benefits of the online community on their website for patients and other health users. While OHCs offer can valuable health-related informational support, community managers should use the 'About Us' or other community introduction pages to stress on the importance of and the potential for connecting with like-minded peers and exchanging emotional support as a result of joining an OHC.

This, as per OCASA, can help more properly setting the expectation of new members and making an alignment between their expectations and the community management activities and initiatives. Second, our results inform health organisations in their policymaking and advocacy efforts towards strengthening the online support for cancer patients and other health users (e.g. carers). Results of this study encourage health organisations to take advantage of OHCs to supplement their existing health support services. For instance, while Cancer Council NSW is currently hosting one of the most active and vibrant online health forums in the NSW state of Australia, their forums are increasingly attracting people from around the country and overseas. This is because cancer health advice and peer support can be used and shared by patients across the globe.

21.7 Conclusion

OHCs are increasingly being used for health-related information and support exchanges. In line with previous studies [35], this research revealed a strong presence of peer exchanges on request for support and support provision topics. Furthermore, we also found a considerable level of interest and exchanges on self-reflection and disclosure, and conversational cues in the online cancer community under study. Our findings revealed that users were more likely to exchange information support rather than emotional support. New users frequently reflect on their personal circumstances and often use these initial conversations as a mechanism to connect to others and feel part of the community.

The OCASA theory puts emphasis on the difference between online communities and traditional information systems, and describes them as 'emergent sociotechnical systems whose design and operation requires an understanding of multilevel social processes.... As a kind of networked IS, online discussion communities are inherently evolutionary, as technology choices and user behaviours interact to shape their emergent character, resources, and capabilities' [14, p. 723]. Yet, despite its specialised focus on online communities, this theory is currently under-utilised in the literature.

Future research needs to incorporate other cohorts of OHCs users, particularly carers of patients, into consideration. A carer is one who gives personal care and help to a loved one who needs help due to some condition they have, someone who shares the care recipient's ailment experiences and manages their emotions. In the process of helping their loved one, they feel stressed and strained by the daily responsibilities of caring as well as isolation from family and friends because they spend all their time caring. As a result, many carers use OHCs to find social support and gather the knowledge they need to tackle carer burden. Yet, despite the importance and uniqueness of caring job, much of extant information systems literature on health has neglected a distinction between different cohorts of health users (e.g. patients vs. their carers) and their unique needs. Thus, we call for future research to examine in what ways various cohorts of health users may use information systems such as OHCs to exchange support, and particularly to understand their attraction, selection and attrition to these communities.

Acknowledgements

This study has been jointly funded by Cancer Council NSW and University of Technology Sydney (grant # PRO18-6515). The authors particularly would like to thank Annette Beattie, Kate Fenerty and Rhiannon Davies from the Cancer Council for their continuous feedback and support in this study.

References

[1] Johnston A. C., Worrell J. L., Di Gangi P. M., and Wasko, M. 'Online health communities: An assessment of the influence of participation on patient empowerment outcomes'. *Information Technology & People*. 2013;**26**(2):213–235.

[2] Priharsari D., Abedin B., and Mastio E., 'Orchestrating firm sponsored communities of interest: A critical realist case study', *PACIS 2019 Proceedings. 32*. Association for Information Systems, Xi'an, China, June 2019.

[3] Beydoun G., Abedin B., Merigó J. M., and Vera M. 'Twenty years of information systems frontiers'. *Information Systems Frontiers*. 2019;**21**(2):485–494.

[4] Sillence E., Hardy C., and Briggs P. 'Why don't we trust health websites that help us help each other? An analysis of online peer-to-peer healthcare'. In: *Proceedings of the 5th Annual ACM Web Science Conference*. Paris, France. May 2013; pp. 396–404.

[5] Fox S., and Jones S. *The Social Life of Health Information*. Washington, DC: Pew Internet and American Life Project; 2009.

[6] Erfani S. S., and Abedin B. 'Impacts of the use of social network sites on users' psychological well-being: A systematic review'. *Journal of the Association for Information Science and Technology*. 2018; **69**(7):900–912.

[7] Webb M., Burns J., and Collin P. 'Providing online support for young people with mental health difficulties: Challenges and opportunities explored'. *Early Intervention in Psychiatry*. 2008;**2**(2):108–113.

[8] Erfani S. S., Abedin B., and Daneshgar F. 'A qualitative evaluation of communication in Ovarian Cancer Facebook communities'. *International Conference on Information Society (i-Society 2013)*. Toronto, Canada. June 2013; pp. 270–272.

[9] Erfani S. S., Abedin B., and Daneshgar F. 'Investigating the impact of Facebook use on cancer survivors' psychological well-being'. *19th Americas Conference on Information Systems (AMCIS)*. Association for Information Systems, Chicago, USA, 2013.

[10] Fan H., and Lederman R. 'Online health communities: How do community members build the trust required to adopt information and form close relationships?'. *European Journal of Information Systems*. 2018;**27**(1),62–89.

[11] Yan Z., Wang T., Chen Y., and Zhang H. 'Knowledge sharing in online health communities: A social exchange theory perspective'. *Information & Management*. 2016;**53**(5),643–653.

[12] Abedin B. 'Investigating the trend of non-task social interactions in online collaborative learning environments'. *44th Hawaii International Conference on System Sciences*. IEEE, Kauai, Hawaii, USA, 2011; pp. 1–8.

[13] Wainwright DW, Oates BJ, Edwards HM, and Childs S. 'Evidence-based information systems: A new perspective and a road map for research-informed practice'. *Journal of the Association for Information Systems*. 2018;**19**(11):1035–63.

[14] Butler B. S., Bateman P. J., Gray P. H., and Diamant E. I. 'An attraction-selection-attrition theory of online community size and resilience'. *MIS Quarterly*. 2014;**38**(3):699–728.

[15] Xing W., Goggins S., and Introne J. 'Quantifying the effect of informational support on membership retention in online communities through large-scale data analytics'. *Computers in Human Behavior*. 2018;**86**:227–234.

[16] Abedin B, Daneshgar F, and D'Ambra J. 'Underlying factors of sense of community in asynchronous computer supported collaborative learning environments'. *MERLOT Journal of Online Learning and Teaching*. 2010; **6**(3):585–596.

[17] Wasko M. M., and Faraj S. 'Why should I share? Examining social capital and knowledge contribution in electronic networks of practice'. *MIS Quarterly*. 2005;**29**:35–57.

[18] Devine P., and Lloyd K. 'Internet use and psychological wellbeing among 10-year-old and 11-year-old children'. *Child Care in Practice*. 2012; **18**(1):5–22.

[19] Erfani S. S., Blount Y., and Abedin B. 'The influence of health-specific social network site use on the psychological well-being of cancer-affected people'. *Journal of the American Medical Informatics Association*. 2016; **23**(3):467–476.

[20] Erfani S. S., Abedin B., and Blount Y. 'The effect of social network site use on the psychological well-being of cancer patients'. *Journal of the Association for Information Science and Technology*. 2017;**68**(5):1308–1322.

[21] Birks D. F., Fernandez W., Levina N., and Nasirin S. Grounded theory method in information systems research: its nature, diversity and opportunities. *European Journal of Information Systems*. 2013;**22**(1):1–8.

[22] Ghapanchi A. H., Ghapanchi A. R., Talaei-Khoei A., and Abedin B. 'A systematic review on information technology personnel's turnover'. *Lecture Notes on Software Engineering*. 2013;**1**(1):98.

[23] Abedin B., Babar A., and Abbasi A., 'Characterization of the use of social media in natural disasters: A systematic review'. *IEEE Fourth International Conference on Big Data and Cloud Computing*, IEEE, Sydney, Australia, December 2014; pp. 449–454.

[24] Blount Y., Abedin B., Vatanasakdakul S., and Erfani S. 'Integrating enterprise resource planning (SAP) in the accounting curriculum: a systematic literature review and case study'. *Accounting Education*. 2016;**25**(2): 185–202.

[25] Wiljer D., Urowitz S., Barbera L., *et al.* 'A qualitative study of an internet-based support group for women with sexual distress due to gynecologic cancer'. *Journal of Cancer Education*. 2011;**26**(3):451–458.

[26] Gill P. S., and Whisnant B. 'A qualitative assessment of an online support community for ovarian cancer patients'. *Patient Related Outcome Measures*. 2012, **3**(51):51–58.

[27] Fahy P. J. 'Addressing some common problems in transcript analysis'. *The International Review of Research in Open and Distributed Learning*. 2001;**1**(2):1–6.

[28] Meier A., Lyons E., Frydman G., Forlenza M., and Rimer, B. 'How cancer survivors provide support on cancer-related Internet mailing lists'. *Journal of Medical Internet Research*. 2007;**9**(2):e12.

[29] Zheng Q., Yao T., and Fan X. 'Improving customer well-being through two-way online social support'. *Journal of Service Theory and Practice*. 2016; **26**(2):179–202.

[30] Green M., Bobrowicz A., and Ang C. S. 'The lesbian, gay, bisexual and transgender community online: Discussions of bullying and self-disclosure in YouTube videos'. *Behaviour & Information Technology*. 2015;**34**(7):704–712.

[31] Abedin B, Daneshgar F, and D'Ambra J. 'Pattern of non-task interactions in asynchronous computer-supported collaborative learning courses'. *Interactive Learning Environments*. 2014;**22**(1):18–34.

[32] Abedin B., Erfani Sh., Milne D., Beattie A., and Fenerty K. 'Unpacking support types in online health communities: An application of attraction-selection-attrition theory'. *Pacific Asia Conference on Information Systems*. Association for Information Systems, Xi'an, China. 2019.

[33] Jefferson G., and Lee JRE. 'The rejection of advice: Managing the problematic convergence of a "troubles-telling" and a "service encounter"'. *Journal of Pragmatics*. 1981;**5**:399–422.

[34] Smithson J., Sharkey S., Hewis E. *et al.* 'Problem presentation and responses on an online forum for young people who self-harm'. *Discourse Studies*. 2011;**13**(4):487–501.

[35] Abedin B., and Babar A. 'Institutional vs. non-institutional use of social media during emergency response: A case of twitter in 2014 Australian bush fire'. *Information Systems Frontiers*. 2018;**20**(4):729–740.

Chapter 22

Business and legal framework for the exchange of mHealth data for aged care across countries

Koel Ghorai[1], Jan M. Smits[3], Maarten Kluitman[4] and Pradeep K. Ray[1,2]

22.1 Executive summary

Innovations in Information Technology has paved the way for easier and more efficient online health data sharing and transfer. However, this has also led to data oriented challenges around privacy, authentication and authorisation. While transfer of sensitive health as well as personal data between organizations and countries requires high level of protection and privacy, most people involved in business processes in the service industry, especially one as complex as healthcare, are generally oblivious of the legal responsibilities and implications of data privacy regulations. This chapter presents the legal and business analysis based on a use case that deals with exchange of mHealth data of an aged care facility across countries. A conceptual framework is developed for legal and business analysis that can be applied to analyse similar use cases. The conceptual framework involves three elements: actors, activities and impact of activities on factors such as risk, cost, quality and productivity. Actors can be classified as subjects, controllers, processors, third party or third country. They can be individuals or organisations. Activities can be categorised as goals, touch-points and resources. This framework is applied to legal and business analysis as summarised in the next two paragraphs.

The legal analysis involves two components: the evolving regulatory environment in the countries involved and their implications for the e-Authentication and e-Authorisation related to sensitive information of the AU2EU use cases in general. Sensitive information, also referred to as data in this chapter, have been classified as regulated data, confidential data and public data. These data may belong to individuals, organisations or government bodies.

[1]School of Public Health and Community Medicine, University of New South Wales, Sydney, Australia
[2]Centre for Entrepreneurship, University of Michigan-Shanghai Jiao Tong University, Shanghai, China
[3]Industrial Engineering & Innovation Sciences Department, Eindhoven University of Technology (TU/e), Eindhoven, The Netherlands
[4]PLM Architect, ASML, Eindhoven, The Netherlands

While the actors and activities relate to the handling of these different types of data, the impact mostly relates to the risk assessment and mitigation in the context of the specific use case.

The business analysis uses the conceptual framework to analyse in detail the value proposition for introducing an electronic platform with e-Authentication and e-Authorisation to replace an existing process. It compares the current situation (e.g. manual record handling) with the proposed e-Authentication and e-Authorisation strategy. The value proposition has been analysed mainly from the perspectives of cost, productivity and risk.

22.2 Conceptual frameworks

Online data sharing and transfer has become easier and more efficient than ever before, but at the same time this has brought about new challenges for the protection of personal data. Technology has transformed both the economy and social life and requires to further facilitate the free flow of data within the European Union and the transfer to third countries and international organisations while ensuring a high level of protection of personal data. The use of e-Authentication and e-Authorisation processes is of great importance in this regard.

To be able to map the e-Authentication and e-Authorisation requirements in the context of data sharing across organisations, a general conceptual framework involving a business process and its components has been developed. This framework will be used for analysing the business and legal aspects of a use case throughout this chapter.

22.2.1 Identifying business process components for e-Authentication and e-Authorisation

A business process is a set of logically related business activities that combine to deliver something of value (e.g. products, goods, services or information) to a customer. A business process can also be seen as a set of activities that create a value chain for an organisation and associate the value chain with the requirements of the subjects involved in the process. Thus, it is important to identify the various components of the process to be able to successfully understand and analyse the value chain and map it to the required level of e-Authentication and e-Authorisation.

To achieve this goal, a general business process model with its various components has been developed. The model provides three main concepts of a business process:

- Actors,
- Activity and
- Impact of activity on business process factors.

The model has been depicted in Figure 22.1.

Actors

An actor is a person or an organisation or a legal entity that can participate in an activity. Four types of actors have been identified in the business process model. For ease of the legal analysis, actors in the biosecurity use case have been identified

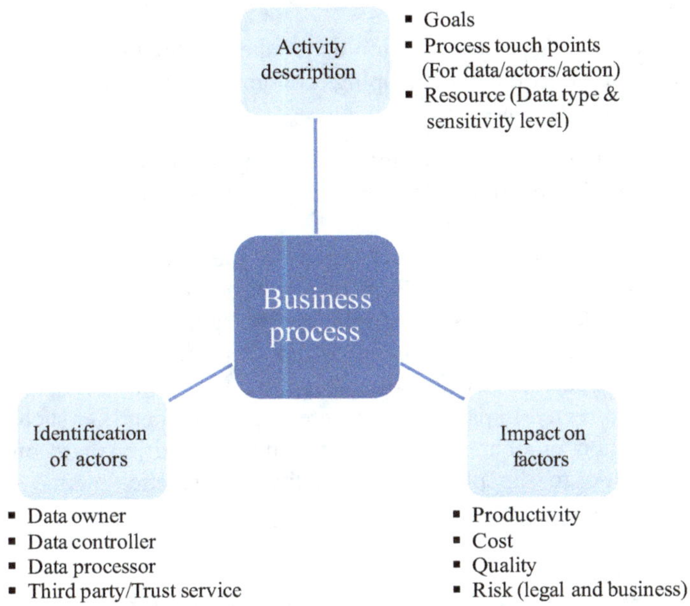

Figure 22.1 Business process model and its components

according to the following categories. However, the actors have been mapped as per Australian regulations and legislations.

- **Data subject**: A data subject is a natural person that can be identified, directly or indirectly, in particular by reference to an identifier, such as a name, an identification number, location data, to a unique identifier, or to one or more factors specific to the physical, physiological, genetic, mental, economic, cultural, social or gender identity of that person.
- **Data controller**: A data controller is a natural or legal person, public authority, agency or any other body which alone or jointly with others determines the purposes and means of the processing of personal data, where the purposes and means of processing are determined by European Union law or Member State law. The controller or the specific criteria for this nomination may be designated by Union law or by Member State law.
- **Data processor**: 'Processing' means any operation or set of operations which is performed upon personal data or sets of personal data, whether or not by automated means, such as collection, recording, organisation, structuring, storage, adaptation or alteration, retrieval, consultation, use, disclosure by transmission, dissemination or otherwise making available, alignment or combination, erasure or destruction. According to applicable laws, a data processor can be a legal person, a public authority, an agency or an electronic platform that carries out the operation or set of operations detailed under 'processing'.
- **Third party**: A third party is any natural or legal person, public authority, agency or any other body other than the data subject, the controller, the processor and the persons who, under the direct authority of the controller or the processor, are authorised to process the data.

Activity

An activity can be described as an action undertaken by the involved actors for the purpose of generating profits or developing economic opportunities. An activity has three main components. These are:

- **Goals**: Goals are the objectives for undertaking an activity.
- **Touch point**: Touch point describes all activities with involvement of the components (actors and their actions).
- **Resource (data)**: Resource is a component of the business process that can be shared physically or electronically between the actors. In this context, resource applies to any kind of data, most importantly, 'personal data', which can be defined as any information relating to an identified or identifiable natural person ('data subject'); an identifiable person is one who can be identified, directly or indirectly, in particular, by reference to an identifier such as a name, an identification number, location data, unique identifier or to one or more factors specific to the physical, physiological, genetic, mental, economic, cultural or social or gender identity of that person.

Impact on factors

Each business process has an impact on various factors that determine the growth of a business or an organisation. We have identified four factors that are impacted by a business process.

- **Productivity**: Productivity is a measure of the efficiency of a person or a process involved in an activity.
- **Cost**: A business process has a major impact on costs.
- **Quality**: Business processes are implemented to improve the quality of output of an organisation.
- **Risk**: In any business process, various kinds of risks are involved. Some of the risks in the context of e-Authorisation and e-Authentication can involve loss of or risk to privacy of personal data.

22.2.2 *Data type and assurance level*

In the context of e-Authentication and e-Authorisation, a business process involves exchange of data which can be personal, organisational, national as well as international. Whenever transaction of data is concerned, there are legal issues which are involved in the process. In order to map the data transactions to legal aspects, data have been categorised into three types according to the level of sensitivity. This will pave the way for mapping data to the legal framework later on in this chapter.

22.2.3 *Application of the business process model and AU2EU legal framework to use cases*

The legal framework (as mentioned in Table 22.2), in combination with the business process model (refer to Figure 22.1), can be used for analysing the use case for the AU2EU project mentioned later in this chapter. Analysis of the use case has been carried out using the following steps.

	Sensitivity	Assurance level	Examples	Requirements	Risks and access
Regulated data	High	High	Social Security Numbers, credit card numbers, bank accounts, driver's license, **health information**, donors, pseudonymous data	Protection of data is required by law or policy	High level of harm to reputation with financial costs, access for only those individuals with explicit authorisation, or designated for approved access. Information provides access to resources, physical or virtual
Confidential data	Medium	Substantial	Research details, library transactions, personnel information, information covered by non-disclosure agreements, financial information, contracts, facilities, management information	Contractual obligation to protect	Medium level of harm to reputation with financial costs, access for employees and non-employees who have a business need to know, delegated access privileges. Smaller subset of restricted data at a school, department or unit level
Public data	Low	Low	Directory information that is not suppressed, campus maps, web pages intended for public use, anonymous data	At the discretion of the data custodian	Low level risk to privacy and reputation and general public with a need to know

Figure 22.2 Types of data and level of sensitivity

Step 1: Identifying the actors and activities

- Identify actor: Actors of the use case have been identified as a 'data subject', 'data controller', 'data processor' or 'third party'.
- Identify resource: The resource, in this context, is data. It can be public, confidential or regulated data with varying levels of sensitivity associated with it (refer to Figure 22.2 for details).
- Identify action: In this context, the activity involves 'data sharing' and all processes associated with it.

Step 2: Validation of data sensitivity

Following the activity description, the level of sensitivity of the transferred data is validated, based on the content of the data. The data, which are exchanged between actors in the business process, are classified as having three levels of sensitivity, as portrayed in Figure 22.2. The three levels of sensitivity are low, medium and high.

Step 3: Identification and application of appropriate regulations for e-Authentication and e-Authorisation

The third step involves the identification and application of appropriate legislations and regulations. These regulations and legislations are specific to each country or union.

Step 4: Business and legal assessment of impact on factors

After the business process components are identified, the impact of the process on factors like productivity, cost, quality and risk (legal and business) will be analysed and presented in this chapter. Figure 22.3 presents a general overview of the business process and mapping of its components to the legal framework.

The above-combined framework has been used throughout the document for analysing the business as well as the legal aspects of the use case. Actors and activities for the use case have been identified and mapped to the framework. Since the use case focuses on e-Authorisation and e-Authentication of sensitive data, regulations and legislations related to electronic identification and trust services for electronic transactions have been considered. Regulations can vary from country to country.

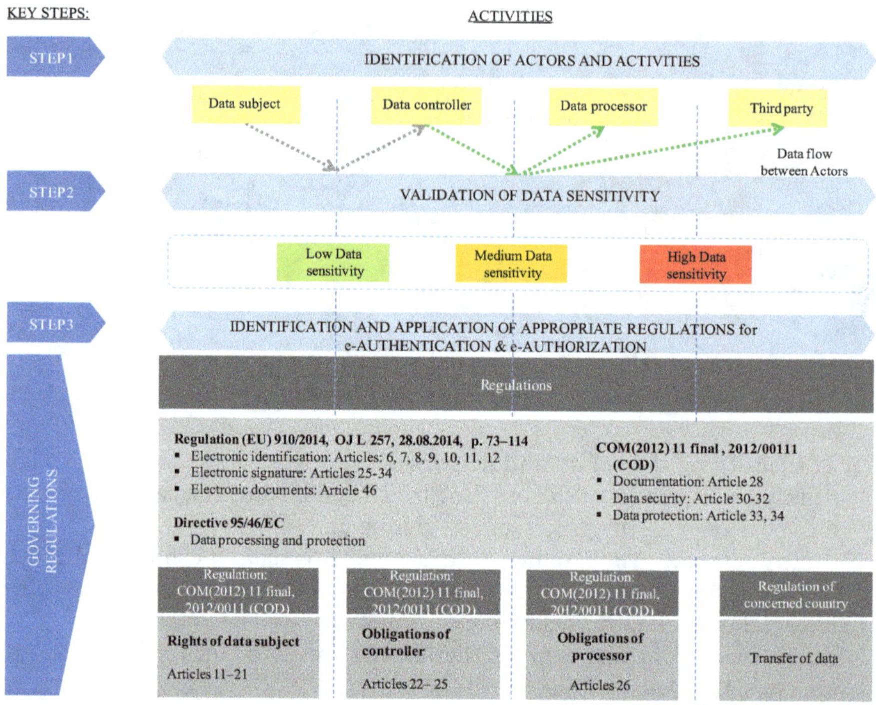

Figure 22.3 Combined business and legal (CBL) framework for e-Authentication and e-Authorisation

22.3 Regulatory framework for the AAL use case

The need for secure and trustworthy cross border online services is steadily on the rise. This need is catalysed by mobility on one hand and flexibility of citizens and businesses on the other. Technological transition is further helping the establishment of digital economies and administrations.

The Digital Agenda for Europe [1] identifies existing barriers to Europe's digital development and proposes legislation on e-Signatures (Key Action 3) and the mutual recognition of e-Identification and authentication (Key Action 16), establishing a clear legal framework so as to eliminate fragmentation and the lack of interoperability, enhance digital citizenship and prevent cybercrime [1].

22.3.1 European approach towards e-Signatures

22.3.1.1 Market fragmentation

According to CROBIES study [2], the European harmonisation brought about by the e-Signatures Directive is imperfect and incomplete, resulting in market fragmentation. Some of the main problems identified include

- Different interpretations of the current Directives leading to cross-border interoperability problems.

- Outdated standards leading to a highly complex standardisation framework.
- Vague Directive on supervision obligations leading to a lack of trust as the effectiveness of supervision regimes is unclear.

22.3.1.2 Interoperability challenges

The usage of electronic identification is stunted by use of different technological solutions leading to interoperability issues. This can also lead to difficulty in exchanging electronically signed documents across organisations as well as across member states/countries with differing regulations and standards.

22.3.1.3 Reliability check

There is no framework of reference for determining the reliability of the entity that issued the electronic identification, the legal certainty on the cross-border use of electronic identification or a clear liability for the correctness of the ID when it is used as electronic representation of a person. It is currently almost impossible for users to use a single electronic identification for accessing cross-border online services. Additionally, electronic identification can be issued by private or public sector parties and may be issued for a specific sector such as e-Banking, eHealth, etc. The absence of a general framework for electronic identification and authentication for recognition and acceptance of the electronic identification outside its context makes it hard, mostly due to liability and data protection challenges.

22.3.1.4 High costs for cross-border legal compliance

Lack of a common European framework can lead to problems such as incurring high costs by related trust service providers for ensuring technical compliance with the rules of the country of destination and obtain guarantees with respect to trustworthiness of foreign electronic identification, authentication and signature tools.

Legislation ensuring the mutual recognition of electronic identification and authentication across the EU and review of the Directive on Electronic Signatures [3] is also a key action in the Single Market Act for the realisation of the digital single market. The roadmap for stability and growth underlines the key role for the development of the digital economy of the future common legal framework for the mutual recognition and acceptance of electronic identification and authentication across borders.

The proposed legal framework, consisting of a ‘Regulation of the European Parliament and of the Council on electronic identification and trust services for electronic transactions in the internal market’ [4], seeks to enable secure and seamless electronic interactions between businesses, citizens and public authorities, thereby increasing the effectiveness of public and private online services, e-business and electronic commerce in the EU.

The existing EU legislation, namely Directive 1999/93/EC on a ‘Community framework for electronic signatures’, essentially covers electronic signatures only. There is no comprehensive EU cross-border and cross-sector framework for secure, trustworthy and easy-to-use electronic transactions that encompasses electronic identification, authentication and signatures. Please refer to the keywords and definitions in Table 22.1.

Table 22.1. Keywords with definitions

Keywords	Definitions
Electronic authentication	An electronic process that allows the validation of the electronic identification of a natural or legal person; or of the origin and integrity of an electronic data
Electronic identification	The process of using person identification data in electronic form unambiguously representing a natural or legal person
Signatory	A natural person who creates an electronic signature
Electronic signature	Data in electronic form which are attached to or logically associated with other electronic data and which are used by the signatory to sign.
Trust service provider	A natural or a legal person who provides one or more trust services
Trust service	Any electronic service consisting in the creation, verification, validation, handling and preservation of electronic signatures, electronic seals, electronic time stamps, electronic documents, electronic delivery services, website authentication and electronic certificates, including certificates for electronic signature and electronic seals
Data subject	An identifiable person who can be identified, directly or indirectly, in particular by reference to an identifier such as a name, an identification number, location data, unique identifier or to one or more factors specific to the physical, physiological, genetic, mental, economic, cultural or social or gender identity of that person
Representative	Any natural or legal person established in the Union who, explicitly designated by the controller, represents the controller with regard to the obligations of the controller under this Regulation
Processor	A natural or legal person, public authority, agency or any other body which processes personal data on behalf of the controller
Controller	The natural or legal person, public authority, agency or any other body which alone or jointly with others determines the purposes and means of the processing of personal data, where the purposes and means of processing are determined by Union law or Member State law, the controller or the specific criteria for his nomination may be designated by Union law or by Member State law
Third party	Any natural or legal person, public authority, agency or any other body other than the data subject, the controller, the processor and the persons who, under the direct authority of the controller or the processor, are authorised to process the data
Third country	Any country outside of the EU either under EU Commission decision as a country that has equivalent data protection or, under an agreement dictated by Safe Harbour Principles
Electronic delivery service	A service that makes it possible to transmit data by electronic means and provides evidence relating to the handling of the transmitted data, including proof of sending or receiving the data, and which protects transmitted data against the risk of loss, theft, damage or any unauthorised alterations
Processing	Any operation or set of operations which is performed upon personal data or sets of personal data, whether or not by automated means, such as collection, recording, organisation, structuring, storage, adaptation or alteration, retrieval, consultation, use, disclosure by

(Continues)

Table 22.1. (Continued)

Keywords	Definitions
	transmission, dissemination or otherwise making available, alignment or combination, erasure or destruction
Personal data	Any information relating to an identified or identifiable natural person ('data subject'); an identifiable person is one who can be identified, directly or indirectly, in particular by reference to an identifier such as a name, an identification number, location data, unique identifier or to one or more factors specific to the physical, physiological, genetic, mental, economic, cultural or social or gender identity of that person
Validation data	Data which are used to validate an electronic signature or an electronic seal
Product	Hardware or software, or relevant components thereof, which are intended to be used for the provision of trust services
Personal data	Any information relating to an identified or identifiable natural person ('data subject'); an identifiable person is one who can be identified, directly or indirectly, in particular by reference to an identifier such as a name, an identification number, location data, unique identifier or to one or more factors specific to the physical, physiological, genetic, mental, economic, cultural or social or gender identity of that person
Anonymous data	Anonymous data is defined as information that does not relate to an identified or identifiable natural person
Pseudonymous data	'Pseudonymous data' means personal data that cannot be attributed to a specific data subject without the use of additional information, as long as such additional information is kept separately and subject to technical and organisational measures to ensure non-attribution
Encrypted data	'Encrypted data' means personal data, which through technological protection measures is rendered unintelligible to any person who is not authorised to access it
Processing	'Processing' means any operation or set of operations which is performed upon personal data or sets of personal data, whether or not by automated means, such as collection, recording, organisation, structuring, storage, adaptation or alteration, retrieval, consultation, use, disclosure by transmission, dissemination or otherwise making available, alignment or combination, erasure or destruction
Profiling	'Profiling' means any form of automated processing of personal data intended to evaluate certain personal aspects relating to a natural person or to analyse or predict in particular that natural person's performance at work, economic situation, location, health, personal preferences, reliability or behaviour
Recipient	'Recipient' means a natural or legal person, public authority, agency or any other body to which the personal data are disclosed
Genetic data	'Genetic data' means all personal data relating to the genetic characteristics of an individual which have been inherited or acquired as they result from an analysis of a biological sample from the individual in question, in particular by chromosomal, deoxyribonucleic acid (DNA) or ribonucleic acid (RNA) analysis or analysis of any other element enabling equivalent information to be obtained
Biometric data	'Biometric data' means any personal data relating to the physical, physiological or behavioural characteristics of an individual which allow their unique identification, such as facial images, or dactyloscopic data

(Continues)

Table 22.1. (*Continued*)

Keywords	Definitions
Data concerning health	'Data concerning health' means any personal data which relates to the physical or mental health of an individual, or the provision of health services to the individual

The aim is to enhance existing legislation and to expand it to cover the mutual recognition and acceptance at EU level of notified electronic identification schemes and other essential related electronic trust services. Table 22.2 summarises the EU policy approach towards e-Signatures, e-Authentication as well as e-Identification [5].

e-Signatures transpose the rich semantics of handwritten signatures into the electronic world. Because a signature is a symbolic representation of an individual, the keystone of the e-Signature Directive is a strong intertwining between electronic signatures, authentication and identification. E-Signature is defined as data in electronic form logically associated with other electronic data, which in turn serves as a method of authentication. An 'advanced' signature is an e-Signature capable of identifying the signatory. The intertwining is reinforced by the reliance of e-Signature and e-Identification on the same technology.

New rules are proposed to enable cross-border and secure electronic transactions in Europe. The Regulation on electronic identification and trust services for electronic transactions in the internal market was adopted by the Commission in June 2012. On 3rd April 2014, the European Parliament adopted its position at first reading and communicated it to the Council for approval and adoption by the co-legislators [6].

Electronic identification (e-ID) and electronic trust services (e-TS – namely electronic signatures, electronic seals, time stamp, electronic delivery service and website authentication) are inseparable by essence when analysing the requirements needed to ensure legal certainty, trust and security in electronic transactions.

In this regard, the draft regulation proposes to:

- ensure that people and businesses can use their own national electronic identification schemes (e-IDs) to access public services in other EU countries where e-IDs are available.
- create a European internal market for e-TS by ensuring that they will work across borders and have the same legal status as traditional paper-based processes. Only by providing certainty on the legal validity of all these services, businesses and citizens will use the digital interactions as their natural way of interaction.

e-ID and e-TS, both elements of the Regulation, will create a predictable regulatory environment to enable secure and seamless electronic interactions between businesses, citizens and public authorities. This will increase the effectiveness of public and private online services, e-Business and electronic commerce in the EU.

An Action Plan on e-Signatures and e-Identification has been adopted in 2008 with the aim to remove interoperability barriers.

22.3.2 Legal keywords and definitions

For the purposes of the legal analysis of the case studies, the following keywords have been shortlisted from various EU legal documents. These keywords have been defined and later categorised and mapped to the respective Regulations. For the full list of keywords and definitions, refer to (Table 22.1).

22.3.3 Identifying and mapping legal actors to corresponding roles and regulations: legal framework

With the introduction of evolving new technologies in the electronic space, online and electronic services will soon be integrated into all kinds of service delivery, be it for government or private organisations. Electronic delivery has the potential to underpin all other delivery channels, providing consistent services within as well as across borders. The legal framework will provide guidance to government and private agencies, sectors as well as jurisdictions in authenticating the identity of a party to a needed or desired level of acceptance and confidence, notably aimed at (public) eHealth issues.

22.3.3.1 Legal framework

Objectives

Objectives of the framework:

- To ensure that approaches to e-Authentication of identity and e-Authorisation balance the underlying risk with the need for ease of use on behalf of both parties;
- To enhance confidence of parties (government or private) in electronic dealings;
- To provide consistency in processes for e-Authentication and e-Authorisation of identity in order to increase efficiency;
- Maximise the ease-of-use for all parties involved in terms of e-Authentication and e-Authorisation processes;
- To provide agencies with the tools to determine the most appropriate approach to the e-Authentication of identity and e-Authorisation and
- To ensure application of due diligence when determining authentication and authorisation approaches.

Table 22.2. Mapping of actors to roles and regulations

Actors	Rights/responsibilities	Associated regulation
Data subject	The rights include: • The provision of clear and easily understandable information regarding the processing of his or her personal data • The right of access, rectification and erasure ('right to be forgotten') of their data • The right to obtain data • The right to object to profiling • The right to lodge a complaint with the competent data protection authority and to bring legal proceedings • The right to compensation and damages resulting from an unlawful processing operation • The right to data portability	**As per Regulation (EU) 910/2014, OJ L 257, 28.08.2014, pp. 73–114** • Electronic identification: Articles 6–12 • Electronic signature: Articles 25–34 • Electronic documents: Article 46 **As per COM(2012) 11 final, 2012/0011 (COD)** • Data protection: Article 23 • Data security: Article 30
Data controller	The controller shall adopt appropriate policies and implement appropriate and demonstrable technical and organisational measures to ensure and be able to demonstrate in a transparent manner that the processing of personal data is performed in compliance with this Regulation, having regard to the state of the art, the nature of personal data processing, the context, scope and purposes of the processing, the risks for the rights and freedoms of the data subjects and the type of the organisation, both at the time of the determination of the means for processing and at the time of the processing itself: • The controller shall be able to demonstrate the adequacy and effectiveness of the measures	**As per COM(2012) 11 final, 2012/0011 (COD)** • Controller: Articles 22–24 **As per COM(2012) 238 final, 2012/0146 (COD)** • Electronic identification: Articles 5–8 • Electronic signature: Articles 20–27 • Electronic documents: Article 34 • Data protection: Article 23 • Data security: Article 30

(Continues)

	• The controller shall have the right to transmit personal data inside the Union within the group of undertakings the controller is part of, where such processing is necessary for legitimate internal administrative purposes between connected business areas of the group of undertakings and an adequate level of data protection as well as the interests of the data subjects are safeguarded by internal data protection provisions or equivalent codes of conduct as referred to in Article 38	
Data processor	• Where processing is to be carried out on behalf of a controller, the controller shall choose a processor providing sufficient guarantees to implement appropriate technical and organisational measures and procedures in such a way that the processing will meet the requirements of this Regulation and ensure the protection of the rights of the data subject, in particular in respect of the technical security measures and organisational measures governing the processing to be carried out and shall ensure compliance with those measures • The carrying out of processing by a processor shall be governed by a contract or other legal act binding the processor to the controller. The controller and the processor shall be free to determine respective roles and tasks with respect to the requirements of this Regulation, and shall provide that the processor shall: (a) Process personal data only on instructions from the controller, unless otherwise required by Union law or Member State law (b) Employ only staff who have committed themselves to confidentiality or are under a statutory obligation of confidentiality (c) Take all required measures pursuant to Article 30 (d) Determine the conditions for enlisting another processor only with the prior permission of the controller, unless otherwise determined	**As per COM(2012) 11 final, 2012/0011 (COD)** • Processor: Articles 26–29 **As per COM(2012) 238 final, 2012/0146 (COD)** • Electronic identification: Articles 5–8 • Electronic signature: Articles 20–27 • Electronic documents: Article 34 • Data protection: Article 23 • Data security: Article 30

(Continues)

Table 22.2. (*Continued*)

Actors	Rights/responsibilities	Associated regulation
	(e) Insofar as this is possible given the nature of the processing, create in agreement with the controller the appropriate and relevant technical and organisational requirements for the fulfilment of the controller's obligation to respond to requests for exercising the data as per subject's rights laid down in Chapter II (f) Assist the controller in ensuring compliance with the obligations pursuant to Articles 30–34 (g) Return all results to the controller after the end of the processing, not process the personal data otherwise and delete existing copies unless Union or Member State law requires storage of the data (h) Make available to the controller all information necessary to demonstrate compliance with the obligations laid down in this Article and allow on-site inspections • The controller and the processor shall document in writing the controller's instructions and the processor's obligations • If a processor processes personal data other than as instructed by the controller or becomes the determining party in relation to the purposes and means of data processing, the processor shall be considered to be a controller in respect of that processing and shall be subject to the rules on joint controllers laid down in Article 24	
Third party	Any party that does not have access to (personal) data except on the basis of either a public legal obligation or a contract between authorised parties	**As per COM(2012) 238 final, 2012/0146 (COD)** • Electronic identification: Articles 5–8 • Electronic signature: Articles 20–27 • Electronic documents: Article 34 • Data protection: Article 23 • Data security: Article 30

22.4 Use case: eHealth/ambient-assisted living

22.4.1 Use case: ambient assisted living (AAL) efficient care coordination

22.4.1.1 Business analysis

Situational analysis

The care coordinator at the HEC provides tele-care and AAL services to home-based patients. The care coordinator has to respond whenever a patient explicitly (by pushing an emergency button) or implicitly (via an alert notification of the AAL-system) requests a home/health-care service. He is then obliged to provide third party home and health care services (e.g. nursing, first aid, medical services, etc.). The care coordinator does so by selecting a third party home/health-care service provider who dispatches a mobile care giver (CG) based on availability and circumstances. The current 'care coordination process' is described below, and has been compared with a new process where the e-Authentication and e-Authorisation platform has been implemented.

- *As-Is Process*

  In the as-is process (as depicted in Figure 22.4), the patient presses the home emergency call button. The HEC operator gets notified of the emergency service request through a message pop-up on his/her computer screen and can see all the patient information on various pages of the customer profile as stored on the database. The operator contacts the customer via the home emergency call system in order to assess the customer's actual situation and status. Depending on the individual case, the operator determines/delegates a dedicated third party home/healthcare service provider (or any pre-registered caregiver with that customer) in order to take care of the customer. The operator informs the care giver by phone and passes on customer details necessary for the required care action, including address as well as highly sensitive health information. The HEC keeps protocol of names and mobile numbers of caregivers.

  The CG then goes to the customer's house and presses the home emergency call button to inform the HEC that they have reached the venue. After the CG provides the service, he/she presses the home emergency call button for the second time to inform HEC of the successful provision of the service. Except for ambulance drivers, no other CGs update any patient information to the HEC. Ambulance drivers submit a paper document including the customer name, cost and reason of attendance, afterwards. This document is neither scanned nor uploaded to the database and is physically stored for 3 years (Figure 22.4).
- *To-Be Process*

In the new process, the e-Authentication and e-Authorisation platform is adopted in order to provide the care giver with the necessary and relevant AAL customer data on a mobile device via a secured channel. Figure 22.5 shows the new AAL care coordination process employed by the DRK HEC. So when the

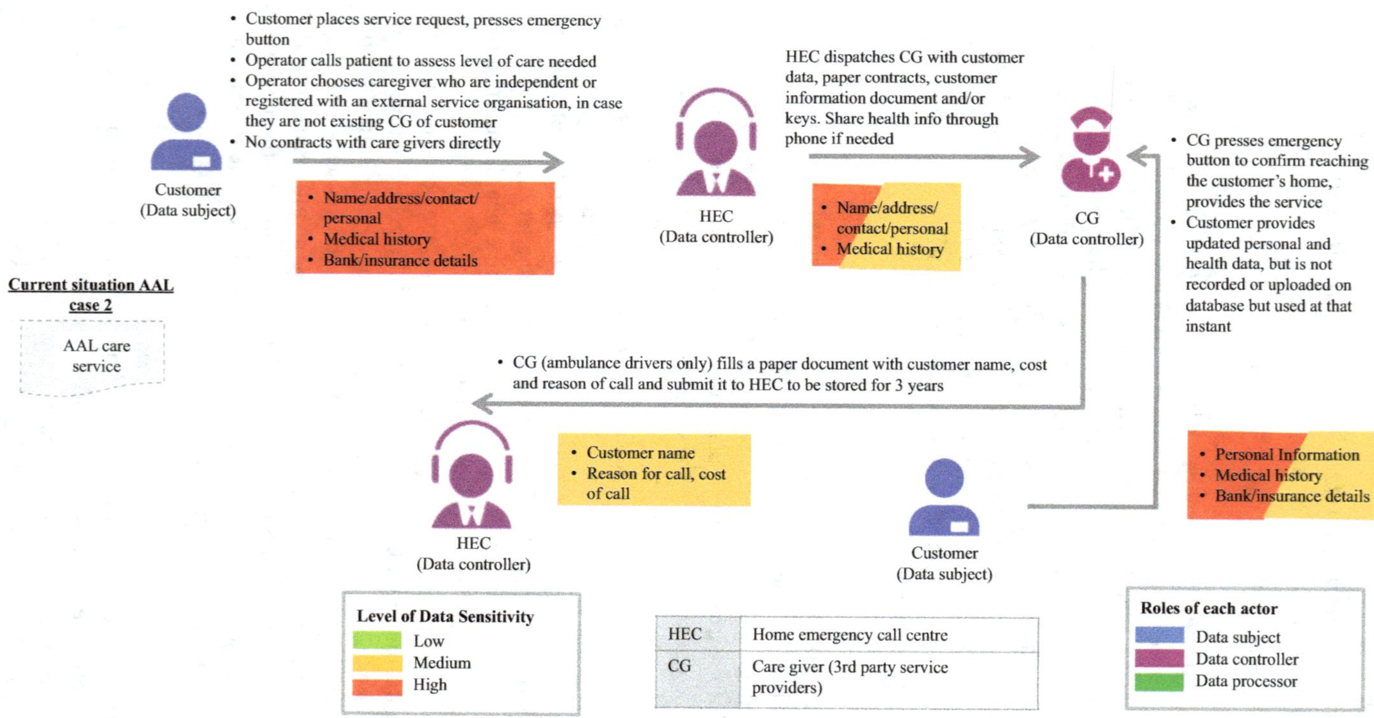

Figure 22.4 AAL case 2 As-Is process mapping

third party home/healthcare service provider dispatches a mobile care giver, most of the times, the care giver does not have to physically appear at the care coordinator's location since the customer data are accessible on his mobile device directly. However, only when the patient is unable to open the door, the care giver might have to go via the HEC since he still has to pick up the patient's home key. Additionally, Table 22.3 provides an overview of the roles the actors play in relation to the handling of data.

To establish a secure connection between care coordinators' patient database and care giver, the care coordinator first has to obtain connection details of the care giver from the third party home/health-care service provider as well as appropriate identification mechanisms that identify the request from the care coordinator to the care giver as valid. Thus, some type of authentication credential has to be obtained from the care provider and presented to the care giver. Then, the care giver is granted access to the patient's data for a limited amount of time, that is, after the completion of the assignment the access to the patient's data records is revoked. The access to the data is controlled by the AU2EU e-Authentication/e-Authorisation platform. Optionally, the data retrieved via the AU2EU e-Authentication/e-Authorisation platform is updated with data from external data sources (e.g. hospitals for medical records and the municipality for housing and general contact details) every time care is requested.

Impact on factors that drive business process management

The AAL use case presents the process of providing third party care givers with remote access to sensitive customer data content-wise and time-wise using the AU2EU e-Authentication/e-Authorisation platform to control the access and secure the data exchanged. The use of the platform will have an impact on productivity, cost, quality and risk.

Productivity/cost: In most cases, the care giver does not need to physically appear at the care coordinator's location since the customer data are accessible on the care giver's mobile device directly. This will save time and money. Moreover, the AU2EU e-Authentication/e-Authorisation platform will allow organisations and customers to communicate and collaborate more efficiently and effectively. In the end, the AU2EU e-Authentication/e-Authorisation platform will help to deliver high-quality healthcare at a lower cost.

Quality: The AU2EU e-Authentication/e-Authorisation platform will allow care givers across different organisations to collaborate more closely with each other and with customers. This makes it easier to maintain customer relationships and to work closely with customers to ensure that the quality of treatment is maintained. Moreover, the collection of data and subsequent analysis will enhance clinical decision making by professionals. Also it will enable customers to take a more active role in managing their personal health. All this is expected to have a positive impact on the service quality.

Risk: Security is of major importance whenever health data is concerned. Maintaining paper documentation of highly sensitive personal data of customers

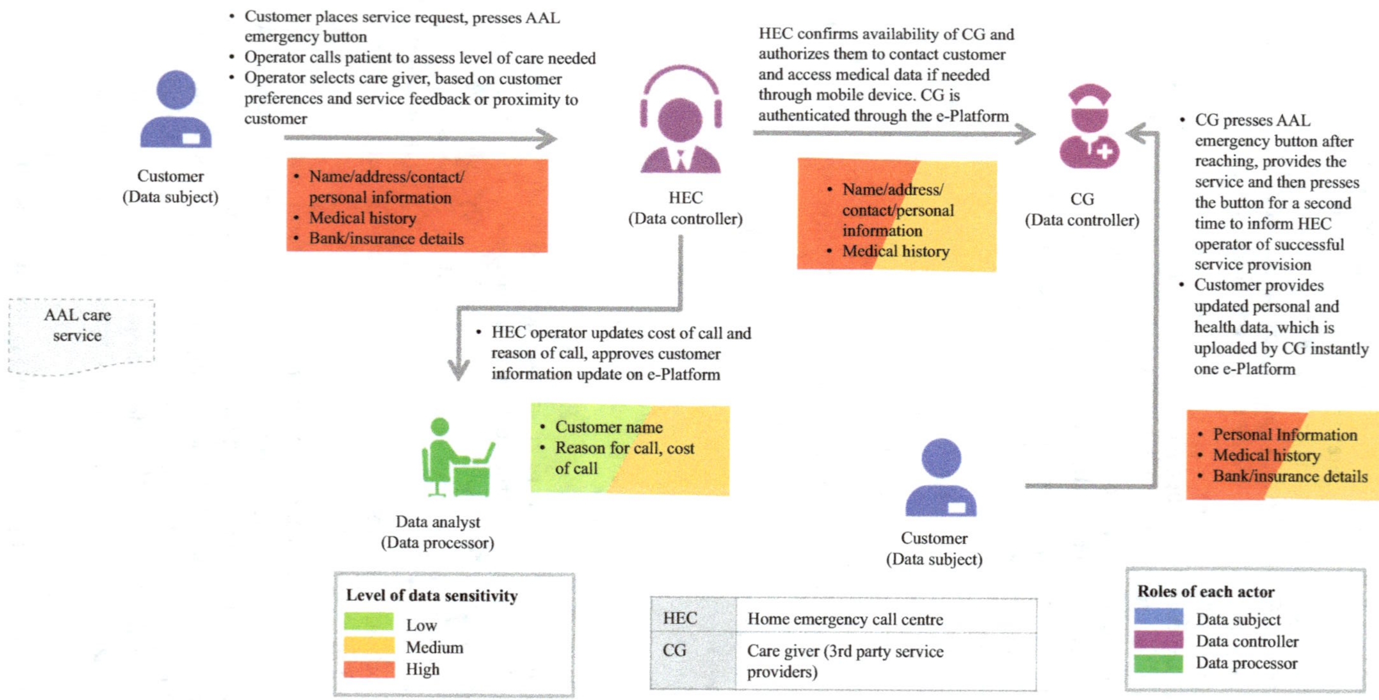

Figure 22.5 AAL case 2 new scenario

Table 22.3. Actors' data role

Sr. no	Actors	Data owner	Data controller	Data processor
1	Customer/patient	x		
2	Care giver		x	x
3	AU2EU e-Authentication/ e-Authorisation platform			x
4	External data sources		x	x
5	AAL service provider		x	x

can raise serious concerns related to data protection and data security risks. An electronic platform can replace paper-based processes and make the transaction and data sharing more secure and protected through adequate e-Authentication and e-Authorisation procedures. In addition to this, the AU2EU e-Authentication/ e-Authorisation platform also provides improved transparency, increased visibility and allows identification of the legally responsible person in the process.

Value proposition

The implementation of the AU2EU e-Authentication/e-Authorisation platform will provide some major advantages in the care coordination process when comparing it to the current process of physically collecting and delivering the customer's data by the care giver.

- **Increased practice efficiencies and cost savings**: With the AU2EU e-Authentication/e-Authorisation platform, the patient is provided with a quicker response to his help requests. This is valuable for patients since they don't have to plan ahead as much, especially in critical situations where a quick response is required for a patient's safety and health. Moreover, future cost reductions can be expected since the AU2EU e-Authentication/ e-Authorisation platform will allow home/health-care organisations and customers to communicate and collaborate more efficiently and effectively.
- **Improved security**: The e-Authentication and e-Authorisation platform provides better ways to safeguard and secure the customer's personal information. In the as-is process, HEC operator provides highly sensitive customer data including medical information over the phone without proper authentication checks or authorisation of care givers. With the AU2EU e-Authentication/ e-Authorisation platform, the care giver is legally authenticated and authorised to access patient data. It creates transparency and patient update can be traced back. Additionally, the AU2EU e-Authentication/e-Authorisation platform allows the patient's data to be treated confidential since no physical copy of the patient's data has to be made. The data are solely and temporarily obtained by the care giver and properly secured by means of e-Authentication and e-Authorisation mechanisms.

Other opportunities for value creation

- Selling anonymised data/statistics/benchmarks to:
  - Healthcare solution providers,
  - Research organisations and
  - Government (policy-making).
- Use data/statistics/benchmarks to optimise business processes and services (internal/external: consultancy):
  - Personalised health care,
  - More active role for customers to manage their personal health records,
  - Enhance clinical decision making,
  - Measure and improve customer service,
  - Measure and improve business processes,
  - Enhance services and
  - Drive sales and marketing.

22.4.1.2 Legal analysis

Mapping actors to regulations for rights and obligations:

In the AAL use case, actors have been categorised into data subjects, data controllers and data processors. The customer or patient is the data subject. Data

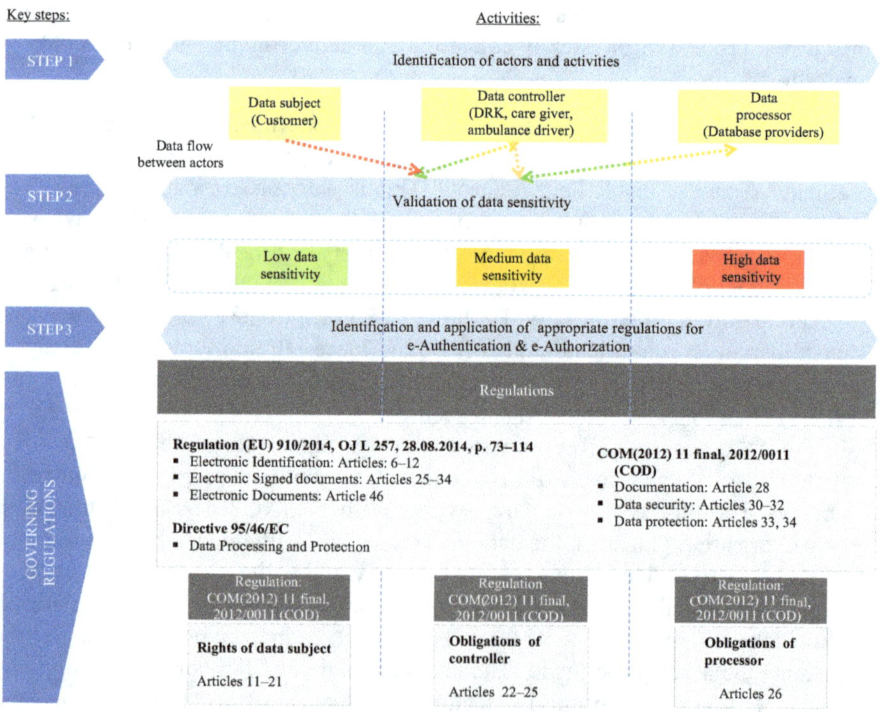

Figure 22.6 AAL use case 2 – Mapping actors to rights and obligations

subjects have rights and responsibilities. These have been mapped to the regulations in Figure 22.6. The DRK HEC operator, who receives the call from the patient, is considered as a data controller since the operator is an employee of DRK HEC. The care giver in this scenario is considered as a data controller since they are assigned by DRK for their services. Thus, all the three categories of actors are bound by specific regulations (Figure 22.6). The database service provider, which is hired by DRK HEC, is the data processor.

All the actors in this use case are governed by regulations and legislations which are portrayed in Figure 22.6. These regulations are exclusive to data protection. The legislations and regulations applicable to the data subject involve articles on electronic identification, electronic signatures, electronic documents, data protection and data security. Refer to Regulation (EU) No 910/2014 of the European Parliament and of the Council of 23 July 2014 on electronic identification and trust services for electronic transactions in the internal market and repealing Directive 1999/93/EC for more details on the governing legislations. Additionally, data controllers and data processors are governed by the same regulation. However, the regulation clearly mentions the different obligations and rights of each actor.

22.5 Conclusion

Business and legal analysis of the use case brought to the forefront the impact of e-Authentication and e-Authorisation platform on a business process. The biggest impact was in the form of risk reduction through the AU2EU e-Authentication/e-Authorisation platform. This combined business and legal framework will provide guidance to organizations in identifying the responsibilities and liabilities of the parties involved in a business process, notably aimed at public health data exchange related issues. The framework presented in this chapter has some noteworthy contributions provided below

1. Ensure that approaches to electronic data privacy and security balance the underlying risk with the need for ease of use on behalf of all parties involved,
2. Enhance confidence of parties (government or private) in electronic data dealings,
3. Provide consistency in processes for electronic data security and privacy through authentication and authorization in order to increase efficiency,
4. Provide agencies with the tools to determine the most appropriate approach to the data privacy and security in a business process
5. Ensure application of due diligence when determining authentication and authorization approaches.

Acknowledgement

This work was partly supported by the European Union Project Authentication and Authorisation for Entrusted Unions (AU2EU) as part of https://cordis.europa.eu/programme/id/FP7-ICT/en and Grant agreement ID: 611659 from December 2013 to November 2015.

References

[1] Digital agenda for Europe. [Online]. Available from http://ec.europa.eu/digital-agenda/digital-agenda-europe [Accessed 27 Aug 2014].
[2] Study on cross-border interoperability of e-Signatures. [Online]. Available from https://ec.europa.eu/digital-agenda/en/news/crobies-study-cross-border-interoperability-esignatures-2010 [Accessed 2 Jun 2014].
[3] Directive 1999/93/EC on a 'Community framework for electronic signatures'.
[4] Proposal for a regulation of the European Parliament and of the Council on electronic identification and trust services for electronic transactions in the internal market. [Online]. Available from http://eur-lex.europa.eu/LexUriServ/LexUriServ.do?uri=COM:2012:0238:FIN:en:PDF [Accessed 27 Aug 2014].
[5] See http://ec.europa.eu/digital-agenda/en/trust-services-and-eid [Online]. Available from http://ec.europa.eu/digital-agenda/en/trust-services-and-eid [Accessed 22 Aug 2014].
[6] Regulation (EU) 910/2014, OJ L 257, 28.08.2014, pp. 73–114 on electronic identification and trust services for electronic transactions in the internal market and repealing Directive 1999/93/EC.

Chapter 23

Applications of machine learning techniques in the diagnosis of Parkinson's disease: promises and challenges

Farhan Mohammed[1], Xiangjian He[2] and Yiguang Lin[3]

Parkinson's disease (PD) is the second most common neurodegenerative disorder, after Alzheimer's disease, affecting approximately 1% of the population aged 55 or older. Major symptoms of PD include tremor, bradykinesia and freezing of gait. The precise diagnosis of PD, at its early stages, remains a challenge for modern clinicians. The difficulty to differentiate PD from other neurodegenerative disorders is high due to the similarity of symptoms with other disorders. Although clinical diagnosis primarily rests on the presence of typical clinical manifestations such as bradykinesia, tremor and other cardinal motor features, PD is associated with a plethora of non-motor symptoms adding to its overall disability.

Recent research into early diagnosis of PD has taken advantage of technological advancements in machine learning. In the stream of applying machine learning for data analysis, several studies have been shown to accurately diagnose PD patients using striatal binding ratio (SBR) values. Furthermore, with deep learning techniques, several neuroimaging modalities, such as single photon emission computed tomography (SPECT) and positron emission tomography (PET), have aided early and differential diagnosis of PD. In this chapter, we will shed some light upon relevant machine learning algorithms, their limitations and advantages, and provide new insights on how machine learning techniques can be potentially and clinically utilised in contributing to the ongoing PD diagnostic research and practice.

23.1 Introduction

Parkinson's disease (PD) is chronic and progressive movement disorder, meaning that symptoms continue and worsen over time. Approximately ten million people

[1]Faculty of Engineering and IT, University of Technology Sydney, Australia
[2]Global Big Data Technologies Center, University of Technology Sydney, Australia
[3]School of Life Sciences, University of Technology Sydney, Australia

worldwide are living with PD. In regard to China and its belt and road region, PD is predominant in the elderly population as China has the largest elderly population [1,2]. PD mortality rate in China is also quite high. Standard mortality ratio (SMR) is the most frequently used index in PD survival survey. It was seen that, from a 10-year follow-up study, the SMR of PD patients in China is 0.87 (95% confidence interval [CI] 0.59–1.25) [3].

The cause for PD is unknown, and there is presently no cure. All current treatment options, such as medication and surgery, aim at the management of symptoms only. Patho-physiologically, PD involves the malfunction and death of vital nerve cells in the basal ganglia of the brain. These dying neurons produce dopamine, a neurotransmitter that controls movement and coordination. As PD progresses, the amount of dopamine produced in the brain decreases, leading to difficulty in controlling movement normally [4].

PD occurs mostly in the ages of 50 and above and it is difficult to identify in the earlier stages. It is primarily characterised by the cardinal motor impairments like rigidity, tremor and bradykinesia. Tremor is the well-known symptom of PD and it results in an automatic shaking movement of the body, arm, lip and hands. The other symptom is rigidity, that is, the stiffness of muscle. Some other symptoms include problems with walking and slowness of movements. The drug levodopa is used at the early stages of the disease. When the disease worsens, the side effects also increases enormously. When the drugs become ineffective, surgical treatment is the only alternative. Therefore, the diagnosis of PD at an earlier stage is important for improving the quality of patient's life [5].

PD impacts people in many different ways. Not everyone will experience all of the symptoms of PD, and if they do, the patients will not necessarily experience the symptoms in quite the same order, or at the same level of intensity. Even so, there are typical patterns of progression in PD that are defined in stages. PD is classified into five different stages described below as follows.

- Stage One. During this initial stage, the person has mild symptoms that generally do not interfere with daily activities. Tremor and other movement symptoms occur on one side of the body only. Friends and family may notice changes in posture, walking and facial expressions.
- Stage Two. In this stage, the symptoms begin to worsen. Tremor, rigidity and other movement symptoms affect both sides of the body. Walking problems and poor posture may become apparent. In this stage, the person is still able to live alone, but completing day-to-day tasks becomes more difficult and may take longer.
- Stage Three. This stage is considered the mid-stage in the progression of the disease. Loss of balance and slowness of movements are hallmarks of this phase. Falls are more common. Though the patient is still fully independent, symptoms significantly impair activities of daily living such as dressing and eating.
- Stage Four. During this stage, symptoms are severe and limits the bodily movement of the person. It is possible to stand without assistance, but movement may require a walker. The patient needs help with activities of daily living and is unable to live alone.

- Stage Five. This is the most advanced and debilitating stage of PD. Stiffness in the legs may make it impossible to stand or walk. The person requires a wheelchair or is bedridden. Around-the-clock nursing care is required for all activities. The person may experience hallucinations and delusions [6].

The precise diagnosis of PD, at its early stages, has enormous challenges for medical doctors as there are currently no laboratory tests that have been proven to be useful in diagnosing PD. Particularly in early stages, the disease can be difficult to diagnose accurately. Doctors may sometimes request brain scans or laboratory tests in order to rule out other diseases. Blood tests, brain imaging techniques such as magnetic resonance image (MRI), PET scan and single photon emission computed tomography (SPECT) may be used to help doctors exclude other medical conditions, such as stroke or brain tumours, that produce symptoms similar to those of PD. Therefore, there is an urgent need to establish objective measures that can be used for the accurate diagnosis of PD. This initiative will require IT experts working together with clinicians and medical scientists using AI tools that have potential medical applications.

23.2 Machine learning concepts

23.2.1 Data mining concepts

Data mining is defined as the nontrivial extraction of implicit, previously unknown, and potentially useful information from data. The use of classifier systems in medical diagnosis is increasing gradually. Recent advances in the field of artificial intelligence (AI) have led to the emergence of expert systems and decision support systems (DSS) for medical applications. Moreover, in the last few decades, computational tools have been designed to improve the experiences and abilities of doctors and medical specialists in making decisions about their patients.

Without doubt, the evaluation of data taken from patients and decisions of experts are still the most important factors in diagnosis. However, expert systems and different AI techniques for classification have the potential of being good supportive tools for the expert. Classification systems can help in increasing accuracy and reliability of diagnoses and minimising possible errors, as well as making the diagnoses more time efficient [7].

Data mining has been defined by previous authors as the process of analysing large databases to discover meaningful patterns and rules [8,9]. Data mining is a step within the knowledge discovery in databases (KDD) process that involves using data analysis and discovery algorithms to yield particular patterns (or models) based on the data. The traditional method of converting data into knowledge, unlike data mining, relies on manual analysis and interpretation.

The data mining process uses several techniques from statistics and AI in a variety of activities or application areas. The main activities are as follows.

- Classification. Classification involves identifying profiles of classes in terms of their attributes and determining which of these predefined classes a new item belongs to. For example, given particular classes of patients with different medical treatment responses, the classification is used to identify the form of treatment, to which a new patient is most likely to respond [10].
- Clustering. Clustering is used to identify a set of classes in which particular items are grouped according to their characteristics. Clustering is best used to identify groups of items that are similar. For example, based on a patient data set, clustering can be used to identify subgroups of patients with similar treatment schema [11].
- Association. Association is the identification of relationships between items, in which the presence of one pattern implies the presence of another pattern. For example, most patients who receive prescriptions for medication A also receive prescriptions for medication B [12].

23.2.2 Popular classification techniques

Classification is a pattern-recognition task that has applications in a broad range of fields. It requires the construction of a model that approximates the relationship between input features and output categories [13]. Some of the most popular techniques are discussed here in brief.

The Naïve Bayes classifier is based on applying Bayes' theorem with strong independence assumptions between the features. As one of its main features, the Naïve Bayes classifier is easy to implement because it requires a small amount of training data in order to estimate the parameters, and good results can be found in most cases. However, it has class conditional independence, meaning that it causes losses of accuracy and dependency [14].

A decision tree (J48) is a fast algorithm to train and generally gives good results. Its output is human readable so one can see if it makes sense. It has tree visualisers to aid in understanding. It is among the most used data mining algorithms. The decision tree partitions the input space of a data set into mutually exclusive regions, each of which is assigned a label, a value or an action to characterise its data points [15].

A Random Forest is a combination of tree predictors such that each tree depends on the values of a random vector sampled independently and with the same distribution for all trees in the forest [16].

23.2.3 Deep learning techniques

Deep learning is a growing trend in general data analysis and has been one of the ten breakthrough technologies of 2013. Deep learning is an improvement of artificial neural networks (ANNs), consisting of more layers that permit higher levels of abstraction and improved predictions from data. To date, it is emerging as the leading machine-learning tool in the general imaging and computer vision domains [17].

In the stream of applying machine learning for data analysis, meaningful feature extraction or feature representation lies at the heart of its success to accomplish target tasks. Conventionally, meaningful or task-related features were mostly designed by human experts based on their knowledge about the target domains, which thus made it challenging for non-experts to exploit machine learning techniques for their own studies.

However, deep learning [18] has relieved such obstacles by absorbing the feature engineering step into a learning step. That is, instead of extracting features in a hand-designed manner, deep learning requires only a set of data with minor pre-processing, if necessary, and then discovers the informative representations in a self-taught manner [19,20]. Therefore, the burden of feature engineering has shifted from a human-side to a computer-side, thus allowing non-experts in machine learning to effectively use deep learning for their own researches and/or applications.

In particular, convolutional neural networks (CNNs) have proven to be powerful tools for a broad range of computer vision tasks. Deep CNNs automatically learn mid-level and high-level abstractions obtained from raw data (e.g. images). Recent studies indicate that the generic descriptors extracted from CNNs are extremely effective in object recognition and localisation in natural images. Medical image analysis groups across the world are quickly entering the field and applying CNNs and other deep learning methodologies to a wide variety of applications.

A typical CNN architecture for image processing consists of a series of layers of convolution filters, interspersed with a series of data reduction or pooling layers. The convolution filters are applied to small patches of the input image. Like the low-level vision processing in the human brain, the convolution filters detect increasingly more relevant image features, for example, lines or circles that may represent straight edges (such as for organ detection) or circles (such as for round objects like colonic polyps), and then higher order features (such as local and global shape and texture). Figure 23.1 illustrates the architecture of a CNN.

The output of a CNN is typically one or more probabilities or class labels. The convolution filters are learned from training data. This is desirable because it reduces the necessity of the time-consuming hand-crafting of features that would otherwise be required to pre-process the images with application-specific filters or by calculating computable features.

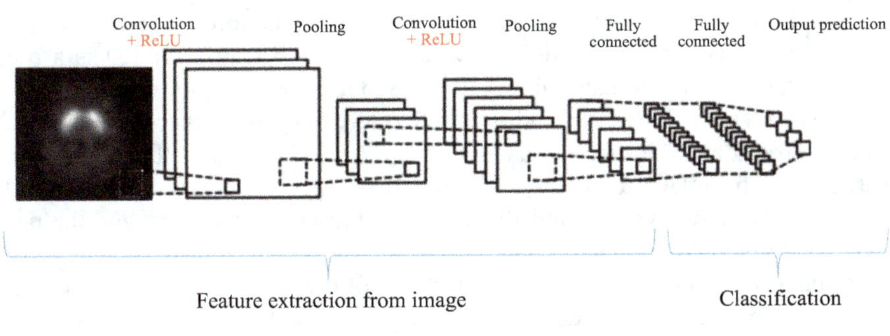

Figure 23.1 Architecture of a convolutional neural network (CNN)

23.3 Prior published studies

In this section, a summary of the research works that have been conducted in classification of PD is provided. These works have been divided according to the features used for classification. These features are vocal features, gait features, striatal binding ratio (SBR) values and SPECT images.

23.3.1 PD classification using vocal attributes

Most of the research in the classification of PD was done by detecting and analysing voice disorders using acoustic tools that record the changes in pressure at lips or inside the vocal tract. One of the earliest classifications of PD using data mining was done by Max Little from University of Oxford. He developed a software that learns to detect differences in voice patterns in order to spot distinctive clues associated with Parkinson's. By using machine learning, a large amount of data were collected at the time when it was known who had the disease or not. A new measure of dysphonia, pitch period entropy (PPE), was introduced, which is robust to many uncontrollable confounding effects including noisy acoustic environments and normal, healthy variations in voice frequency. He collected sustained phonations from 31 people, 23 with PD, and using a kernel support vector machine (SVM), achieved overall correct classification performance of 91.4% [21].

Another study [22] aimed to classify between healthy people and people with PD. The dataset was gathered from the University of California at Irvine (UCI) machine learning repository. The dataset was created by Max Little of the University of Oxford, in collaboration with the National Centre for Voice and Speech, Denver Colorado, who recorded the speech signals. The authors applied fuzzy c-means (FCM) clustering and pattern recognition techniques to the database to classify patients with PD. FCM clustering/classification depends on certain assumptions in order to define the subgroups presented in a dataset. Then, a pattern recognition technique was applied to identify the structure in data by a comparison with the known structure (through clustering). Because of the unbalanced data, FCM clustering resulted in a low classification result of 58.46%. By adding pattern recognition technique, the success rate increased to 68.04%. It was also noted that, through the combination of FCM and pattern recognition, the positive prediction value was 80.88%. This indicated that the classifier prediction of patients with PD was 80.88%. This is a very satisfactory result as classification of PD is a quite complex problem and the data mining tools used are very simple.

A research study [23] was conducted to explore WEKA filters on Naïve Bayes, a data mining tool. The datasets used were of Arrhythmia and PD. The datasets were obtained from UCI repository. At first, Nave Bayes classifier was used on the processed data of Arrhythmia and PD using tenfold cross validation and the parameters were noted down. Then, a supervised filter, Discrete from WEKA, was used on both data sets, and it divided the input values of the datasets to a range of values and their parameters are noted down. Similarly, another filter (unsupervised), numeric transform, was used on both datasets and the results were noted down. To compare the performance, the measures of accuracy, sensitivity and specificity were obtained. It was seen that, before applying any filters, the datasets showed 62.39% accuracy for Arrhythmia and 69.23% for PD. After adding the filter Discrete, the results on the Arrhythmia dataset showed an increased accuracy of 75% and on PD dataset showed an accuracy of 84.62%. Finally, with the filter Numeric Transform, the accuracy on the Arrhythmia dataset reduced to 63.1% and on PD reduced to 78.46%.

Khemphila and Boonjing [7] conducted PD classifications with a reduced number of attributes. They used information gain (IG) to determine the attributes from patients. Then, they used ANNs to classify the presence of PD in the given dataset. The dataset was taken from the UCI machine learning repository. Their experiment was done using WEKA. The dataset was divided into two sets: training and testing datasets. Initially, a pure classification using ANNs was performed resulting in an accuracy of 91.45% on the training set and 80.76% on the testing set. Then, by using IG, the attributes were sorted according to feature importance for classification. After implementing IG, the attributes were reduced to 16 and then the ANNs were implemented. The accuracy rate was 82.05% on the training set and 83.33% on the testing set.

A new data mining algorithm was developed by Suganya and Sumathi [24] and it was named artificial bear optimisation (ABO). The algorithm was designed and implemented to evaluate the performance through the area under the curve (AUC). The dataset was collected from a private healthcare institution. From the dataset, 195 instances were collected for investigation. These 195 instances had 23 characteristic features that were in a wide range of biomedical voice measurements. They utilised voice measurements because majority of reliable studies had shown that PD patients showed vocal deterioration symptoms. They implemented their algorithm and compared it with other algorithms including subtracting clustering features weighing with kernel-based extreme learning machine (SCFW with KELM), FCM, particle swarm optimisation (PSO) and ant colony optimisation (ACO). The performance matrices of accuracy, recall, precision and f-measure were used as evaluation metrics. Based on their results, it was seen that ABO had the highest accuracy (97.5%), recall, precision and f-measure than the other algorithms.

Murat Gok [25] stated that PD was a neuropathological disorder in which motor function disorders were commonly witnessed. He experimented on the dysphonic symptoms of PD (vocal characteristics). The dataset was taken from the UCI machine learning repository. The experiment consisted of two phases. First phase was feature selection (FS). In FS, relevant features were gradually selected from 22 features using a linear SVM for discovering informative features. Thus, out of 22, 10 were selected. Then, those ten were ranked based on their IGs with respect to classes. Six classifiers were selected to perform the comparison analysis. The accuracy of the competing algorithms was evaluated by means of using both the selected 10 and all 22 features. The best result of 98.46% was obtained by k-nearest neighbour (k-NN) on PD dataset using only the ten selected features.

23.3.2 PD classification using gait attributes

Gait analysis plays an important role for obtaining information on motor deficits in PD. Gait information has been widely used for movement studies in healthy controls and also in subjects with PD. Analysis of gait parameters is very useful for a better understanding of the mechanisms of movement disorders, and also has the high potential in presenting automatic non-invasive methods based on gait characteristics for diagnosis of PD.

The authors in [26] proposed a method to classify patients with PD and healthy control subjects using gait analysis via deterministic learning theory. The method consisted of two phases: a training phase and a classification phase. The data were provided by PhysioNet bank [27] and contained measures of gait for 93 idiopathic PD patients and 73 healthy controls. In the training phase, gait characteristics were derived from vertical ground reaction forces under the usual and self-selected pace of the subjects. The patterns of PD patients and healthy controls constituted a training set. In the classification phase, a bank of dynamical estimators was constructed for all the training gait patterns. Prior knowledge of gait dynamics represented by the constant radial basis functions (RBF) networks was embedded in the estimators. By comparing the set of estimators with a testing gait pattern of a certain PD patient to be classified (diagnosed), a set of classification errors were generated. The average of the errors was taken as the classification measure between the dynamics of the training gait patterns and the dynamics of the testing PD gait pattern according to the smallest error principle. With RBF network classification along with five-fold cross-validation method, an accuracy of 96.39% was obtained.

In [28], the authors employed hidden Markov model (HMM) with Gaussian mixtures to classify PD patients from healthy subjects. HMM was a state machine with two layers including state and observation layers, in which a Markovian process controlled the selection of the state in each time. The data were gathered from the PhysioNet bank. The results showed that the HMM classifier performed better than the results obtained from least squared support vector machines (LS-SVM). The HMM method could effectively separate the gait data in terms of stride interval obtained from healthy control and PD patients with an accuracy of 90.3%.

23.3.3 PD classification using imaging features

One of the most well-known databases used for identification in Parkinson disease classification is the Parkinson progression markers initiative (PPMI) [29]. The PPMI repository contains a full set of clinical, imaging and biological data collected as part of this ongoing study along with processed images and bio-specimen analysis results. The PPMI database is an international multi-centre study involving subjects from different countries adding diversity in the database thus making it more robust. The repository is updated regularly as longitudinal follow-up of study subjects continues and the data generated from different analysis techniques are completed. PPMI is sponsored by the Michael J. Fox Foundation (MJFF) for Parkinson's Research [30].

Since 2002, MJFF has been an essential driver for PD biomarker development efforts, and as a result of collaboration and efforts from several researchers, PPMI is the resulting database of these collaborations. Following are some research works done using the PPMI database for Parkinson disease classification.

Oliviera et al. [31] conducted a study to assess the potentiality of SBR features extracted from SPECT images in assisting clinical decision to diagnose PD. Seven features were extracted and tested on dataset of 652 images. Three different classifiers were used and they are: support vector machines (SVM), k-NN and logistic regression. It was observed that SVM outperformed the other classifiers.

In [32], the objective was to develop a fully automated computational solution for computer-aided diagnosis in PD using SPECT. The images were gathered from PPMI and pre-processed using automated template-based registration followed by computation of the binding potential at a voxel level. SVM classifier was used and achieved 97.86% accuracy.

Prashanth et al. [33] performed a study for automatic classification of early PD. The data were gathered from the PPMI database. They used SVM as their classifier for developing automatic classification and prediction/prognostic models for early PD. In their study, it was observed that the accuracy of SVM with RBF provided the highest accuracy.

23.3.4 PD classification using SPECT images

SPECT images have demonstrated the detection of even early stages of the disease [31,34,35]. Dopaminergic imaging discriminates patients with PD from healthy normal and tremor disorders by identifying presynaptic dopaminergic deficits in the caudate and putamen with high sensitivity and specificity [36]. Normal SPECT scans are characterised by intense and symmetric dopamine transporter (DAT) binding in the caudate nucleus and putamen on both hemispheres that appear as two comma-shaped regions. Any asymmetry or distortion of this shape implies an abnormal finding. Figure 23.2(a) and (b) illustrates SPECT images of a non-PD and a PD patient.

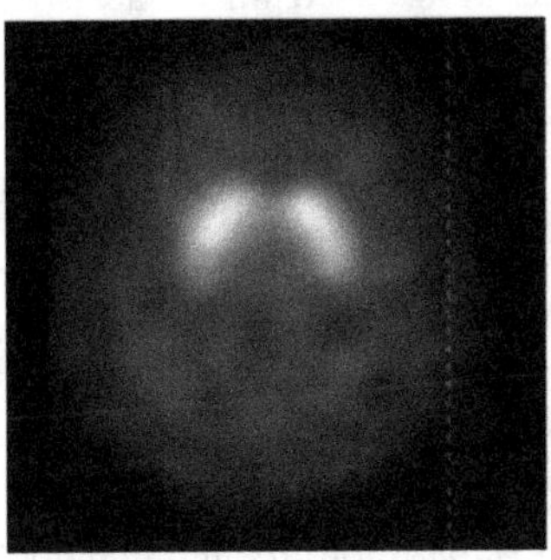

(a)

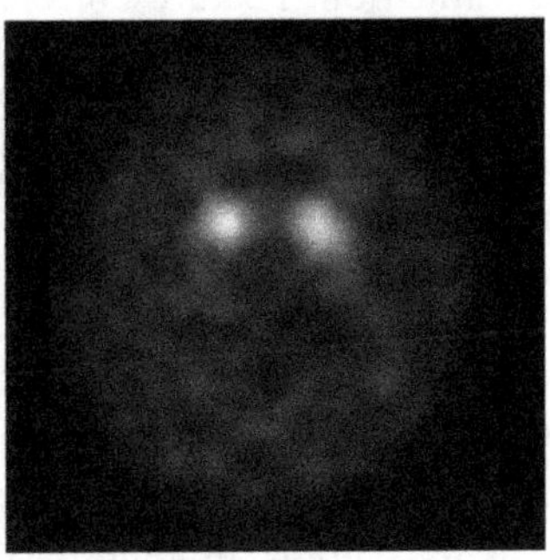

(b)

Figure 23.2 SPECT scans of (a) non-Parkinson's disease (PD) patient and (b) PD patient

Martinez et al. [37] adopted CNNs to classify PD patients from unaffected subjects. The data were gathered from PPMI with a total of 301 subjects. A bounding box was drawn around the regions of interest, which was gathered by calculating the intensity threshold. Once this was applied the rest of the image was obviated. A tenfold cross validation was used for evaluation, from which metrics such as accuracy, sensitivity and specificity, were extracted.

Choi et al. [38] also utilised CNNs for PD classification. In their study, a deep-learning-based SPECT interpretation system to refine diagnosis of PD was developed. The system was trained on the SPECT images obtained from PPMI and showed a high accuracy comparable with the experts' evaluation referring to quantification results. The system achieved an accuracy of 96%.

23.4 New research applications of PD

In this section, new avenues of research that are being conducted in the classification of PD using machine learning technologies are addressed. Recently, studies have shown that analysing handwriting features can be of diagnostic potential in the classification of PD patient from non-PD patient.

According to [39], advances in digitised handwriting technologies have enabled the measurement, quantification and analysis of kinematic handwriting process features, offering the potential for earlier detection and more accurate diagnosis of PD. Generally, PD handwriting and drawing test tasks are recorded using a digitised tablet and/or stylus and stored as a number of raw variables, including x, y and z coordinates, time and relative pressure. Grip angle may also be recorded depending on the capabilities of the data collection platform and software. From these raw variables, features of the final writing output and kinematic handwriting process are calculated for analysis and classification.

In the study, the data were collected from a publicly available spiral drawing PD dataset. Univariate and multivariate analyses were performed on derived features. Classification outcome was determined using logistic regression models with tenfold cross validation. Feature correlation was based on model specificity and sensitivity. Variations in grip angle, instantaneous acceleration and pressure indices were found to have high predictive potential as clinical markers of PD, with combined classification accuracy of above 90%.

Another research topic [40] is the classification of PD patients for surgical treatment. As PD is primarily identified with the onset of cardinal motor symptoms like tremor, bradykinesia and freezing of gait, the initial course of action is to control the symptoms using prescription drugs. However, as PD progresses, pharmacotherapy often fails to provide adequate symptom relief and sometimes causes disabling complications. Additional treatment approaches, such as surgical treatments including deep brain stimulation (DBS), pallidotomy and thalamotomy, were used to manage problems of advanced PD [41,42]. The efficacy of surgical therapy such as DBS has been well established through randomised controlled studies involving a large number of PD patients. The success of DBS is firstly dependent on the selection of appropriate patients as not all PDs are suitable for surgical therapy.

Selection of appropriate patients, in clinical practice, is based on many factors including the age of a patient, disease stage, disease duration, comorbidities and responsiveness to levodopa medication. An interdisciplinary team is usually needed to discuss these factors and then decide if the patient is suitable for surgical treatment. Therefore, there is an urgent need to streamline the process of selecting appropriate PD patients for surgical treatments. In this study, an effective model was proposed to classify PD and select suitable patients for surgery using data mining algorithm and an FS process based on IG with PD patients. The data were gathered from the PPMI database. Initially, a baseline classifier was identified based on the highest accuracy of PD classification. It was observed that multilayer perceptron (MLP) outperformed the other classifiers. Keeping MLP as the classifier, a feature reduction technique was used to determine if all features were necessary to include for achieving a high or equal classification accuracy. IG technique was used and it was observed that, with 60% of the features, an equal accuracy result was achieved to that with all features. This infers that using small number of clinical parameters is sufficient for reliable and accurate classification of PD.

23.5 Challenges of machine learning techniques

One of the most pertinent issues is the availability of data to train and build models based on deep learning without suffering from overfitting. An overfitted model arises when there are too many free parameters resulting in confusing the training data with random noise or other confounds. This is a pervasive problem in machine learning because the complexity of a model can often be set as high as required to get arbitrarily high prediction accuracy [43].

Another challenge is the quality of the data collected [44]. Sampling bias is an unavoidable issue in every machine learning research. The majority of datasets are uneven, resulting in a skewed distribution of data. The dataset may also contain repetitive attribute values or missing values, which tend to be an issue as we may not know whether that specific attribute value holds any importance or not in regard to the machine learning application.

The vast majority of machine learning algorithms make the implicit assumption that the distribution of the training data is static and unchanging. When machine learning algorithms are trained on a particular dataset, they are trained to discover patterns that are specific to those data as if they are samples from the population distribution. However, when new data are gathered, the model trained on the previous data may provide an inaccurate result [45].

The technical implementation of current machine learning algorithms is not modular. This implies that a small change in one parameter can have substantial and large unpredictable effects on the entire model. All of the input data must be in exact same form as it was when used to train the model. These types of dependencies to slight changes imply that small changes can have huge consequences resulting in a very high maintenance [46].

23.6 Conclusion and future direction

Adopting machine learning algorithms for diagnosis and classification of PD shows a very high potential for practical use. Diagnosing PD, in its early stages, is challenging due to many overlapping common clinical manifestations in patients with other neurodegenerative diseases. However, with the challenges mentioned earlier, the road for such technology to fulfil its full potential in PD diagnosis requires several plans. According to [47], several key steps can be undertaken to fulfil such plans. These are clinical validation, open platform standardisation and data sharing. Clinical validation is required for regulatory approval, much like the measurement of, for example, blood pressure. Such approval requires that the information provided is an accurate parameter of a clinically relevant feature of the disease and that there is confirmed evidence of this parameter having a relevant response within some clinical application and having target numerical ranges to measure adequate treatment response. Essentially, for machine learning-based models to be reliable and accurate, the information must be of critical value in relation to its corresponding disease. Such crucial data can only be validated by clinicians/medical specialists.

Platform standardisation requires that the software and algorithms are made publicly available for general and widespread use because technology lives or dies by the scale of its adoption and dissemination in the wider community.

Finally, data sharing is a key aspect for such research area. By sharing data, we can further refine algorithms and provide increasingly extensive and rigorous clinical validation evidence. Incentives encouraging data sharing should be established at institutional and disciplinary levels.

References

[1] Zhang ZX, Roman GC, Hong Z, *et al.* Parkinson's disease in China: Prevalence in Beijing, Xian, and Shanghai. *The Lancet*. 2005;365(9459): 595–597.

[2] Dorsey E, Constantinescu R, Thompson J, *et al.* 'Projected number of people with Parkinson's disease in the most populous nations, 2005–2030'. In: *Movement Disorders*. vol. 21. Hoboken, NJ: John Wiley & Sons; 2006. pp. S483–S483.

[3] Zhang Y, Wang C, Wang Y, *et al.* Mortality from Parkinson's disease in China: Findings from a ten-year follow up study in Shanghai. *Parkinsonism & Related Disorders*. 2018;55:75–80.

[4] Ramani RG, and Sivagami G. Parkinson disease classification using data mining algorithms. *International Journal of Computer Applications*. 2011; 32(9):17–22.

[5] Durga P, Jebakumari VS, and Shanthi D. Diagnosis and classification of Parkinson's disease using data mining techniques. *International Journal of Advanced Research Trends in Engineering and Technology*. 2016;3:86–90.

[6] Foundation NP. The stages of Parkinson's disease; 2017. http://www.parkinson.org/understanding-parkinsons/what-is- parkinsons/The-Stages-of-Parkinson's-Disease

[7] Khemphila A, and Boonjing V. *Parkinson's Disease Classification Using Neural Network and Feature Selection*. Chicago: World Academy of Science, Engineering and Technology, Open Science Index 64; 2012;6(4):377–380.

[8] Berry MJ, and Linoff G. *Mastering Data Mining*. New York: Wiley; 2000.

[9] Shmueli G, Patel NR, and Bruce PC. *Data Mining for Business Intelligence: Concepts, Techniques, and Applications in Microsoft Office Excel with XLMiner*. New Jersey: John Wiley and Sons; 2011.

[10] Han J, Pei J, and Kamber M. *Data Mining: Concepts and Techniques*. Massachusetts: Morgan Kaufman (Elsevier); 2011.

[11] Verma M, Srivastava M, Chack N, *et al.* A comparative study of various clustering algorithms in data mining. *International Journal of Engineering Research and Applications (IJERA)*. 2012;2(3):1379–1384.

[12] Larose DT, and Larose CD. *Discovering Knowledge in Data: An Introduction to Data Mining*. New Jersey: John Wiley & Sons; 2014.

[13] Bouktif S, Hanna EM, Zaki N, *et al.* 'Ant colony optimization algorithm for interpretable Bayesian classifiers combination: Application to medical predictions'. *PloS One*. 2014;9(3).

[14] Wu X, Kumar V, Quinlan JR, *et al.* Top 10 algorithms in data mining. *Knowledge and Information Systems*. 2008;14(1):1–37.

[15] Nasa C, and Suman S. Evaluation of different classification techniques for web data. *International Journal of Computer Applications*. 2012;52(9):34–40.

[16] Breiman L. Random forests. *Machine Learning*. 2001;45(1):5–32.

[17] Greenspan H, Van Ginneken B, and Summers RM. 'Guest editorial: Deep learning in medical imaging: Overview and future promise of an exciting new technique'. *IEEE Transactions on Medical Imaging*. 2016;35(5):1153–1159.

[18] Schmidhuber J. Deep learning in neural networks: An overview. *Neural Networks*. 2015; 61:85–117.

[19] Bengio Y Learning deep architectures for AI. *Foundations and Trends in Machine Learning*. 2009;2(1):1–127.

[20] LeCun Y, Bengio Y, and Hinton G. Deep learning. *Nature*. 2015;521 (7553):436.

[21] Little MA, McSharry PE, Hunter EJ, *et al.* Suitability of dysphonia measurements for telemonitoring of Parkinson's disease. *IEEE Transactions on Biomedical Engineering*. 2009;56(4):1015–1022.

[22] Rustempasic I, and Can M. Diagnosis of Parkinson's disease using fuzzy c-means clustering and pattern recognition. *Southeast Europe Journal of Soft Computing*. 2013;2(1): 42–49.

[23] Shaikh TA, and Chhabra A. Effect of WEKA filters on the performance of the NaïveBayes data mining algorithm on Arrhythmia and Parkinson's

datasets. *International Journal of Computer Science and Engineering*. 2014;2(5):45–51.

[24] Suganya P, and Sumathi C. A novel metaheuristic data mining algorithm for the detection and classification of Parkinson disease. *Indian Journal of Science and Technology*. 2015;8(14):1–9.

[25] Gök M. An ensemble of k-nearest neighbours algorithm for detection of Parkinson's disease. *International Journal of Systems Science*. 2015;46(6): 1108–1112.

[26] Zeng W, Liu F, Wang Q, *et al.* Parkinson's disease classification using gait analysis via deterministic learning. *Neuroscience Letters*. 2016; 633:268–278.

[27] Goldberger AL, Amaral LAN, Glass L, *et al.* PhysioBank, PhysioToolkit, and PhysioNet: Components of a new research resource for complex physiologic signals. *Circulation*. 2000;101(23):e215–e220. http://circ.ahajournals.org/content/101/23/e215.full.

[28] Khorasani A, and Daliri MR. HMM for classification of Parkinson's disease based on the raw gait data. Journal of Medical Systems. 2014;38(12):147.

[29] Parkinson's Progression Markers Initiative; 2017. http://www.ppmi-info.org/

[30] The Michael J Fox Foundation for Parkinson's Research; 2017. https://www.michaeljfox.org/

[31] Oliveira FP, Faria DB, Costa DC, *et al.* Extraction, selection and comparison of features for an effective automated computer-aided diagnosis of Parkinson's disease based on [123 I] FP-CIT SPECT images. *European Journal of Nuclear Medicine and Molecular Imaging*. 2018;45(6):1052–1062.

[32] Oliveira FP, and Castelo-Branco M. Computer-aided diagnosis of Parkinson's disease based on [123I] FP-CIT SPECT binding potential images, using the voxels-as-features approach and support vector machines. *Journal of Neural Engineering*. 2015;12(2):026008.

[33] Prashanth R, Roy SD, Mandal PK, *et al.* Automatic classification and prediction models for early Parkinson's disease diagnosis from SPECT imaging. *Expert Systems with Applications*. 2014;41(7):3333–3342.

[34] Booth T, Nathan M, Waldman A, *et al.* The role of functional dopamine-transporter SPECT imaging in parkinsonian syndromes, part 1. *American Journal of Neuroradiology*. 2015;36(2):229–235.

[35] Cummings JL, Henchcliffe C, Schaier S, *et al.* The role of dopaminergic imaging in patients with symptoms of dopaminergic system neurodegeneration. *Brain*. 2011;134(11):3146–3166.

[36] Prashanth R, Roy SD, Mandal PK, *et al.* High-accuracy classification of Parkinson's disease through shape analysis and surface fitting in 123I-Ioflupane SPECT imaging. *IEEE Journal of Biomedical and Health Informatics*. 2017;21(3):794–802.

[37] Martinez-Murcia FJ, Ortiz A, Górriz JM, *et al.* A 3D convolutional neural network approach for the diagnosis of Parkinson's disease. In: *International Work-Conference on the Interplay Between Natural and Artificial Computation*. Cham: Springer; 2017. p. 324–333.

[38] Choi H, Ha S, Im HJ, *et al.* Refining diagnosis of Parkinson's disease with deep learning-based interpretation of dopamine transporter imaging. *NeuroImage: Clinical.* 2017;16:586–594.

[39] Poon C, Gorji N, Latt M, *et al.* Derivation and Analysis of dynamic handwriting features as clinical markers of Parkinson's disease. In: *Proceedings of the 52nd Hawaii International Conference on System Sciences (HICSS).* Manoa: IEEE Computer Society Press; 2019.

[40] Mohammed F, He X, Lin Y, *et al.* A novel model for classification of Parkinson's disease: Accurately identifying patients for surgical therapy. In: *Proceedings of the 52nd Hawaii International Conference on System Sciences (HICSS).* Manoa: IEEE Computer Society Press; 2019.

[41] Surgery for Parkinson's Disease; 2018. https://www.webmd.com/parkinsons-disease/guide/parkinsonssurgical-treatments

[42] Mohammed A, Bayford R, and Demosthenous A. Toward adaptive deep brain stimulation in Parkinson's disease: A review. *Neurodegenerative Disease Management.* 2018;8(2):115–136.

[43] Hastie T, Tibshirani R, and Friedman J. The Elements of Statistical Learning: Data Mining, Inference, and Prediction. Springer Series in Statistics. New York: Springer; 2009.

[44] Cortes C, Mohri M, Riley M, *et al.* Sample selection bias correction theory. In: *International Conference on Algorithmic Learning Theory.* Berlin: Springer; 2008. pp. 38–53.

[45] Hand DJ. Classifier technology and the illusion of progress. *Statistical Science.* 2006;21(1):1–15.

[46] Sculley D, Holt G, Golovin D, *et al.* Hidden technical debt in machine learning systems. In: *Advances in Neural Information Processing Systems.* Montreal: Curran Associates, Inc; 2015. pp. 2503–2511.

[47] Fox Insight Clinical Trials NCT0266835 and NCT02474329; 2017. https://foxinsight.michaeljfox.org/

Chapter 24

Assessment of vulnerability to natural disasters for emergency management in Victoria, Australia

Arni Ariani[1], John Lewis[1], Padmanesan Narasimhan[1,2], Soegijardjo Soegijoko[3] and Pradeep K. Ray[1,4]*

24.1 Introduction

Substantial environmental, demographic, political and socio-economic changes are taking place in most parts of the world [1]. According to the latest United Nations report on World Population Prospects, the world population will reach 9.7 billion by 2050 and will continue to grow to 11.2 billion by 2100 [2]. In the twenty-first century, it will be a time of unprecedented expansion in human activity, and this may increase pressure on resources, such as natural resources and renewable resources. The incidence of natural disasters in such crowded living areas may result in unsafe situations where a high degree of vulnerability may increase significantly. Such a vulnerable population would be a perfect choice to examine how closely the medical and social vulnerability indexes are related.

Victoria is one of the south-eastern states of Australia most affected by natural disasters. The unique geographical characteristics of Victoria have increased the likelihood of destruction from natural disasters, such as bushfires, floods, storms and tornadoes [3]. These natural disasters have resulted in huge financial losses to the Victorian Government and the surrounding communities, with losses totalling about $19.937 billion during the decade from 2003 to 2013 [4]. In addition, Victoria is the second-most densely populated state in Australia, with an estimated population of 5.94 million people in 2016 [5]. By 2050, it is projected that the population of Victoria will be 8.4 million, an increase of 50% from 2012 [6].

[1]WHO Collaborating Centre on eHealth, University of New South Wales, Sydney, Australia
[2]Faculty of Medicine, School of Public Health and Community Medicine, University of New South Wales, Sydney, Australia
[3]Department of Electrical Engineering, Institut Teknologi Nasional, Bandung, Indonesia
[4]Centre for Entrepreneurship, University of Michigan-Shanghai Jiao Tong University Joint Institute, China
[*]John Lewis has passed away on Sunday night, 7 April 2019

One of the recommended solutions to reduce disaster impacts and risks on the communities is to perform a vulnerability assessment. A vulnerability assessment can be defined as 'the process of identifying and quantifying vulnerabilities in a system' [7]. This type of assessment may be used as a primary guide when preparing the emergency response and recovery plans following natural disasters and is an effective tool to improve the public awareness of natural disaster risks. An assessment will likely answer important questions, including which community is more susceptible to the impact of these hazards and what needs to be done to reduce the toll of natural disasters. The results of vulnerability assessments are measured in vulnerability indexes and displayed by ArcGIS application.

The main contribution of geographical information systems to disaster management is that the integrated system can help conduct accurate (spatial) decision making particularly for areas where they are critical [8]. With the ability of simulating different natural disaster scenarios, ArcGIS application may also enable researchers to create evacuation routes [8], particularly for areas with higher level of medical and social vulnerabilities.

For the first stage of this research, we would like to argue that the current set of integrated social vulnerability measures are not well-tuned enough to take into account other factors such as more complex health-related factors which increase overall population vulnerability. Therefore, the objective of this research is to investigate the connection between the medical and social vulnerability indices in Victoria, Australia.

24.2 Geographical information system (GIS)

24.2.1 Definition of GIS

Dymon has provided the closest definition for geographical information system (GIS), affirming that 'GIS as a powerful set of tools for acquiring, storing, retrieving, analysing, transforming and displaying spatial data from the real world for a particular set of purposes' [9]. While in another study by Longley et al., the term GIS has been defined based on the user group [10]:

- People in general consider GIS as digital map storage.
- Decision-makers, government, institutions and planners perceive GIS as a spatial decision-support system (SDSS). The SDSS uses the fusion of heterogeneous spatial data to solve environmental issues.
- Management scientists view GIS as an advanced Geospatial Decision Support System (GDSS). The extensive modelling capabilities of this system allow the users to solve complex spatial decision problems.

In the last 10 years, tremendous advances in computer technology have given an essential contribution to the evolution of GIS technology [11]. There are four major stages in GIS technology evolution [11].

The pioneering stage of GIS technology happened from 1960 to 1975, to which the future strategies of GIS technology development have carefully designed by individual institutions such as Canadian government, United Kingdom Ordinance Survey and United States Census Bureau [11]. At that period, the powerfulness of digital mapping technology has been the key reason behind the adoption of GIS technology by several world-mapping agencies [11].

The commercialisation stage of GIS technology occurred from 1975 to 1990, to which the GIS technology first launched by a private company called Environmental System Research Institute (ESRI) [11]. At that time, ESRI has released the first version of ARC/INFO desktop product [11].

The third stage took place between 1990 and 2010, to which the introduction and integration of information communication technology (including high-speed computers, remote sensing technology and various types of software) have indeed contributed to the increase use of GIS technology [11].

The fourth and the final stages were from 2010 to now, to which the source code is openly shared to enable massive collaboration among researchers in the fields of GIS technology [11]. Through the years, there has been substantial transformation of GIS technology from traditional mainframe-based solution to wireless-based solution [12].

24.2.2 ArcGIS as a system for emergency/disaster management

There are four stages of disaster management activities when considering time and the functional state of the affected community, namely mitigation, preparedness, response and recovery [13].

Below are the detailed explanations of each disaster management phase [13]:

- Mitigation refers to preventive steps for minimising or completely avoiding the adverse effects of natural disasters. The preventive activities in this stage include the disaster risk assessment (DRA) and disaster risk reduction (DDR) either to reduce the potential disaster impacts on society or to minimise the disaster damage and losses in the future.
- Preparedness refers to the planning activities aimed at ensuring resources are appropriately allocated to the needs of affected population and actions are specifically tailored to effectively respond to the various types of disasters.
- Response refers to the set of procedural activities that would come into effect once disaster strikes. This procedural manual is a guideline for providing emergency assistance to disaster-affected communities as well as for decreasing the possibility of secondary damage.
- Recovery refers to the last stage of disaster cycle. Recovery activities will be carried out until all systems reach the desired state (normal or near-normal operation).

The biggest commercial company in the world for GIS technology (ESRI) has created and maintained ArcGIS, which is an umbrella term covering many different types of GIS technologies [14]. Geographic information system (GIS) provides high-speed, efficient data exchange, management and analysis solutions that not only give improved urban disaster management but also accommodate a better way to make reliable decisions [13]. Hence, GIS can be considered as an ideal solution in the disaster management lifecycle, as shown in Figures 24.1 and 24.2 [13,15,16].

24.2.2.1 Desktop GIS

The capacity of a desktop-based GIS to perform spatial analysis and modelling means that the GIS professionals will be able to obtain an accurate risk and hazard assessment [16]. Some of the advantages of a desktop-based GIS include data (i.e. community, infrastructure and property) from the affected disasters areas can be quickly analysed and plotted, and GIS modelling tool can be used to minimise future disaster-related consequences and losses [17]. Moreover, the GIS desktop is still regarded as an ideal solution in disaster management because it provides high-computing power for handling such massive amount of disaster data [14].

According to a report by Tomaszewski [14], demand for a powerful, flexible thin-client GIS platform (such as mobile and web-based platforms) started to grow rapidly since 2004. This is mainly due to falling demand for specialised desktop GIS software as well as growing demand of lightweight software tools for GIS and location-based services (LBS) [14].

24.2.2.2 Web GIS

A web-GIS interactive mapping application combines data from base map layers and dynamic layers to enable operational personnel to perform operational analysis, for instance, demographic analysis, plume modelling, road closures and others [16]. Furthermore, dynamic data and services from other systems (i.e. emergency call, GPS, surveillance system and weather) can be consumed and published through a web-based GIS platform [16].

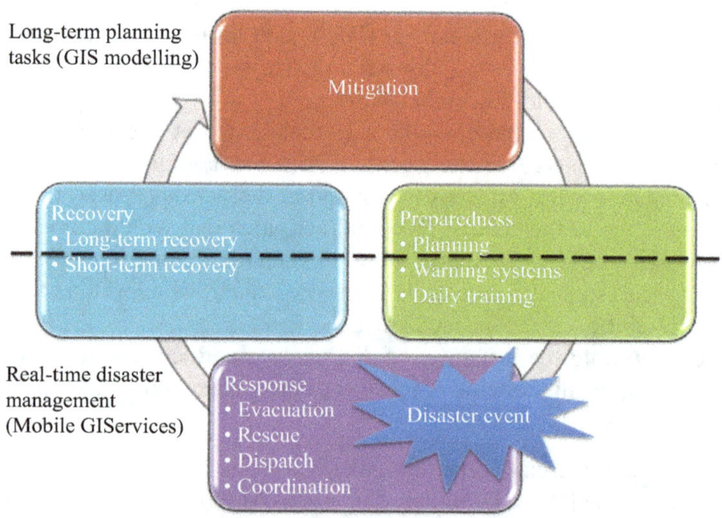

Figure 24.1 Use of GIS technologies in all four stages of emergency/disaster management lifecycle. Reprinted, with permission, from [15]. Copyright 2007 by the CRC Press (Taylor & Francis)

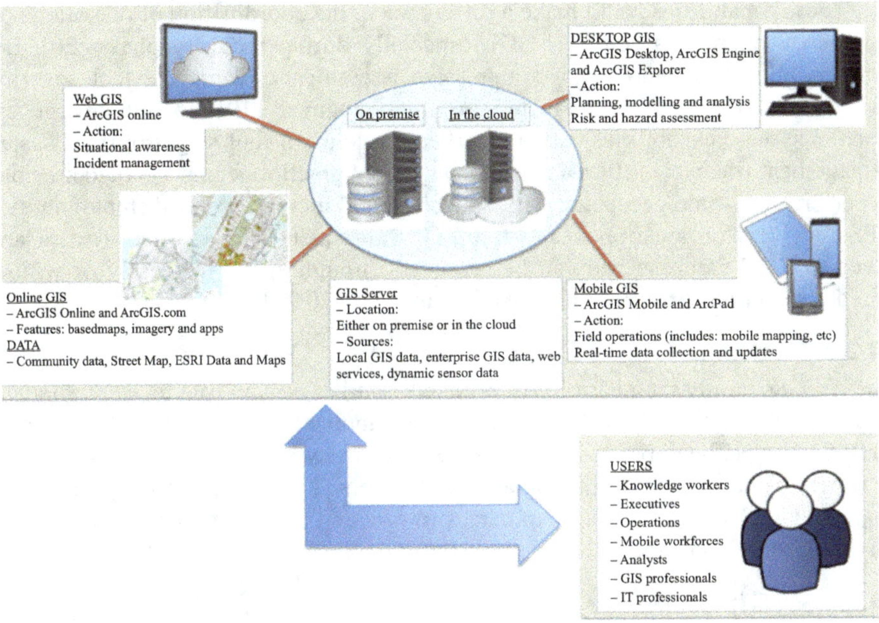

Figure 24.2 Solutions offered by ArcGIS for emergency/disaster management. Adapted from [16]. Copyright 2012 by ESRI India Magazine

Further advantages of using web-based GIS are the application is accessible from anywhere anytime as long as connected to the Internet and by any current web browser, operating systems or plug-ins as long as the platform conforms to W3C standards for coding HTML pages [14].

The rapid dissemination of information via web-based GIS application is allowing both authorities and scientists to access crucial data shared by civilians, engineers, security forces, etc., in real time [18]. Thus, security solutions must be tailored to ensure the confidentiality of information exchanged and prevent unauthorised access [18]. These solutions include the following: the use of secure and encrypted gateway for data collection and transmission, the assignment of specific access rights and privileges based on the role of the users [18].

24.2.2.3 Mobile GIS

Mobile GIS (MGIS) as defined by Ming-Hsiang Tsou [19] – 'an integrated software/hardware framework for the access of geospatial data and services through mobile devices via wireline or wireless networks'. The ArcGIS for Windows Mobile has been specifically designed to allow easy configuration with minimal training [16]. In terms of emergency management, the capabilities offered by mobile GIS technology are the provision of access to the field common operating pictures (FCOPs), the ability of updating changes in tactical and administrative operation of the site, the transmission of either GIS or non-GIS data to COP for geo-visualisation [16].

These capabilities could make a difference in the coordination of operations of emergency operations centre (EOC), especially during recovery phase [20]. By using mobile GIS technology, a compressive assessment of damage extent, severity and significance can be conducted in timely manner [19]. In non-emergency situations, these capabilities play a significant role in all four stages of the disaster management life cycle [20]. Disaster management practitioners in the field are able to perform real-time geospatial data collection and modification by employing the GPS receivers on smartphones [14,20,21]. Subsequently, the collected data are saved to EOC database and can be retrieved through either wirelessly or with a wired connection for further insights and analysis [20,22].

24.2.2.4 Online GIS and data

The ArcGIS family member of GIS products that has a main role to accommodate access to all types of GIS data, imagery and applications is ArcGIS Online and ArcGIS.com [17]. Global base maps come in a variety of types include community base maps, imagery, streets, topography and others [17]. The emergency staffs can share and exchange data (i.e. map data, projects and presentations) through either private or public channels [17].

24.2.2.5 GIS server

There are two deployment options for GIS server, either installed in one of the emergency management servers, on-premise environment or hosted in a completely virtual, cloud-based environment [17]. As the core component of the GIS system, the ArcGIS for Server has important roles in emergency/disaster management [16]. Some of the vital roles of GIS server can be enumerated as follows [17]: (1) establishing GIS data organisation and management platform for desktop for a better decision support and situational analysis, (2) allowing GIS users to store, manipulate and visualise spatial data over a mobile data connection and (3) ensuring that only authorised people gain access to dynamic data, services and other online GIS data.

24.2.3 GIS limitations and constraints

The widespread use of GIS technology for the assessment of hazard still comes with limitations and constraints [23]. The quality and availability of geospatial data are limited in the least developed countries when compared to the developed countries (such as Australia, Japan, Singapore and the United States) and some developing countries (such as Indonesia and Malaysia). This is due to the fact that the acquisition of spatial data can be quite costly and very expensive to maintain [23].

The levels of input data heterogeneity and quality have a direct impact on the capability of GIS technology [23]. The provision of high-quality, reliable and valid data is critical because the risk analysis process and future decision-making processes cannot be done automatically [24]. GIS experts will still be needed to examine the relation between hazards over time and space [25].

Moreover, in emergency situations, most of the humanitarian staffs are not familiar with GIS or ArcGIS services and do not have a technical background

[26,27]. Therefore, it is crucial to train them in how to apply GIS technologies to support disaster management and preparedness [27]. This will help them to comfortably use GIS technologies even when dealing with difficult and stressful environment [27].

Finally, another challenge in emergency/disaster situations is extensive damage to communication infrastructure, which leads to the failure of data transmission [27]. Therefore, offline solutions are needed to ensure the continuity of work in disconnected environment and to update information without access to digital resources [27]. Also, the standard equipment in the field must be easy to use without technical knowledge and available locally without the need to import special and expensive foreign equipment [27].

24.3 Two types of vulnerability

Previous literature studies have demonstrated that the vulnerability concept in disasters can often be interpreted in different ways, depending on the nature of research [28–30]. The three research orientations on vulnerability were: (a) an exposure model, this refers to the recognition of conditions that may exacerbate vulnerability in people and places in case of an extreme natural hazard [31,32]; (b) a social resilience to natural hazards model, this was done under the assumptions that vulnerability is viewed as a measure of disaster resilience [33,34] and (c) the combined model between the potential exposures and the social resilience in terms of specific regions [35,36].

Vulnerability is defined as the population's characteristics that affect the community's ability to prevent, prepare, respond to and recover (PPRR) from natural disasters [37]. Here, we will focus on vulnerabilities based on socio-economic and medical variables.

24.3.1 Vulnerability based on socio-economic variables

Several published papers have reported that people with low socio-economic status living in disaster-prone areas have a higher risk of harm from natural hazards [38,39]. These populations may not be able to access basic services after extreme disasters, especially accommodation, food, medical care and transportation [40]. Hence, the assessment must be undertaken to investigate who would be most affected by natural disasters and what types of vulnerabilities are likely to persist [41].

By having a deep understanding of social vulnerability, we can understand why communities and individuals respond differently when struck with the same natural hazard [42].

24.3.2 Vulnerability based on medical variables

Some studies have highlighted that the two major factors that affect medical vulnerabilities are health needs and healthcare access [43,44]. We further divided the health needs into three subgroups, namely physical, psychological and complex social health needs [43].

Healthcare access can be defined as the ability of individual and/or community to acquire medical services [44]. Healthcare access indicators are associated with the availability of medical facilities and experienced medical staffs providing affordable and high-quality care services. It also must be noted that health insurance status can also be counted as one of the indicators [44].

In this chapter, the authors recommend the inclusion of unhealthy lifestyle practices for measuring medical vulnerability index (MedVI) [45]. The unhealthy lifestyle behaviours in populations include populations with sleep loss and sleep-related disorders, populations with poor work-life balance, populations that fail to meet dietary guidelines and physical activity guidelines and populations who consume high sugar-content beverages on daily basis [45].

This recommendation was based on the following research studies:

- *Sleep loss and sleep-related disorders*: Findings have shown that sleeping less than 7 hours per night is associated with increased physical health risk (cardiovascular disease and hypertension, diabetes and impaired glucose tolerance, obesity in both adults and children) and increased physiological health risk (alcohol use, anxiety and depressed mood) [46].
- *Poor work-life balance*: Research has shown that personal life and work-life imbalance may lead to negative consequences such as conflict at work/home, feeling of overwork/burnout, frequent acute illness, lengthy sick leave due to chronic illness and stress [47].
- *Meet dietary guidelines and physical activity guidelines*: The three leading causes of death for people aged above 18 years old are cancer, heart disease and stroke [48]. These chronic diseases can be prevented or lessened by implementing healthy eating habits and performing exercise regularly. Moreover, poor diet and lack of exercise among young generation can lead to an increased risk of developing high blood pressure, type 2 diabetes and obesity [49].
- *Consume sugar-sweetened soft drinks daily*: Findings from several studies have pointed out that the negative consequences of consuming sugary drinks daily are type 2 diabetes, dental carriers and hypertension [50].

24.4 Methodology

In order to build an effective emergency response plan, assessing medical vulnerability in relation to social vulnerability will be carried out in three steps: (a) creating vulnerability metrics; (b) evaluating statistical analysis results and (c) interpreting spatial analysis results [43]. This study relies on socio-economic and medical data derived from Department of Health & Human Services, State Government of Victoria, Australia [51]. The time period of the data was 2012.

24.4.1 Metric construction and preliminary mapping

In this stage, two vulnerability metrics are generated for verifying the association of medical vulnerability with social vulnerability [44]. Those metrics were social vulnerability index (SoVI) and medical vulnerability index (MedVI). The metric construction process involved four phases: (1) the z-score standardisation is applied to the datasets; (2) the principal component analysis (PCA) with rotation method is selected to extract macro factors from the large dataset; (3) the cardinality of each factor is further investigated to determine whether the related factor has a likelihood to intensify social vulnerability or to enhance social resilience and (4) the calculation of composite score for vulnerability index is performed for each local government areas (LGA) by summing up all extracted factors [44].

The original input variables for SoVI and MedVI metrics were 42 and 36 variables, respectively [44,52]. The selection of these original target variables can be found in more details in Cutter [52] and Morath [44]. However, based on the data available, this study selected 19 target variables for SoVI metric (Table 24.1) and 44 target variables for MedVI metric (Tables 24.2–24.4). These factors were selected because of their scalability, which enables the comparison of either social

Table 24.1 SoVI target variables

Name	Description	Name	Description
MVALOO12	Average value of the owned homes (in dollars), 2012	PCTPOV12	Percentage living in poverty – low-income households, 2012
MEDRENT12	Average cost of the rental properties (in dollars), 2012	PCTNOHS12	Percentage of population 25 years or older with no high school diploma, 2012
GPRACTS12	Number of general practitioners per 100,000 population, 2012	NDAFC12	New dwellings approved for construction per 1,000 population
PCTFARMS12	Farm lands in percentage of total land, 2012	HOSPTPC12	Per capita number of community hospitals, 2012
PCTATSI12	Percentage Aboriginal or Torres Strait Islander, 2012	TOTMAL12	Total males, 2012
PCTNIP12	Percentage non-indigenous population, 2012	TOTFEM12	Total females, 2012
PCTKIDS12	Percentage of population under 14 years old, 2012	PCTM_HH12	Percentage male-headed households, no spouse present, 2012
PCTOLD12	Percentage of population over 65 years, 2012	PCTF_HH12	Percentage female-headed households, no spouse present, 2012
PCTVLUN12	Percentage of civilian labour force unemployed, 2012	PCTURB12	Percentage urban population, 2012
PCTHH2012	Percentage of households earning more than $20,800, 2012		

Table 24.2 Unhealthy lifestyle variables for MedVI metric

QLowPhysicalActivities	Persons who fail to meet the physical activity guidelines
QLowVeggies	Persons who do not meet the dietary guidelines for fruit and vegetables consumption
QSleepingLess7Hours	Persons sleeping less than 7 hours per day
Qsoftdrinks	Persons who drink soft drink every day
QLifeBalance	Persons with adequate work-life balance

Table 24.3 Health need variables for MedVI metric

Physical and/or physiological needs		Physical need	
QAlcohol	Consumed alcohol at least weekly, at levels likely to cause short-term harm – persons aged 18+	LBW	Low birth weight babies
QBullied-adolescent	Adolescents who report being bullied	QArthritis	Persons reporting arthritis
QDevdis1/more-child	Children who are developmentally vulnerable on one or more domains	QAsthma	Persons reporting asthma
QDevdis2/more-child	Children who are developmentally vulnerable on two or more domains	QCancer	Malignant cancers diagnosed per 100,000 pop
QEmotional-child	Children with emotional or behavioural problems at school entry	QCoreActivity Assistance	Persons with core activity need for assistance
QIOHC-child	Rate of children in out of home care per 1,000 population	QDental	Poor dental health
QSpeech-child	Children with speech or language problems at school entry	QDiabetic	Persons reporting type 2 diabetes
Physiological need		QDisability65+	People with severe and profound disability living in the community (aged 65+)

(Continues)

Table 24.3 (Continued)

Physical and/or physiological needs		Physical need	
QAbuse-child	Rate of substantiated child abuse per 1,000 population	QDisabilityAllAges	People with severe and profound disability living in the community (all ages)
QDrug	Drug usage and possession offences per 1,000 population	QHeart	Persons reporting heart disease
QDrug&AlcoholTreatments	Clients who received Alcohol and Drug treatment services in 2011–12, per 1,000 population	QHypertension	Persons reporting high blood pressure
QMentalDisability	Persons who have a high degree of psychological distress	QObese	Persons who are obese
QProtection-child	Rate of children on child protection orders per 1,000 population	QOsteoporosis	Persons reporting osteoporosis
QSocialInteractions	Social networking used to organise time with family/friends	QOverweight	Persons who are overweight
QPoorHealthStatus	Persons reporting fair or poor health status	QSmoker	Persons 18+ who are current smokers

Table 24.4 Healthcare access variables for MedVI metric

AliedHealthSites	Allied health sites per 1,000 population
Clinics	General practice clinics per 1,000 population
DentalServices	Dental services per 1,000 population
GP	GPs per 1,000 population
HighCareBeds	Aged care High-Care beds per 1,000 eligible population
Hospital	Number of hospitals/health services
Insurance	Population with private health insurance
LowCareBeds	Aged care Low-Care beds per 1,000 eligible population
MentalClinics	Registered mental health clients, per 1,000 population
Pharmacies	Pharmacies per 1,000 population

or medical vulnerabilities between different local governments in Victoria, Australia.

Following that, ArcGIS 10 (ESRI) is used to map the aggregate scores based on their vulnerability level [44]. Victoria comprises 79 LGAs [5]. Figure 24.3(a) shows the map of Regional Victoria while Figure 24.3(b) shows the map of metropolitan Melbourne [53].

24.4.2 Correlation, reliability and regression analysis

In this stage, a series of statistical analyses are performed to assess statistical significance of overlap of medical and social vulnerabilities [44]. The components of the assessment include correlation and partial correlation analyses, simple and multiple linear regression [44]. The interpretation of the correlation coefficient can be found in Box 24.1 [54].

Box 24.1: The interpretation of correlation coefficient [54]

The correlation coefficient is used to determine the strength and direction of a relationship between two variables.

- rs $= \pm 1$: perfect linear and monotone relationship.
- rs $= 0$: no linear or monotone relationship.
- rs < 0: negative, inverse relationship.
- rs > 0: positive relationship.

The Spearman's rank correlation coefficient is selected to examine the strength of a monotonic relationship between MedVI, SoVI and their compositional components. The addition of control variables is the main difference between partial correlation and the Spearman's rank [55]. In this chapter, we would only pick out the one that has a Spearman correlation score 'rs' above 0.5 for control variable [45]. We believed that this approach is much more effective than using all combinations of compositional components of both vulnerability metrics [45].

The Cronbach's coefficient alpha is used to calculate the reliability within or between quantitative metrics. The reliability score is equal to one in the absence of random errors [55]. Results were considered significant at $\alpha > 0.700$ [55].

The investigation of linear relationship of the two metrics proceeds to access the feasibility of using vulnerabilities based on social aspects to forecast vulnerabilities based on medical variables [44]. In a simple linear regression model, the aggregate SoVI and MedVI scores are used as independent and dependent variables, respectively [44]. Meanwhile, the compositional SoVI components were selected as a replacement of aggregate SoVI score in the multiple regression analysis [44]. Then, the evaluation of predictive power must also be performed for all independent variables [44]. For positive statistical congruence between MedVI and SoVI scores to occur, the p-value needs to be below 0.05 for all components and the adjusted r^2 value needs to be above 0.

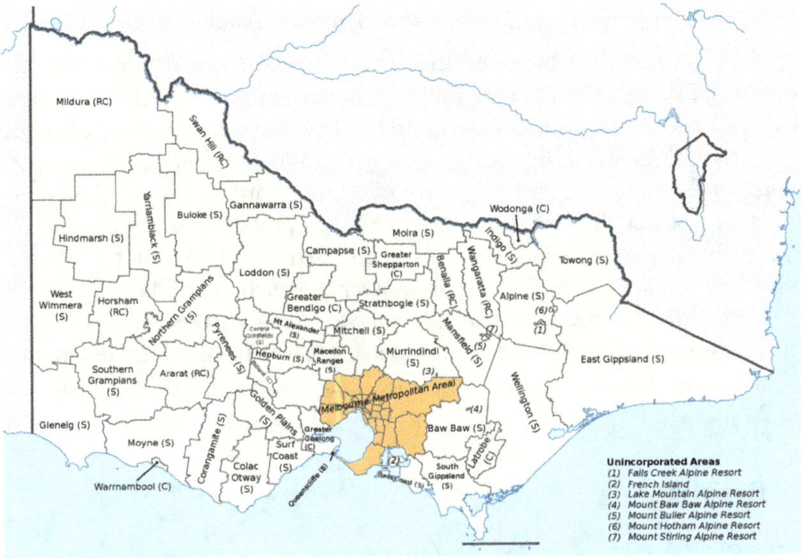

(a)

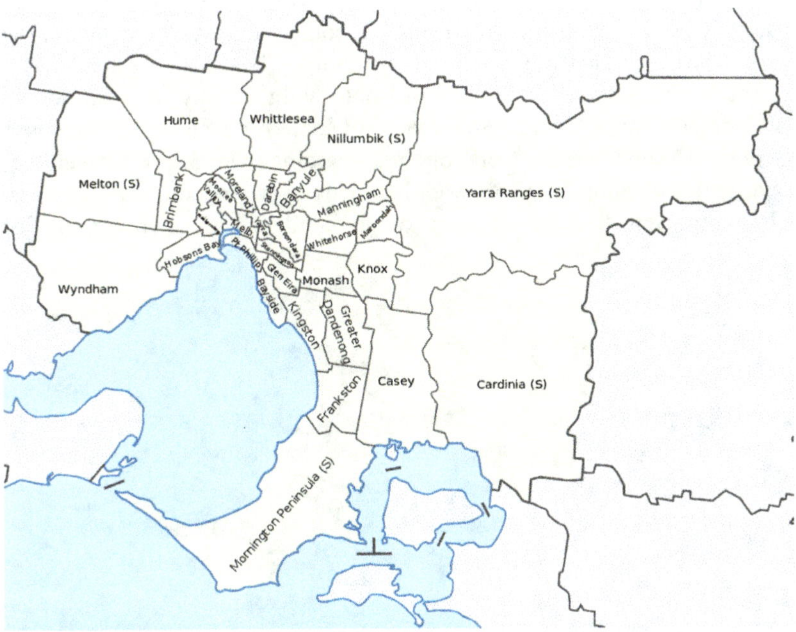

(b)

Figure 24.3 (a) Regional Victoria is comprised of 48 LGAs and (b) Melbourne Metropolitan is comprised of 31 LGAs. Adapted from [53]

24.4.3 Bivariate and residual mapping analysis

The aim of constructing a bivariate map is to illustrate two vulnerability indexes concurrently [44]. This kind of map provides better visualisation than a comparison map of the two vulnerability indexes [44]. The aggregate scores obtained are converted to the vulnerability grades using a range of statistical classification techniques [44]. Each of LGAs is colour-coded in accordance to the dominant type and the level of the vulnerability severity (e.g. low, medium or high) [44].

The residual mapping analysis has been carried out in order to have more understanding in the SoVI's explanatory power representation [44]. In this chapter, the residuals were classified into three groups: an adequate prediction was obtained when the score fall within a 95% confidence interval (CI), while under- or over-predictions were achieved when the score lies below or above a 95% CI [44] (Figure 24.4).

24.5 Results

24.5.1 Social vulnerability index (SoVI)

At the end of the PCA, three composite principal components were obtained from the 19 computed target variables and the extraction process was completed based on Kaiser's Rule (i.e. choosing only principal components with eigenvalues greater than one). The researcher adjusted each component based on the tendency of the component to either decrease or increase social vulnerability. An additional equation was created to measure an aggregate SoVI score for each LGA. The equation is SoVI score = Component 1 − Component 2 + Component 3. We derived the SoVI score without assigning a priori weights. However, we did assign cardinality to each component to take account of its tendency to increase or decrease

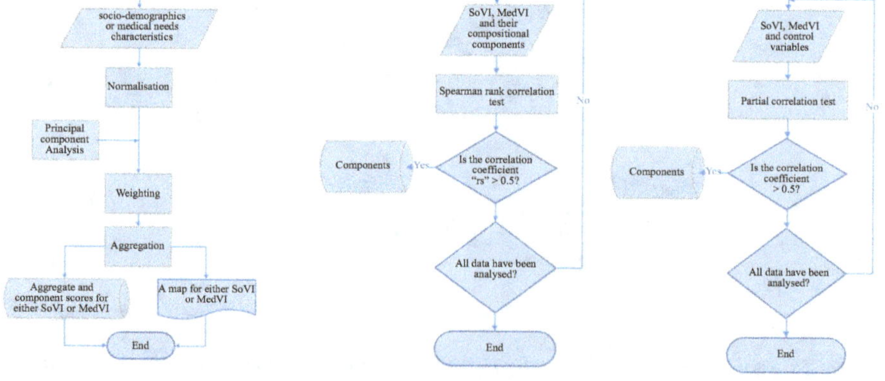

Figure 24.4 (a) Vulnerability metrics construction flowchart and (b) correlation analysis tests. Reprinted, with permission, from [45]. Copyright 2016 by IEEE.

vulnerability. The cardinality of each component will be explained in detail below. The three latent components illustrated the relationships between all variables to 75.494% of the cumulative variance (as shown in Table 24.5). While the representation of SoVI aggregate score for each LGA can be found in Figure 24.5.

The first and third components of SoVI were assigned a positive (+) cardinality due to the likelihood of increasing social vulnerability. This decision made was due to the following reasons. High levels of unemployment in communities would certainly increase poverty and homelessness thus increasing the risk of social vulnerability [56]. Furthermore, many studies have confirmed that low-income

Table 24.5 Summary of social vulnerability PCA

Component	Cardinality	Description	Dominant Variables	Component loading	% variance explained
1	+	Unemployment and socio-economic status	PCTATSI12	−0.136	28.017
			PCTVLUN12	0.795	
			PCTNOHS12	−0.461	
			NDAFC12	0.437	
			TOTFEM12	0.823	
			TOTMAL12	0.834	
2	–	Elderly and living costs	MVALOO12	0.79	24.35
			MEDRENT12	0.753	
			GPRACTS12	0.854	
			PCTOLD12	−0.113	
3	+	Rural working class poor	PCTFARMS12	−0.348	23.127
			PCTNIP12	0.904	
			PCTHH2012	0.651	
			PCTM_HH12	0.255	
Total variance explained					75.494

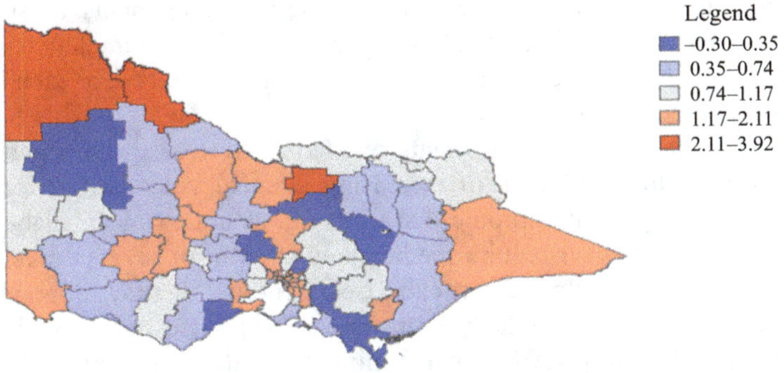

Figure 24.5 Overall, the four LGAs with the highest SoVI scores are found in Swan Hill (RC) (3.92), Mildura (RC) (2.85), Greater Shepparton (C) (2.75) and Monash (C) (2.11)

earners are the most affected population when disaster strikes [57,58], for example, a low-income family will be less likely to be able to secure alternate short-term accommodation if their home is destroyed by a bushfire. According to a 2012 report by Australian Council of Social Service, approximately one-third of sole-parent families were identified as poor families or low-income earners in Australia [59]. Hamilton et al. have confirmed that the modest family income for a couple with one or more children in Australia was $45,000.00 in 2007 [60]. Howlett et al. confirmed that the average income for non-indigenous women was $37,400.00 in 2011 [61].

The second component was assigned a negative (–) cardinality to designate the tendency to decrease social vulnerability. This decision was made for the following reasons. First, higher incomes within communities would enable individuals to recover faster from the impact of disasters [57]. Improved housing and rental affordability reflect an improvement in economic wellbeing among people in Victoria [62] thus improving community resilience. Second, the healthcare resources have a crucial role in the initial medical response to natural disaster and the onsite rescue [63]. The effect of the elderly proportion in the population was not significant (–0.113).

24.5.2 Medical vulnerability index (MedVI)

At the end of the PCA, nine composite principal components were obtained from the 44 computed target variables and the extraction process was completed based on Kaiser's Rule (i.e. choosing only principal components with eigenvalues greater than one). The researcher adjusted each component based on the tendency of the component to either decrease or increase medical vulnerability. A simple addition equation was created to measure an aggregate MedVI score for each LGA. We derived the MedVI score without assigning a priori weights. However, we did assign cardinality to each component to take account of its tendency to increase or decrease vulnerability. The cardinality of each component will be explained in detail below. The equation is MedVI score = Component 1 + Component 2 + Component 3 + Component 4 + Component 5 + Component 6 + Component 7 – Component 8 – Component 9. The nine latent components illustrated the relationships between all variables to 75.561% of the cumulative variance (Table 24.6). While the representation of MedVI aggregate score for each LGA can be found in Figure 24.6.

The first to the seventh components of MedVI were assigned a positive (+) cardinality due to the likelihood of increasing medical vulnerability for the following reasons. People with chronic diseases (e.g. asthma, cancer, diabetes, high blood pressure and obesity) require medications or even in severe cases, hospitalisation or may need to follow a particular treatment and therapy program such as using supplemental oxygen or dialysis machines [44]. Also people with physical disabilities face difficulties when performing their daily activities [44]. There is also a need to include populations with complex social health needs (e.g. intellectually disabled people or domestic violence victims), since their disabilities and needs may require medical care or other therapies [43,44]. People with

Table 24.6 Summary of medical vulnerability PCA

Component	Cardinality	Description	Dominant variables	Component loading	% variance explained
1	+	Low health perception and medical dependence	QHypertension	0.583	12.713
			QArthritis	0.601	
			QObese	0.734	
			QSpeech-child	0.78	
			QBullied-adolescent	0.605	
			QLowVeggies	0.504	
			QSoftDrinks	0.589	
2	+	Chronic diseases	QSocialInteractions	0.241	11.772
			QDiabetic	0.704	
			QOsteoporosis	0.497	
			QDental	0.54	
			QSmoker	0.574	
			QDisability65+	0.748	
			QPoorHealthStatus	0.753	
			QMentalDisability	0.706	
			QSleepingLess7Hours	0.468	
3	+	Disabilities	QCancer	0.819	11.463
			QCoreActivityAssistance	0.769	
			QDisabilityAllAges	0.689	
4	+	Domestic violence propensity	QEmotional-child	0.461	10.958
			QAbuse-child	0.721	
			QProtection-child	0.815	
			QIOHC-child	0.503	
			QDrug&AlcoholTreatments	0.802	
			MentalClinics	0.75	

(Continues)

Table 24.6 (Continued)

Component	Cardinality	Description	Dominant variables	Component loading	% variance explained
5	+	Special needs institution	Hospital	0.603	10.412
			GP	0.09	
			Clinics	0.88	
			AliedHealthSites	0.875	
			DentalServices	0.839	
			Pharmacies	0.747	
			LowCareBeds	0.496	
6	+	Developmental vulnerability issue	LBW	0.757	6.557
			QDevdis1/more-child	0.711	
			QDevdis2/more-child	0.647	
7	+	Weight issues	QOverweight	0.841	4.125
8	-	Lifestyle choices	QLowPhysicalActivities	0.601	4.103
			Insurance	0.023	
			QLifeBalance	0.692	
9	-	Alcohol abuse	QAlcohol	0.527	3.458
Total variance explained					75.561

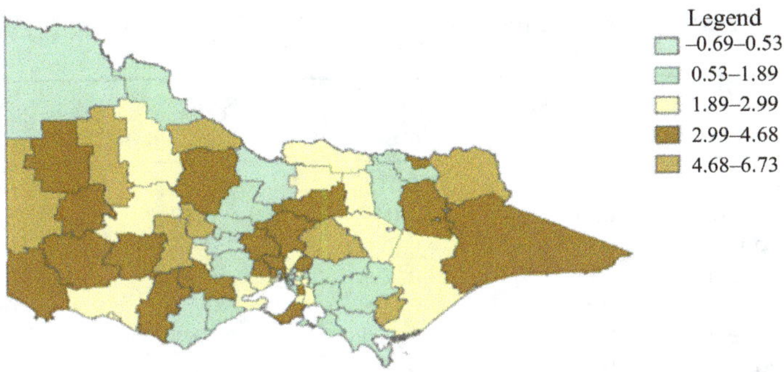

Figure 24.6 Overall, the four LGAs with the highest MedVI scores are found in Murrindindi (S) (6.73) Central Goldfields (S) (6.58), Gannawarra (S) (6.58) and West Wimmera (S) (6.38)

psychosomatic disorders (e.g. drug and alcohol addiction, depression and mental illness) or mental limitations usually need more support from their loved ones and also require professional mental health treatment or in acute cases, institutionalisation [43,44]. Some studies also highlighted that damage to healthcare infrastructure and shortages in medical supplies and essential equipment may affect the medical team's abilities to provide care for victims of a large-scale disaster [64,65]. To conclude, we believed that these populations are more vulnerable to the consequences of natural disasters due to their fragile health conditions and the lack of access to healthcare services.

Some studies have shown the negative effects of alcohol and unhealthy lifestyles to the health status of individuals and populations [47,49]. Research has shown that personal life and work-life imbalance may lead to negative consequences such as conflict at work/home, feeling of overwork/burnout, frequent acute illness, lengthy sick leave due to chronic illness and stress [47]. The three leading causes of death for people aged above 18 years old are cancer, heart disease and stroke [66]. These chronic diseases can be prevented or lessened by implementing healthy eating habits and performing exercise regularly. Moreover, poor diet and lack of exercise among the younger generation are associated with increased risk of getting high blood pressure, type 2 diabetes and obesity [49]. However, since these groups do not represent the majority of the population, a negative (–) cardinality is applied to components 8 and 9 to designate their tendency to decrease medical vulnerability.

24.5.3 Correlation, reliability and regression analyses

As shown in Table 24.7, the correlation between the aggregate SoVI and MedVI scores proved to be quite weak (rs = 0.045) when compared with the correlation between individual components.

For example, the correlation between the SoVI Component 2 and the MedVI Component 5, significant at the 0.01 level (two-tailed), demonstrated a strong

Table 24.7 Spearman's rank correlations for MedVI, SoVI and their component

	SoVI score	SoVI component 1	SoVI component 2	SoVI component 3
MedVI score	0.045	0.105	0.281*	0.145
MedVI component 1	−0.167	−0.017	0.182	−0.001
MedVI component 2	−0.075	0.204	0.367**	0.098
MedVI component 3	−0.006	0.05	0.234*	0.191
MedVI component 4	−0.151	−0.038	0.230*	−0.012
MedVI component 5	−0.059	0.124	0.584**	.427**
MedVI component 6	−0.08	−0.038	0.280*	0.124
MedVI component 7	−0.08	−0.024	−0.004	−0.1
MedVI component 8	0.105	0.239*	0.300**	.288*
MedVI component 9	−0.395**	−0.252*	0.087	−0.193

*Correlation is significant at the 0.05 level (two-tailed).
**Correlation is significant at the 0.01 level (two-tailed).

Table 24.8 Partial correlation summary

Variables held constant	Partial correlation (SoVI and MedVI scores)
SoVI component 2	0.038
MedVI component 5	0.011
SoVI component 2 and MedVI component 5	0.012

positive association at rs = 0.584. The second moderately strong association is prevalent between the SoVI component 3 and the MedVI Component 5 with rs = 0.427. The third strong association was achieved between the SoVI Component 2 and the MedVI Component 2 at rs = 0.367. A correlation score that greater than 0.5 indicates a strong influence on the relationship between the two components [55].

Based on the acquired results from a Spearman rank correlation, we selected a pair of components (SoVI Component 2 and MedVI Component 5) as control variables for partial correlation. As shown in Table 24.8, there is a weak positive relationship between SoVI and MedVI scores if we select either SoVI Component 2 (0.038), MedVI Component 5 (0.011) or the combination of SoVI Component 2 and MedVI Component 5 (0.012) as a control variable.

The researchers reported that Cronbach's alpha scores were −0.058 and 0.514 for the overall aggregate scores and the complete combination of compositional components, as shown in Table 24.9. These were graded as the unacceptable level of internal consistency, indicating that the social vulnerability cannot be used to predict medical vulnerability

Table 24.9 Reliability score for aggregate scores and compositional components

Cronbach's alpha for MedVI and SoVI aggregate scores		
Cronbach's alpha	**Cronbach's alpha based on standardised items**[a]	**No. of items**
−0.058	−0.082	2
Cronbach's alpha for MedVI and SoVI compositional components		
Cronbach's alpha	**Cronbach's alpha based on standardised items**	**No. of items**
0.514	0.681	12

[a]The value is negative due to a negative average covariance among items. This violates reliability model assumptions. You may want to check item codings.

Table 24.10 Results from simple and multiple regression analyses

Model	**Adjusted R^2**	***F***	***F* sig.**	***t***	**Beta**	**Sig.**
SoVI score	−0.11	0.119	0.731	−0.345	−0.039	−0.731
Adjusted R^2	*F*	*F* sig.	Model	*t*	Beta	Sig.
0.047	2.293	0.85	SoVI component 1	−0.208	−0.27	0.836
			SoVI component 2	−2.227	−0.268	0.029
			SoVI component 3	0.558	0.072	0.579

As shown in Table 24.10, the aggregate SoVI score had a negative effect on MedVI score (adjusted $r^2 = -0.11$ or equal to 0), while the three components of SoVI had a positive effect on MedVI score (adjusted $r^2 = 0.047$). Furthermore, a small improvement in r^2 (i.e. from 0 to 0.047) showed that weak predictive capability between the three components of SoVI and the aggregate MedVI score. Approximately 95.3% of the variance in MedVI remains unexplained. Of the three SoVI components, only one variable is statistically significant: Component 2, an indicator of Elderly Population and Living Costs, with Sig. = 0.029. Finally, a lower score of adjusted r^2 demonstrated the fact that there was significant incongruence between the two vulnerabilities scores. In other words, the researchers need to find another aspect of population characteristics to explain the remaining variance in the MedVI score.

24.5.4 Bivariate and residual mapping analysis

Green hues demonstrated LGAs, which were highly affected by the medical vulnerability while orange hues illustrated LGAs, which were highly affected by the social vulnerability. Examining the map in Figure 24.7, most of the LGAs exhibiting the combination of low SoVI and low MedVI classification (16.5%), the combination of medium SoVI and medium MedVI classification (18.99), and the combination of low SoVI and medium MedVI classification (36.7%).

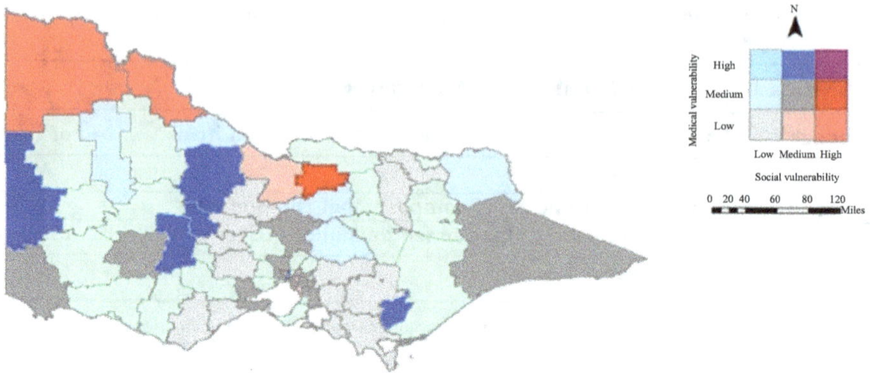

Figure 24.7 Social vulnerability index (SoVI)–medical vulnerability index (MedVI) bivariate map

Analysing the map, nearly three-fourths of the LGAs in Victoria (70.89%) presented the same mapped category for both vulnerability indexes, with 62.03% representing low to high MedVI classifications when compared with Figure 24.6 and 8.86% representing medium to high SoVI classifications when compared with Figure 24.5.

The results showed that 2 LGAs (2.53%) exhibited under-prediction, 4 LGAs (5.06%) displayed over-prediction and 73 LGAs (92.41%) showed adequate prediction (as shown in Figure 24.8(a)). In other words, the obtained results showed that SoVI and MedVI capture separate sections of the vulnerable population.

24.6 Discussion

The differences between our work and the work by Morath [44] are that our work also investigates the effects of unhealthy lifestyle behaviours on medical vulnerability metrics. As shown in Section 24.5, unhealthy lifestyle behaviours were less likely to impact the medical vulnerability of people in vulnerable areas. This could be because the individual's vulnerability depends not only on lifestyle choices but also maybe significantly impacted by genetic, environmental and complex factors.

In addition to that, our findings coincide with previous findings that people with medical dependence/health needs are more susceptible to the impacts of disasters than the other population groups. The comorbidity of chronic physical diseases and mental illness may affect people's ability to look after themselves [56]. Special assistance is required for frail people with complex needs during and after disasters [56].

While indicators of medical and social vulnerability are useful predictors of community resilience in the face of natural disasters, more research is needed to assess how each indicator may influence the other. The relatively surprising finding that social vulnerability is not related to medical vulnerability warrants further

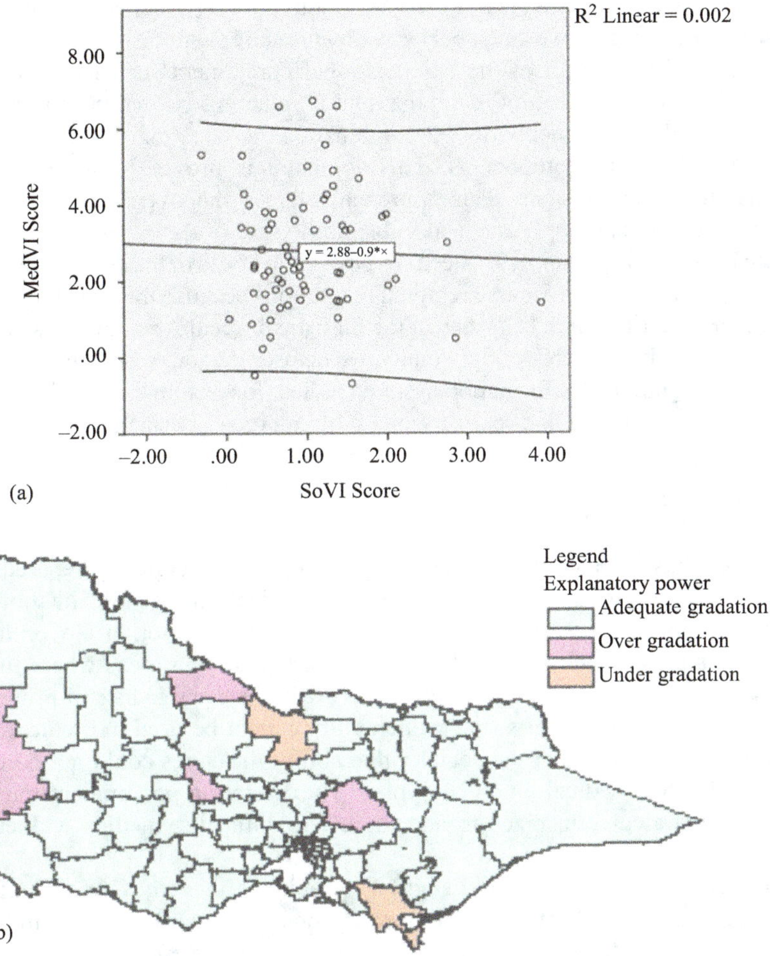

Figure 24.8 *(a) Scatter plot has been produced using SoVI score as independent variable and MedVI score as dependent variable with regression line and 95% confidence interval and (b) a regression residual map with SoVI score as independent variable*

investigation. Such factor like the level and extent of community connectedness, either through social media or face to face interaction may play a part in influencing vulnerability to disasters. This could be done, for example, neighbour warning each other, either electronically or by phone of approaching fires or flooded roads, local arrangements to provide emergency accommodation. The study did not assess these other factors and we acknowledge this is a limitation and a worthy subject of further research.

Furthermore, one of the main contributions of this chapter was the improvement of indicators for vulnerability assessment. Our approach has proven to efficiently reduce the numbers of iterations required for a partial correlation test. As shown in Section 5.3, we only perform the measurement for partial correlation three times. If we use all of the compositional components of MedVI and SoVI metrics, then we will need 66 combinations if selecting two compositional components from 12 components or 792 combinations if selecting five compositional components from 12 components. This approach is proving to be effective in reducing the iteration steps. This approach reduces the overall time and effort required to create and apply medical vulnerability metrics.

We believed more surveying needs to be done to confirm these results and that it was only possible to do a 'coarse regional resolution' because this is what data were available. Further research is needed at the Statistical Local Area level to confirm or disprove the findings of this study. Finally, we believe that our works may contribute to further geographical information system studies, for example, the role of mobile GIS during the response and recovery phase of emergency management.

24.7 Conclusion

This chapter has revealed the urgency of improving the emergency preparedness of public health system and the management of medical emergency situations. The construction of medical vulnerability metric helps the Victorian Government to improve healthcare access and affordability, particularly in areas where the individuals' and the communities' medical needs are highest and in hazard-prone areas. Our research has found that social vulnerability cannot be used to predict medical vulnerability. It means that the social vulnerability measures could not be used as indicators for the medical emergency plan. The Victorian government must have intervention strategies in place to address LGAs with high medical vulnerability scores.

For future studies, we would suggest to replicate this study in different geographic settings to test for the boundary conditions and expansion of our indicators. Particularly interesting cases may be conducted in emerging economies and disaster-prone countries. According to a recent report, emerging economies such as China, India, Indonesia and the Philippines may suffer disproportionally from natural disasters as they may have relatively high population density and comparatively limited investment in disaster prevention and preparedness [67]. Spatial mapping is an inexpensive but effective tool to visualise and map these populations. This method will provide valuable information to policy makers and healthcare organisations in disaster management that will assist them to rapidly deploy the right resources in a timely manner to assist the more vulnerable.

References

[1] UNEP. *Assessing Human Vulnerability Due to Environmental Change: Concepts, Issues, Methods and Case Studies*. Nairobi, Kenya: United Nations Environment Programme; 2002.

[2] UN DESA. *World Population Prospects: The 2015 Revision, Key Findings and Advance Tables*. New York: The United Nations Department of Economic and Social Affairs; 2015.

[3] Australian Government Disaster Assist. *State and Territories Current Disasters*. Melbourne, Australia: Department of Home Affairs; 2016.

[4] Walker C. Natural disasters cost Victoria almost $ 20 billion over 10 years. 2014.

[5] ABS. *Australian Demographic Statistics, September 2015*. Canberra, Australia: Australian Bureau of Statistics; 2016.

[6] ABS. *Population Projections, Australia, 2012 (Base) to 2101*. Canberra, Australia: Australian Bureau of Statistics; 2013.

[7] Pyles J, and Buechler CM. Fox B, *et al. Sharepoint 2007: The Definitive Guide*. Sebastopol: O'Reilly Media, Inc; 2007.

[8] Merrett HC, and Chen WW. Applications of geographical information systems and remote sensing in natural disaster hazard assessment and mitigation in Taiwan. *Geomatics, Natural Hazards and Risk*. 2013;4(2):145–63.

[9] Dymon UJ. *The Role of Emergency Mapping in Disaster Response*. Colorado, United States: FMHI Publications. 1990; Paper 45. Available from http://scholarcommons.usf.edu/fmhi_pub/45

[10] Longley P, and Goodchild MF. Maguire DJ, and Rhind DW. *Geographic Information Systems and Science*. Chichester: John Wiley & Sons; 2005.

[11] The Remarkable History of GIS [Internet]. *GIS Geography*. 2018. Available from https://gisgeography.com/history-of-gis/ (accessed May 2016).

[12] Mensah-Okantey E. Designing a prototype mobile GIS to support cadastral data collection in Ghana. Master thesis. Enschede, Netherlands: University of Twente; 2007.

[13] Montoya L. 'Geo-data acquisition through mobile GIS and digital video: An urban disaster management perspective'. *Environmental Modelling & Software*. 2003;18(10):869–76.

[14] Tomaszewski B. *Geographic Information Systems (GIS) for Disaster Management*. 1st ed. New York: CRC Press; 2014.

[15] Tsou MH, and Sun CH. Mobile GIServices applications in disaster management. In: *Dynamic and Mobile GIS: Investigating Change in Space and Time*. London: CRC Press; 2007. pp. 213–36.

[16] ArcGIS as a system for emergency/disaster management. *ESRI India Magazine*. 2012;6(1):7.

[17] Geospatial Intelligence for Fusion Centers - Esri [Internet]. 2011. Available from https://www.esri.com/library/whitepapers/pdfs/geospatial_intelligence_fusion_centers.pdf (accessed May 2016).

[18] Grigoriadis VN, Papadopoulou ID. Spyridaki P, Doukas ID, and Tziavos IN, Savvaidis P. Presentation of a Web-Based GIS System for the Management of Natural Disasters. Studying, Modeling and Sense Making of Planet Earth, Mytilene, Greece. 2008. pp. 1–6. University of the Aegean.

[19] Tsou M-H. 'Integrated mobile GIS and wireless Internet map servers for environmental monitoring and management'. *Cartography and Geographic Information Science*. 2004;31(3):153–65.

[20] Geographic Information Systems (GIS) for Disaster Management - ESRI [Internet]. Available from http://www.esriindia.com/~/media/esri-india/files/pdfs/industries/gis-framework-for-disaster-management.pdf?la=en (accessed May 2016).

[21] Maguire D. 'Mobile geographic services'. *GIS Development*. 2001;5(1):28–32.

[22] Mobaraki A, and Mansourian A. Malek M, and Mohammadi H. Application of mobile GIS and SDI for emergency management. *Revue Francaise de Photogrammetric et de Teledetection*. 2007;185(1):95–100.

[23] Eddy. GIS in disaster management: a case study of tsunami risk mapping in Bali, Indonesia. Master thesis. Townsville, Australia: James Cook University; 2006.

[24] Gaspar JL, Goulart C, Queiroz G, Silveira D, and Gomes A. 'Dynamic structure and data sets of a GIS database for geological risk analysis in the Azores volcanic islands'. *Natural Hazards and Earth System Science*. 2004; 4(2):233–42.

[25] Cutter SL, Mitchell JT, and Scott MS. *Handbook for Conducting a GIS-Based Hazards Assessment at the County Level*. Columbia, SC: University of South Carolina; 1997.

[26] Alcántara-Ayala I. 'Geomorphology, natural hazards, vulnerability and prevention of natural disasters in developing countries'. *Geomorphology*. 2002;47(2–4):107–24.

[27] Baehr I. 'Sharing geo-information for humanitarian response and disaster management'. *Geoforum Perspektiv*. 2015;14(26):10–17.

[28] Dow K. 'Exploring differences in our common future(s): the meaning of vulnerability to global environmental change'. *Geoforum*. 1992;23(3):417–36.

[29] Cutter SL. 'Vulnerability to environmental hazards'. *Progress in Human Geography*. 1996;20(4):529–39.

[30] Cutter SL. *American Hazardscapes: The Rgionalization of Hzards and Disasters*. Washington, DC: Joseph Henry Press; 2002.

[31] Burton I, Kates RW, and White GF. *The Environment as Hazard*. New York: Guilford Press; 1993.

[32] Anderson MB. *Vulnerability to Disaster and Sustainable Development: A General Framework for Assessing Vulnerability*. Disaster Prevention for Sustainable Development: Economic and Policy Issues. Washington, DC: World Bank. 1995. pp. 41–59.

[33] Blaikie P, Cannon T, Davis I, and Wisner B. *At Risk: Natural Hazards, People's Vulnerability and Disasters*. London: Routledge; 2004.

[34] Hewitt K. *Regions of Risk: A Geographical Approach to Disaster*. London: Addison Wesley Longman; 1997.

[35] Cutter SL, Mitchell JT, and Scott MS. 'Revealing the vulnerability of people and places: A case study of Georgetown County, South Carolina'. *Annals of the Association of American Geographers*. 2000;90(4):713–737.

[36] Cutter SL, Burton CG, and Emrich CT. 'Disaster resilience indicators for benchmarking baseline conditions'. *Journal of Homeland Security and Emergency Management*. 2010;7(1):1–22.

[37] Tate E. 'Social vulnerability indices: A comparative assessment using uncertainty and sensitivity analysis'. *Natural Hazards*. 2012;63(2):325–247.

[38] Yoon DK. Assessment of social vulnerability to natural disasters: A comparative study. *Natural Hazards*. 2012;63(2):823–843.

[39] Cutter SL. *From Social Vulnerability to Resilience: Measuring Progress Toward Disaster Risk Reduction*. Bonn, Germany: UNU-EHS, United Nations University; 2013.

[40] Leaning J, and Guha-Sapir D. 'Natural disasters, armed conflict, and public health'. *New England Journal of Medicine*. 2013;369(19):1836–1842.

[41] Azad AK, Hossain KM, and Nasreen M. 'Flood-induced vulnerabilities and problems encountered by women in northern Bangladesh'. *International Journal of Disaster Risk Science*. 2013;4(4):190–199.

[42] Armaş I, and Gavriş A. 'Social vulnerability assessment using spatial multi-criteria analysis (SEVI model) and the Social Vulnerability Index (SoVI model) – A case study for Bucharest, Romania'. *Natural Hazards and Earth System Sciences*. 2013;13(6):1481–99.

[43] Aday L. 'Health status of vulnerable populations'. *Annual Review of Public Health*. 1994;15(1):487–509.

[44] Morath DP. 'Social vulnerability and public health: Developing a metric for medical emergency management in Florida'. Master thesis. Columbia: University of South Carolina; 2010.

[45] Ariani A, Lewis J, and Ray PK. 'The vulnerability assessment for emergency response plans'. IEEE International Symposium on Technology and Society (IEEE ISTAS) 2016, Kerala, India. 2016 pp. 1–4. IEEE.

[46] Altevogt BM, and Colten HR. *Sleep Disorders and Sleep Deprivation: An Unmet Public Health Problem*. Washington, DC: National Academies Press; 2006.

[47] Tomazevic N, Kozjek T, and Stare J. 'The consequences of a work-family (im)balance: From the point of view of employers and employees'. *International Business Research*. 2014;7(8):83–100.

[48] HHS. *The Surgeon General's Call to Action to Prevent and Decrease Overweight and Obesity*. Washington, DC: The U.S. Department of Health and Human Services; 2001.

[49] Lichtenstein AH, Appel LJ, Brands M, et al. 'Diet and lifestyle recommendations revision 2006: A scientific statement from the American Heart Association Nutrition Committee'. *Circulation*. 2006;114(1):82–96.

[50] Vartanian LR, Schwartz MB, and Brownell KD. Effects of soft drink consumption on nutrition and health: A systematic review and meta-analysis. *American Journal of Public Health*. 2007;97(4):667–75.

[51] 2013 LGA profiles data [Internet]. Department of Health & Human Services; 2014. Available from https://www2.health.vic.gov.au/about/publications/policiesandguidelines/2013-LGA-profiles-data (accessed February 2016).

[52] Cutter SL, Boruff BJ, and Shirley WL. 'Social vulnerability to environmental hazards'. *Social Science Quarterly*. 2003;84(2):242–261.

[53] Map of local government areas in Victoria & detail of local government areas in and around Melbourne [Internet]. Wikipedia. 2015. Available from https://en.wikipedia.org/wiki/Local_government_in_Victoria (accessed February 2016).

[54] Schneider A, Hommel G, and Blettner M. 'Linear regression analysis'. *Deutsches Aerzteblatt Online*. 2010;107(44):776–782.

[55] Pallant J. *SPSS Survival Manual: A Step by Step Guide to Data Analysis Using SPSS for Windows (version 12)*. Sydney, Australia: Allen & Unwin; 2013.

[56] VCOSS. *Disaster and Disadvantage Social Vulnerability in Emergency Management*. Victoria, Australia: Victorian Council of Social Service, 2014.

[57] Aday LA. *At Risk in America: The Health and Health Care Needs of Vulnerable Populations in the United States*. San Francisco: John Wiley & Sons; 2001.

[58] Yarnal B. 'Vulnerability and all that jazz: Addressing vulnerability in New Orleans after Hurricane Katrina'. *Technology in Society*. 2007;29(2):249–55.

[59] ACOSS. *Poverty in Australia*. Redfern, Australia: Australian Council of Social Service; 2014.

[60] Hamilton C, Downie C, and Lu Y-H. *The State of the Australian Middle Class*. Manuka, Australia: Australia Institute; 2007.

[61] Howlett M, Gray M, and Hunter B. *Unpacking the Income of Indigenous and Non-Indigenous Australians: Wages, Government Payments and Other Income*. Canberra, Australia: Centre for Aboriginal Economic Policy Research; 2015.

[62] BIS Shrapnel. *Australian Housing Outlook 2014–2017*. Sydney, Australia: QBE Insurance (Australia) Limited; 2014.

[63] Pourhosseini SS, Ardalan A, and Mehrolhassani MH. Key aspects of providing healthcare services in disaster response stage. *Iranian Journal of Public Health*. 2015;44(1):111–118.

[64] Ferdinand KC. 'Public health and Hurricane Katrina: Lessons learned and what we can do now'. *Journal of the National Medical Association*. 2006; 98(2):271.

[65] Petterson JS, Stanley LD, Glazier E, and Philipp J. 'A preliminary assessment of social and economic impacts associated with Hurricane Katrina'. *American Anthropologist*. 2006;108(4):643–670.

[66] NCHS. *Health, United States, 2010: With special Feature on Death and Dying*. Hyattsville: National Center for Health Statistics; 2011.

[67] Kinghorn J. Five countries most frequently hit by natural disasters [Internet]. AIR Worldwide. 2015. Available from https://www.air-worldwide.com/Blog/Five-Countries-Most-Frequently-Hit-by-Natural-Disasters/ (accessed June 2017).

Chapter 25
Conclusion and future work

25.1 Conclusion and future work

The book has discussed examples of the use of mobile technologies for healthcare development to help socially disadvantaged populations (e.g. poor, disabled, elderly, etc.) in remote, rural or developing regions. This book brings together examples of large scale, international projects from developing regions of China and countries in the Belt and Road region (Pakistan, Bangladesh, India, Cambodia, Nepal, etc.) from researchers in Australia, Bangladesh, Denmark, India, Norway, Japan, Portugal, Thailand and China. Many of the projects involve collaboration between neighbouring governments, NGOs and/or private enterprises and are discussed from the multi-disciplinary perspective of software development, mobile communications, public health, social welfare and cost effectiveness. The chapters have discussed the challenges presented to those seeking to deploy mobile technologies on a large scale and solutions undertaken in these projects. The book should be of interest to engineers and researchers working in healthcare in sustainable development settings. While healthcare is mainly controlled by governments in developed countries, in developing countries private enterprises have become increasingly involved due to the scarcity of resources (funds, skills and management abilities) in these areas. As well as sections on the use of drones, robots and mHealth applications, the book has also included case studies related to the development of public–private partnerships and the cooperation required to overcome the obstacles associated with deploying technological solutions in developing regions.

The topic of this book has been quite popular given its applications in many parts of the world and hence many groups of researchers, industry and global organisation (e.g. WHO) are working on this topic. As stated earlier, this book has been an outcome of collaborative research across more than ten countries as part of the mHBR (mobile health for Belt and Road region) initiative launched in September 2018 through the Entrepreneurship Week event organised by the University of Michigan-Shanghai Jiao Tong University Joint Institute. As a first such event, it was attended by about 120 participants from 14 countries. This event led to the initial plan of mHBR in consultation with multi-national partners in academia, business and the government and consolidated the organisation of mHBR project. We now discuss some areas of research that mHBR initiative is working on to take these projects forward. These are discussed below in terms of the various mHBR projects that were the foci of the sections of this book.

25.2 Project 1 – Global challenge

This project brings together various stakeholders, such as governments, NGOs, universities, research institutes, healthcare providers, technology providers, incubators, financial organisations across countries in the Belt and Road region to investigate how these stakeholders can cooperate to achieve sustainable development for various issue areas (particularly healthcare) in different sectors of the society.

The instruments under study include the entrepreneurship ecosystem that combines government policies, financial resources, entrepreneurial talents, with innovation from the private sector as well as academia, in order to provide practical support under one umbrella (e.g. incubators). More evaluative case studies are needed regarding the roles and impacts of such ecosystem in bringing sustainable development through mobile health applications, but these case studies will simultaneously aim at bringing more stakeholders into symbiotic relationships within the ecosystems to strength existing mHBR projects.

The Global Challenge project also brings an integrating perspective (umbrella) to the other mHBR projects. While each technology entrepreneurship project focuses on optimising the technology application, the Global Challenge project will continue to focus on stakeholder needs to explore integrative use of technologies or identify a new direction for innovation. Underserved segments of population, including dwellers of remote areas, intra- or trans-regional migrants and generation with different needs along the Belt and Road countries will be a starting point of our enquiry. In doing so, we will focus on carrying out demonstrative trials of technologies including local stakeholders as partners. This will, in turn, broaden the scope of international cooperation and also serve as a point of research on policies, evaluation frameworks and participation of local entrepreneurs through broader entrepreneurship ecosystem.

25.3 Project 2 – Portable health clinic

As portable health clinic (PHC) is disseminated as a strategy to provide healthcare to the poor, it is likely that its customisability will emerge as another major advantage. That is to say, PHC can adapt to the needs of the people in the given region in which it is used. Depending on the most common health-related problems in a given area, the capabilities of PHC can be adjusted. Diseases and illnesses that exist more prominently due to the prevalence of certain industries, for example, can be targeted more closely in that particular iteration of the PHC. PHC treating unreached communities occupied in labour in coal mining, as an example, may focus on preventing the most common health hazards involved in the job, such as silicosis or other respiratory illnesses. Not only can PHC be customised to aid populations suffering from diseases caused by a particular industry but also those related to population trends within the demographic it attempts to treat.

However, PHC project has so far concentrated on several Asian countries and there is substantial scope to extend the benefits of mHealth to people in many other countries. For example, Mobile healthcare technology is exceptionally valuable to reach out to marginalised communities in remote areas and provide quality healthcare services. Their work is correcting two major market failures in Pakistan. First, it enables people living in remote locations to get quality healthcare services using new mediums of technology. Second, online availability of doctors serving the patients creates novel employment opportunities for home-based specialists and professionals and addresses the issues of childcare and women's labour participation.

It is now common knowledge that many sophisticated western technologies, such as telemedicine and personalised health record (PHR) have not been very successful in developing countries and there is a need to understand the reasons and develop better practical solutions. Therefore, it is important for one developing country to help another with appropriate solutions.

25.4 Project 3 – Drones for disaster management

ICT plays an important role in coping with natural disasters in the world. In the acute phase of emergencies, the existing infrastructure such as telecommunication, transportation and health facilities are often damaged. Therefore, this study presented the resilient triage models that can work without relying on the Internet technologies in disaster situations. In the rural areas of developing countries, no matter the occurrence of disasters, the access to the health facilities is the common challenge. This study reviewed the global application of the drone technology for the humanitarian purposes in developing countries. The comparative study on the drone application in the rural areas of Nepal and Japan pointed out the importance of the daily drone uses as the solutions for the social challenges in rural communities. This daily drone use is crucial to build up the capacity to operate drones in sudden onset disasters. The case study in Nepal clearly identified that the entrepreneurship was imperative for the sustainable localisation of drone technologies in developing countries. In addition, in the case study on the community drone uses in Minami, Oguni in Japan presented the ideal drone use model to solve the various challenges in the rural areas.

Based on the outputs of this study, the authors propose 'the Ambulance Drone Concept', which is the combined service of telemedicine and drug delivery by drones. In this concept, the drone with a smartphone delivers the diagnostic devices to the patients in a rural community. A community health worker and the patients will be connected to the medical doctor at a referral hospital using the delivered diagnostic devices. Based on the prescription by the doctor at the referral hospital, another drone delivers the medicines to the patient. These services build up the daily medical service platform which can be used in emergencies.

Toward the realisation of this concept, the authors will conduct the field test of the medical cargo drone to deliver the diagnostic devices, medicines, blood, human specimens and other items for the treatment in the rural areas of Japan, Nepal, India and other countries.

25.5 Project 4 – mHealth for the elderly

This project followed from the EU Victoryahome project where telepresence robots (with medicine dispensation and fall detection) were trialled at more than 20 locations in five countries (Norway, Netherlands, Sweden, Portugal and Australia) to assess their benefits for the emotional health of the elderly. The project was undertaken in collaboration with universities, especially those for the elderly (e.g. University of Third Age, Australia), Aged Care Providers, researchers and Aged Care Technology Providers. It was observed that telepresence robots used in the project were too expensive (approx. $10,000 each) and were unsuitable for the elderly in terms of the technical complexities.

Hence the current mHBR project is aimed at first developing a low cost, simple robot made in the Belt in the Road region so that they can adapt to the local needs. Concurrently, the project group is working with European partners in Norway, Portugal, Italy, etc., funded by EU to develop social robotics applications. For example, the group is working with Lifebots Exchange funded by EU RISE to involve entrepreneurs in the development of services and robots for such social applications.

Researchers of this project are working on a combination of telepresence robots with wearables to bring down the cost of the overall mHealth system for the elderly and trials are planned in a developing country, such as Bangladesh.

25.6 Project 5 – mHealth for chronic illnesses

This project deals with mHealth applications for chronic illnesses, such as cancer, diabetes and Parkinson's disease. Although three chapters of this section of the book discussed collaborative approaches (including geospatial information systems) to the management of chronic illnesses, Chapters 1 and 3 also discussed general issues related to the management of mHealth.

There has been a worldwide, major push towards systemic capabilities to manage non-communicable diseases (NCD). mHealth can play a major role in the management of NCDs that require lifestyle changes (e.g. smoking cessation, regular exercise, diet control, etc.). Hence this project group is working on a multi-disciplinary, multi-country approach in collaboration with various global bodies, such as the WHO Collaborating Centres on eHealth and AeHIN (Asia eHealth Information Network).

Researchers of this project are working across Australia, Bangladesh, China, Europe and India and in many other parts of the world on the development of mHealth apps for the management of chronic illnesses, such as asthma, diabetes and cancer by integrating such apps to involve stakeholder groups through social media interventions.

25.7 Project 6 – mHealth security and controls

The book did not have any section or chapter on this topic though Chapter 22 discussed secure data sharing across jurisdictions as part of EU Project AU2EU, involving five countries (Australia, Netherlands, Germany, France, Switzerland and UK). Some authors of this book have published articles on Security and Control of mHealth services including blockchain techniques in international conferences and journals. This is a growing field and it is important to bring together knowledge from multiple disciplines, such as privacy laws (e.g. evolving applications of GDPR in Europe), evolving network and data security techniques (encryption management) and controls (e.g. smart contracts in blockchains) and healthcare for the trust and management of mHealth services.

It is impossible to cover all aspects of this vast area of information in one book. For example, this book did not cover any major trials on mHealth from the health researchers' perspective, nor did the book delve into the technical details of any of the technologies as available in many technical literatures. However, the authors and editors have tried to provide a balanced view from the perspectives of entrepreneurs, managers and technologist wanting to understand how mobile technologies can make a difference to the healthcare needs of the people in remote, rural or developing regions. Also the book has provided an overview of how entrepreneurs can use mobile technologies for businesses across this fast growing Belt and Road region for healthcare services.

Index

www.ingramcontent.com/pod-product-compliance
Lightning Source LLC
LaVergne TN
LVHW011555200926
848484LV00001B/319